# Head Injury
## A Multidisciplinary Approach

Edited by

**Peter C. Whitfield**
Consultant Neurosurgeon and Honorary Clinical Senior Lecturer
South West Neurosurgery Centre
Derriford Hospital
Plymouth Hospitals NHS Trust
Plymouth, UK

**Elfyn O. Thomas**
Consultant in Anaesthesia and Intensive Care
Derriford Hospital
Plymouth Hospitals NHS Trust
Plymouth, UK

**Fiona Summers**
Consultant Clinical Neuropsychologist
Aberdeen Royal Infirmary
NHS Grampian
Aberdeen, UK

**Maggie Whyte**
Consultant Clinical Neuropsychologist
Aberdeen Royal Infirmary
NHS Grampian
Aberdeen, UK

**Peter J. Hutchinson**
Senior Academy Fellow and Honorary Consultant Neurosurgeon
Academic Neurosurgical Unit
Cambridge University Hospitals NHS Foundation Trust
Cambridge, UK

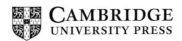

CAMBRIDGE UNIVERSITY PRESS
Cambridge, New York, Melbourne, Madrid, Cape Town,
Singapore, São Paulo, Delhi

Cambridge University Press
The Edinburgh Building, Cambridge CB2 8RU, UK

Published in the United States of America by Cambridge
University Press, New York

www.cambridge.org
Information on this title: www.cambridge.org/9780521697620

First published 2009

Printed in the United Kingdom at the University Press,
Cambridge

*A catalogue record for this publication is available from the
British Library*

ISBN 978-0-521-69762-0 paperback

*This book is dedicated to Hannah and her friends at the Peninsula Medical School.*

# Contents

# Contributors

**Gareth Allen MB BCh FFARCSI DIBICM**
Consultant in Anaesthesia and Intensive
Care Medicine, Belfast City Hospital,
Belfast, UK

**Rowan Burnstein MBBS FRCA PhD**
Consultant in Intensive Care
Medicine and Anaesthesia, SDU Director,
Neurocritical Care, Cambridge
University Hospitals
NHS Foundation Trust, Cambridge, UK

**Mick Cafferkey**
Senior Illustrator, Medical Photography
and Illustration, Addenbrooke's Hospital,
Cambridge, UK

**Joseph Carter MBBS FRCA**
Consultant in Anaesthesia, Queen Elizabeth
Hospital, King's Lynn, UK

**Jonathan Cole MB ChB DA
FRCA PhD**
Honorary Consultant & Academy of
Medical Sciences/Health Foundation
Clinician Scientist, Cambridge University
Department of Anaesthesia, Cambridge
University Hospitals NHS Foundation
Trust, Cambridge, UK

**Giles Critchley MA MD
FRCS (Surg Neurol)**
Consultant Neurosurgeon and Honorary
Clinical Senior Lecturer, Hurstwood Park
Neurological Centre, Brighton and Sussex
University Hospitals NHS Trust, Haywards
Heath, UK

**Marek Czosnyka PhD**
Reader in Brain Physics, Neurosurgical
Unit, Department of Clinical
Neurosciences, Cambridge University
Hospitals NHS Foundation Trust,
Cambridge, UK

**Egidio J. da Silva MB ChB DA FRCA
PGCME**
Honorary Senior Lecturer, University of
Birmingham; Consultant in Anaesthesia
and High Dependency Care, The Royal
Orthopaedic Hospital, Birmingham, UK

**Bruce Downey MA (Hons) DClinPsychol**
Clinical Psychologist, Woodend Hospital,
Aberdeen, UK

**Susan Dutch MA (Hons) MSc**
Consultant Clinical Psychologist, Royal
Aberdeen Children's Hospital,
Aberdeen, UK

**Jonathan J. Evans BSc (Hons)
DipClinPsychol PhD**
Professor of Applied Neuropsychology and
Honorary Consultant Clinical Psychologist,
Section of Psychological Medicine,
University of Glasgow, Glasgow, UK

**Peter Farling FFARCSI FRCA**
Consultant in Neuroanaesthesia, Royal
Victoria Hospital, Belfast, UK

**Judith Fewings Bsc (Physiotherapy) PG
Cert (Neurological Physiotherapy) MCSP**
Consultant Therapist in Neurosurgery and
Honorary University Fellow, South West
Neurosurgery Centre, Derriford Hospital,
Plymouth Hospitals NHS Trust,
Plymouth, UK

**Clare N. Gallagher MD PhD FRCS(C)**
Division of Neurosurgery, Department of
Clinical Neurosciences, University of
Calgary, Calgary, Alberta, Canada

**Helen M. K. Gooday MB ChB MRCPsych**
Consultant in Rehabilitation Medicine,
Woodend Hospital, Aberdeen, UK

**Arun K. Gupta MBBS MA PhD FRCA**
Consultant in Anaesthesia and Neuro
Intensive Care, Director of Postgraduate
Medical Education, Associate Lecturer,
Cambridge University Hospitals NHS
Foundation Trust, Cambridge, UK

**Adel Helmy MA MB BChir(Cantab) MRCS**
Specialist Registrar and Academic Clinical
Fellow, Academic Neurosurgery Unit,
Cambridge University Hospitals NHS
Foundation Trust, Cambridge, UK

**Camilla Herbert MA MSc DClin Psych
AFBPsS**
Consultant in Neuropsychology and
Rehabilitation, Kerwin Court, Brain Injury
Rehabilitation Trust, Horsham, UK

**David A. Hilton MBBCh MD FRCP
FRCPath**
Consultant Neuropathologist and
Honorary Clinical Senior Lecturer,
Derriford Hospital, Plymouth Hospitals
NHS Trust, Plymouth, UK

**Peter J. Hutchinson BSc MBBS PhD
FRCS (Surg Neurol)**
Senior Academy Fellow and Honorary
Consultant Neurosurgeon, Academic
Neurosurgical Unit, Cambridge University
Hospitals NHS Foundation Trust,
Cambridge, UK

**Roisin Jack BSc (Hons) DClinPsychol**
Clinical Psychologist, Aberdeen Royal
Infirmary, Aberdeen, UK

**Thérèse Jackson Dip COT**
Consultant Occupational Therapist,
Grampian, Scotland, UK

**Deva S. Jeyaretna BM MRCS**
Research Fellow, Brain Tumour Research
Center, Massachusetts General Hospital and
Harvard Medical School, Boston, MA, USA

**Peter J. Kirkpatrick BSc MBChB MSc
FRCS (Surg Neurol) FMedSci**
Consultant Neurosurgeon and Honorary
Lecturer, Academic Neurosurgical Unit,
Cambridge University Hospitals NHS
Foundation Trust, Cambridge, UK

**W. Hiu Lam BMedSci(Hons) BM BS
MRCP FRCA**
Consultant in Neuroanaesthesia & College
Tutor, Honorary University Fellow, Deputy
Director of Medical Education (postgradu-
ate), Derriford Hospital, Plymouth
Hospitals NHS Trust, Plymouth, UK

**Fiona Lecky MB ChB DA MSc FRCS(Ed)
PhD FCEM**
Senior Lecturer in Emergency Medicine/
Honorary Consultant Research, Director,
Trauma Audit and Research Network
(TARN), Salford Royal Hospital,
Salford, UK

**Paul McArdle FDS FRCS FRCS(OMFS)**
Consultant Oral and Maxillofacial Surgeon,
Derriford Hospital, Plymouth Hospitals
NHS Trust, Plymouth, UK

**Duncan McAuley MA MRCP FRCS(A&E)
FCEM DipIMC**
Consultant in Emergency Medicine,
Cambridge University Hospitals NHS
Foundation Trust, Cambridge, UK

**William W. McKinlay BA (Hons) MSc PhD**
Consultant Clinical Neuropsychologist,
Case Management Services Ltd,
Edinburgh, UK

**Chris Maimaris FRCS FCEM**
Consultant in Emergency Medicine,
Cambridge University Hospitals NHS
Foundation Trust, Cambridge, UK

**Alexander R. Manara FRCP FRCA**
Consultant in Anaesthesia and Intensive
Care Medicine, Frenchay Hospital,
Bristol, UK

**Anjum Memon MBBS DPhil (Oxon) FFPH**
Senior Lecturer and Hon Consultant in
Public Health Medicine, Division of
Primary Care and Public Health, Brighton
and Sussex Medical School and Brighton
and Hove City Teaching PCT, Brighton, UK

**Patrick Mitchell FRCS Eng FRCS
(Surg Neurol)**
Senior Lecturer in Neurosurgery,
Department of Neurosurgery, Newcastle
General Hospital, Newcastle upon
Tyne, UK

**H. C. Patel PhD FRCS (Surg Neurol)**
Clinical Lecturer, University Department of
Neurosurgery, Cambridge University
Hospitals NHS Foundation Trust,
Cambridge, UK

**Brian Pentland BSc MB ChB FRCPE
FRCSLT**
Consultant Neurologist, Astley Ainslie
Hospital, Edinburgh, UK

**Puneet Plaha MBBS MS FRCS**
Neurosurgical Specialist Registrar, South
West Neurosurgery Centre, Derriford
Hospital, Plymouth Hospitals NHS Trust,
Plymouth, UK

**Ann-Marie Pringle MA (Hons) Dip PhD**
Consultant Speech and Language Therapist,
Astley Ainslie Hospital, Edinburgh, UK

**Richard Protheroe FRCA MRCP MRCS**
Consultant in Intensive Care Medicine,
Salford Royal NHS Foundation Trust,
Salford, UK

**Heinke Pülhorn BSc MRCS**
Trust Grade Registrar in Neurosurgery,
Morriston Hospital, Swansea, UK

**Robert Redfern MBBS FRCS**
Consultant Neurosurgeon, Morriston
Hospital, Swansea, UK

**Jane V. Russell BSc (Hons)**
Assistant Psychologist, Case Management
Services Ltd, Edinburgh, UK

**Ayan Sen MB BS**
Post-doctoral Fellow, Program in Trauma,
R. Adams Cowley Shock Trauma Center,
University of Maryland School of Medicine,
Baltimore, MD, USA

**Martin Smith MBBS FRCA**
Consultant in Neuroanaesthesia and
Neurocritical Care, Honorary Reader in
Anaesthesia and Critical Care, Department
of Neuroanaesthesia and Neurocritical
Care, The National Hospital for Neurology
and Neurosurgery, University College
London Hospitals NHS Foundation Trust,
London, UK

**Fiona Summers BSc MA (Hons)
DClinPsychol**
Consultant Clinical Neuropsychologist,
Aberdeen Royal Infirmary, NHS Grampian,
Aberdeen, UK

**Matthew J. C. Thomas FRCA MRCP**
Consultant in Anaesthesia
and Intensive Care Medicine, Bristol Royal
Infirmary, Bristol, UK

**Elfyn O. Thomas**
Consultant in Anaesthesia
and Intensive Care, Derriford Hospital,
Plymouth Hospitals NHS Trust,
Plymouth, UK

**I. Timofeev MB BS (Hons) MRCS(Glas)
MRCS(Eng)**
Clinical Research Fellow, Academic
Neurosurgery Unit, Cambridge University
Hospitals NHS Foundation Trust,
Cambridge, UK

**Lorna Torrens BA (Hons) DClinPsychol**
Consultant Clinical Neuropsychologist,
Scottish Neurobehavioural Rehabilitation
Service, The Robert Fergusson Unit, Royal
Edinburgh Hospital, Edinburgh, UK

**Rikin A. Trivedi MRCP(UK) MRCS PhD**
Specialist Registrar in Neurosurgery,
Cambridge University Hospitals NHS
Foundation Trust, Cambridge, UK

**Martin B. Walker MB BS FRCA**
Consultant in Intensive Care Medicine
and Anaesthesia, Derriford Hospital,
Plymouth Hospitals NHS Trust,
Plymouth, UK

**Laurence Watkins MA FRCS (Surg Neurol)**
Consultant Neurosurgeon, National
Hospital for Neurology & Neurosurgery,
London, UK

**Ruwan Alwis Weerakkody MA MB
BChir(Cantab)**
Department of Neurosurgery, Cambridge
University Hospitals NHS Foundation
Trust, Cambridge, UK

**Peter C. Whitfield BM (Dist) PhD
FRCS(Eng) FRCS (Surg Neurol)**
Consultant Neurosurgeon and Honorary
Clinical Senior Lecturer, South West
Neurosurgery Centre, Derriford Hospital,
Plymouth Hospitals NHS Trust,
Plymouth, UK

**Maggie Whyte BSc (Hons) DClinPsychol**
Consultant Clinical Neuropsychologist,
Aberdeen Royal Infirmary, NHS Grampian,
Aberdeen, UK

**Maralyn Woodford BSc**
Executive Director, Trauma Audit and
Research Network (TARN), Salford Royal
Hospital, Salford, UK

# Foreword

There are many types of head injury, they affect many people and their care demands input from many disciplines. No one person can know everything needed to provide effective comprehensive management, yet this is the key to improving outcome – in acute and late phases. This book provides a much-needed, coherent but concise account that sets out the principles and practice of management within a discipline and also what each discipline needs to know about each other. This reflects the wide spread of expertise in its multi-disciplinary authorship – encompassing pathology, neurosurgery, maxillofacial surgery, anaesthesia, intensive care, emergency medicine, neuropsychology, neurology, rehabilitation specialists, public health physicians and basic science. Most come from the UK, in particular from the Cambridge 'school', but the perspective is international and integrated. It will benefit all kinds of personnel involved in caring for head-injured people – from the site of the injury, through acute assessment, investigation and intervention to recovery, rehabilitation and dealing with long-lasting sequelae. These are disturbingly frequent after either an apparently mild or a severe initial injury, so the expectation that their impact will be reduced through the clinical application of the knowledge and wisdom set out here is greatly valued.

**Sir Graham M Teasdale**

Emeritus Professor of Neurosurgery, University of Glasgow,
Chairman NHS Quality Improvement Scotland
Editor in Chief of *Acta Neurochirurgica*, the European Journal of Neurosurgery

Past President of the Royal College of Physicians and Surgeons of Glasgow,
Chairman of the European Brain Injury Consortium and of the
International Neurotrauma Society
MB, BS Dunelm, FRCS Edinburgh,
FRCPS Glasgow, FRCP London, FRCP Edinburgh

Honorary FRCS England, Ireland
MD Hon Causae, Athens,
Honorary International Fellow, American College of Surgeons
Fellow of the Academy of Medical Sciences
Fellow of the Royal Society of Edinburgh

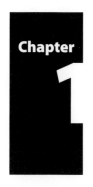

# Epidemiology of head injury

Giles Critchley and Anjum Memon

## Introduction

Head injury is a major cause of morbidity and mortality in all age groups. Currently, there is no effective treatment to reverse the effects of the primary brain injury sustained, and treatment is aimed at minimizing the secondary brain injury that can occur due to the effects of ischaemia, hypoxia and raised intracranial pressure. An understanding of the epidemiology of head injury is essential for devising preventive measures, to plan population-based primary prevention strategies and to provide effective and timely treatment including provision of rehabilitation facilities to those who have suffered a head injury.

Epidemiology is the basic science of public health and clinical medicine. It describes the occurrence of health-related states or events, quantifies the risk of disease and its outcome and postulates causal mechanisms for disease in populations. The main function of epidemiology is to provide an evidence-based public health policy thereby guiding clinical practice to protect, restore and promote health. Epidemiological studies have highlighted three important aspects of head injury: (i) socio-demographic factors (age, gender, ethnicity, socio-economic status, geographic location, legislation and enforcement, physical/psychological condition, use of alcohol and drugs); (ii) mechanism of injury (nature of accident or trauma – road traffic accident (RTA), fall, violence, sport injury); and (iii) efficiency of the healthcare system (emergency rescue/ambulance service, in- and out-patient medical care, rehabilitation services). Thus, for devising a prevention programme, we need to identify the risk factors for head injury, the mechanisms and patterns of head injury, possible methods for prevention and the relationship between brain injury and outcome. The aim of this chapter is to describe the descriptive epidemiology of traumatic brain injury (TBI), its causes and preventive measures targeted at the 'at-risk' population.

## Definition and classification of traumatic brain injury

While studying the epidemiology of TBI, it is important to realize that definitions, coding practices, inclusion criteria for patients and items of data collected have varied between studies. This has made it difficult to draw meaningful comparisons of rates and risk factors between populations. The term 'head injury' is commonly used to describe injuries affecting not just the brain but also the scalp, skull, maxilla and mandible and special senses of smell, vision and hearing. Head injuries are also commonly referred to as brain injury or traumatic brain injury, depending on the extent of the head trauma. TBI is usually considered an insult or trauma to the brain from an external mechanical force, possibly leading to temporary or permanent impairments of physical, cognitive and psychosocial functions with an associated diminished or altered state of consciousness. It is also important to consider TBI in the context of the skull and other structures above the neck, as well as to identify those with

*Head Injury: A Multidisciplinary Approach*, ed. Peter C. Whitfield, Elfyn O. Thomas, Fiona Summers, Maggie Whyte and Peter J. Hutchinson. Published by Cambridge University Press. © Cambridge University Press 2009.

**Table 1.1.** List of ICD-10 codes and categories for injuries to the head

| ICD Code | Category |
| --- | --- |
| S00 | Superficial injury of head |
| S01 | Open wound of head |
| S02 | Fracture of skull and facial bones |
| S03 | Dislocation, sprain and strain of joints and ligaments of head |
| S04 | Injury of cranial nerves |
| S05 | Injury of eye and orbit |
| **S06** | **Intracranial injury** |
| S06.0 | Concussion |
| S06.1 | Traumatic cerebral oedema |
| S06.2 | Diffuse brain injury |
| S06.3 | Focal brain injury |
| S06.4 | Epidural haemorrhage |
| S06.5 | Traumatic subdural haemorrhage |
| S06.6 | Traumatic subarachnoid haemorrhage |
| S06.7 | Intracranial injury with prolonged coma |
| S06.8 | Other intracranial injuries |
| S06.9 | Intracranial injury, unspecified |
| S07 | Crushing injury of head |
| S08 | Traumatic amputation of part of head |
| S09 | Other and unspecified injuries of head |

*Source: International Statistical Classification of Diseases and Related Health Problems, 10th Revision,* Version for 2007 published by the WHO http://www.who.int/classifications/apps/icd/ icd10online/. Reproduced with permission from the World Health Organization, © 2007.

'isolated' head injuries and those with multisystem polytrauma where other injuries may contribute to secondary brain injury. The severity of TBI is usually classified according to the Glasgow Coma Scale (GCS) scores as mild (13–15), moderate (9–12) and severe (3–8).

The International Classification of Diseases (ICD) is the standard diagnostic classification for clinical, epidemiological and health service data and is used to classify diseases and other health problems recorded on many types of health and vital records (e.g. hospital records, death certificates).[1] It is used for compilation of morbidity and mortality statistics and comparison of health data collected in different countries at different times. In ICD-10, which was implemented in 1994, 'accidents, poisonings and violence' are classified according to their 'external cause' in the interests of strategic planning of preventive policy and action. The codes for recording injuries to the head (S00–S09) include injuries of ear, eye, face, gum, jaw, mandibular joint area, oral cavity, palate, periocular area, scalp, tongue and tooth (Table 1.1). This excludes burns, corrosions and effects of a foreign body. As with all coding systems, they may be applied in different ways and the use of general codes (e.g. S09, other and unspecified injuries of the head) may underestimate more specific injuries.[2] One of

**Table 1.2.** Sources of data on accidents and injury in the UK

- Hospital records/statistics (including A&E departments): presentation to health services is dependent on severity of head injury and proximity/access to services.
- Mortality data: the most reliable and complete source of information on deaths due to external causes (http://www.statistics.gov.uk).
- HASS and LASS (Home and Leisure Accident Surveillance System): a reliable source of information on home and leisure accidents, dependent on data from A&E departments (http://www.hassandlass.org.uk).
- Health and Safety Executive: collects data on serious employment-related injuries and accidents (http://www.hse.gov.uk).
- Police services: collate data on RTAs and their causes (speeding, traffic law violations, drink-driving, use of illicit drugs, etc.).
- Surveys such as the General Household Survey and Labour Force Survey (http://www.statistics.gov.uk).

the problems of head injury research is case ascertainment. The most reliable sources of data on head injury and its outcome include hospital records (i.e. in- and out-patient records, hospital discharge register, radiology reports, accident and emergency department attendance records), prospective observational studies and death certification (Table 1.2).[3]

While studying the epidemiology of head injury, it is important to understand that patients with TBI may not survive before reaching hospital or may even present after a delay to primary care; they may present to an accident and emergency department, with subsequent admission to an observation or neurosurgical ward or a neurosurgical intensive care. Following admission, they may not survive the injury or may be discharged home or to a rehabilitation facility or long-term institutional care. This information is essential for planning, resource allocation and efficient delivery of treatment and rehabilitation services to patients with TBI.

## Burden of traumatic brain injury

TBI is an important global public health problem. It is a major cause of disability. Survivors often suffer cognitive, mood and behavioural disorders. The societal cost of the disability following TBI can be substantial due to loss of years of productive life and a need for long-term or lifelong services. Worldwide, it has been estimated that around 10 million TBIs serious enough to result in hospitalization, long-term or lifelong disability, or death occur annually.[4] In the USA, an average of 1.4 million TBIs occur each year, including 1.1 million A&E department visits, 235 000 hospitalizations and 50 000 deaths.[5] In a recent report, it was estimated that about 5.3 million people have some TBI-related disability, impairment, complaint, or handicap in the USA.[5] Similarly, it has been estimated that about 6.2 million people in the European Union have some form of TBI-related disability.[6]

## Incidence of TBI

*Incidence* is a count of *new cases* of TBI in the population during a specified time period. The *incidence rate* is the number of *new cases* of TBI in a defined population within a specified time period (usually a calendar year), divided by the total number of persons in that population (usually expressed as per 100 000 population). Like most conditions, the incidence of TBI varies according to age, gender and geographic location. Most of the published reports are from developed countries in Europe and North America, and there is little

3

**Table 1.3.** Incidence of traumatic head injury in different populations (selected studies)

| Population | Annual incidence per 100 000 population | Male : female ratio |
|---|---|---|
| *Africa* | | |
| South Africa, Johannesburg (Nell & Brown, 1991) | 316 | 4.8:1 |
| *Asia* | | |
| India (Gururaj *et al.* 2004) | 160 | NR |
| Taiwan, Taipei City (Chiu *et al.* 2007) | 218 | 1.9:1 |
| *Europe* | | |
| Spain, Cantabria (Vazquez-Barquero *et al.* 1992) | 91 | 2.7:1 |
| Finland (Alaranta *et al.* 2000) | 95 | 1.5:1 |
| Portugal (Santos *et al.* 2003) | 137 | 1.8:1 |
| Denmark (Engberg & Teasdale, 2001) | 157 | 2.2:1 |
| Italy, Northeast (Baldo *et al.* 2003) | 212 | 1.6:1 |
| Norway, Tromso (Ingebrigtsen *et al.* 1998) | 229 | 1.7:1 |
| UK, England (Tennant, 2005) | 229 | NR |
| Sweden (Kleiven *et al.* 2003) | 259 | 2.1:1 |
| Italy, Romagna (Servadei *et al.* 2002) | 297 | 1.6:1 |
| UK, Staffordshire (Hawley *et al.* 2003) | 280[a] | 1.8:1 |
| France, Aquitaine (Tiret *et al.* 1990) | 282 | 2.1:1 |
| Italy, Trentino (Servadei *et al.* 2002) | 332 | 1.8:1 |
| Germany (Steudel *et al.* 2005) | 337 | NR |
| Germany (Firsching & Woischneck, 2001) | 350 | NR |
| Sweden, Northern (Styrke *et al.* 2007) | 354 | 1.2:1 |
| UK, Southwest England (Yates *et al.* 2006) | 453 | 1.6:1 |
| Sweden, Western (Andersson *et al.* 2003) | 546 | 1.4:1 |
| *North America* | | |
| USA, Alaska (Sallee *et al.* 2000) | 105 | 2.3:1 |
| USA, Utah (Thurman *et al.* 1996) | 109 | 2.2:1 |
| USA (Guerrero *et al.* 2000) | 392 | 1.6:1 |
| USA (Jager *et al.* 2000) | 444 | 1.7:1 |
| *Oceania* | | |
| Australia, NSW (Tate *et al.* 1998) | 100 | NR |
| Australia, South (Hillier *et al.* 1997) | 322 | 2.3:1 |

[a] In children aged ≤15 years. NR, not reported
This table is adapted from data reviewed by Tagliaferri *et al.*, 6 with permission.

information on epidemiology of head injury from most developing countries. The annual incidence rates of TBI range from a low of 91 per 100 000 population in a province in Spain to a high of 546 per '100 000 in western Sweden (Table 1.3). The rate from Spain included only hospitalized patients, while the rate from Sweden included hospital admissions, A&E attendances and deaths. Most rates are in the range of 150–450 new cases per 100 000 per year. The variation observed could be partly explained by differences in criteria used to define TBI or identify patients. In a recent study from England, the incidence rates of head injury varied by a factor of 4.6 across different health authorities (range 91–419 per 100 000).[7] Similarly, in the USA incidence rates of TBI vary from a low of 101 per 100 000 in Colorado to a high of 367 per 100 000 in Chicago.[8] In a recent review of TBI epidemiology in the European Union (EU), an overall average rate of 235 per 100 000 per year was obtained. Considering the EU population of about 330 million, this accounts for about 775 500 new cases of TBI per year.[6]

## Variation by age

In most studies, three distinct peaks in the incidence of TBI are noted. The risk of having a TBI is particularly high among children, young adults and the elderly population.[9] The highest incidence, in most studies, is reported in adolescents and young adults. For A&E visits, hospitalizations and deaths combined, children aged 0–4 years and adolescents aged 15–19 years are more likely to sustain a TBI than persons in other age groups.[5] For hospitalizations only, persons aged ≥75 years have the highest incidence of TBI.[5] In a study of hospital admissions due to TBI in the UK, 30% were children aged <15 years.[10] Among those attending A&E departments in the UK with head injuries the highest rates are observed in urban males aged 15–19 years.[10] In the European Brain Injury Consortium (EBIC) study of patients admitted to neurosurgical centres in 12 European countries, the median age of the subjects was 38 years with a higher preponderance of male patients.[3]

## Variation by gender

Almost all studies show a male preponderance. Overall, males are about twice as likely as females to experience a TBI. For studies from Europe and North America, the male : female ratio varies from 1.2:1 in Sweden to 2.7:1 in Spain. Males in developing countries apparently have a much higher risk of TBI compared with those in developed countries. In a study from South Africa, the male : female ratio was 4.8 : 1 (Table 1.3). In the UK study of TBI-related hospital admissions, 72% were male patients.[10] In the EBIC study of severe head injuries, 74% of the patients were males.[3] In the Traumatic Coma Data Bank of patients with severe head injury, about 77% were males.[11] In the CRASH study of the effect of corticosteroids on death within 14 days, which included 10 008 patients with clinically significant head injury, 81% were males.[12] The male excess of TBI is attributed to greater exposure and more risk-taking behaviour. At younger ages the exposure of males to violence and RTAs leads to a male : female ratio of head injury incidence of about 4:1.

## Mortality from TBI

The *mortality rate* is the number of deaths from TBI in a defined population within a specified time period (usually a calendar year), divided by the total number of persons in that population (usually expressed as per 100 000 population). The mortality rate varies considerably in different countries. In the UK, the mortality rate from head injury is 6–10 per 100 000 population per year.[13] For France, a mortality rate of about 22 per 100 000 has been reported.[14] In the EU, the mortality from TBI varies from a low of 9.4 per 100 000 in

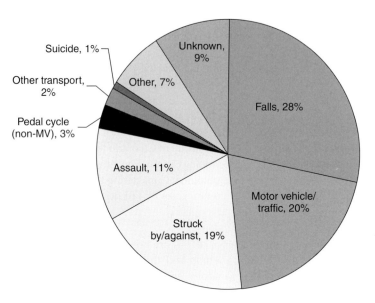

**Fig. 1.1.** Percentage of average annual TBI-related A&E department visits, hospitalizations, and deaths, by external cause, USA, 1995–2001.
[Source: Centre for Disease Control, USA.]

Germany to a high of 24.4 per 100 000 in Ravenna, Italy, with an overall average rate of about 15 deaths per 100 000 population per year.[6] In the USA, the overall mortality rate is 20–30 per 100 000 with half of the patients dying out of hospital.[15] For the Bronx area in New York, a rate of 28 per 100 000 has been reported.[16] Among adults in Johannesburg, South Africa, a much higher mortality rate of 138 per 100 000 for males and 24 per 100 000 for females has been reported, with 20% of TBIs resulting in death.[17]

## Causes of head injury

The most common causes of TBI are RTAs, falls, 'struck by' or 'struck against' events, assault/violence and sporting or recreation activities (Fig. 1.1). The majority of reports show RTAs as the leading cause of TBI followed by falls (which is reported as the leading cause in a few studies). In a review of studies from the EU, 21%–60% of TBIs were caused by RTAs (from a low of 21% in Norway and UK to a high of 60% in Sweden and Spain); 15%–62% were caused by falls (15% in Italy, 62% in Norway).[6] One study from Glasgow, Scotland, reported violence/assault (28%) as the second most common cause after falls (46%).[18] Overall, it has been estimated that, in the EU, 40% of TBIs are caused by RTAs, 37% are caused by falls, 7% are caused by violence/assault and 16% by other causes.[6]

It may be realized that the cause–effect relationships between the mechanisms of injury and TBI is confounded by age, gender, car ownership, urban residence and socioeconomic factors. For example, elderly people who have a relatively high incidence of falls are more likely than other age groups to be pedestrian victims of RTAs. The contributing factors may include side effects of medication, poor vision/hearing, slow reaction time and impairment of balance and mobility. In a study of TBI in children, the most common cause of injury was accidents involving children as pedestrians (36%), followed by falls (24%), cycling accidents (10%), as motor vehicle occupants (9%) and assault (6%).[19] In a UK study of minor head injury in adults, the common causes of injury were assault (30%–50%), RTA (25%) and falls (22%–43%).[10] It was reported that alcohol might be involved in 65% of adult head injuries. In a study from the USA, RTAs accounted for 50%, falls for 23%–30% and assaults for 20% of head injuries.[9] In the USA gunshot wound to the head is now a more frequent cause of serious head injury than RTA with a case fatality of about 90%.[9] In a study from Canada, RTAs accounted for 43% and assault for 11% of head injuries. In the EBIC study of patients admitted to neurosurgical units (with GCS ≤ 12), 51% were involved in a RTA, 12% in falls and 5% in assaults.[3] In the CRASH trial, the RTAs accounted for 64% and falls 13% of all head injuries.[12]

## Sporting head injuries

The study of the epidemiology of traumatic brain injury in sports is an area where significant advances in the prevention of head injuries by alteration of rules of participation and protective equipment have been made. Epidemiological studies are difficult to interpret, as they may be reported as relative frequencies compared to other mechanisms of head injuries, other types of sports injuries, injuries in other sports or often reported as incidence of injury per participant exposure within the sport. Media reporting of high profile sports injuries may give the perception of a much higher incidence rate than actually occurs both within the sport and compared to other sports. In certain sports such as boxing where there may be repetitive head injuries, epidemiological studies of chronic traumatic brain injury are important to inform opinion.

Overall, sports and recreation may account for up to 5%–10% of head injuries in studies of mechanism. Non-fatal traumatic brain injuries from sports and recreational activities are reported for hospital emergency department presentations in the USA from 2001–2005 as part of the National Electronic Injury Surveillance System – All Injury Program. An estimated 207 830 patients with sports- and recreation-related TBIs accounted for 5.1% of sports-related emergency department visits. Approximately 10.3% of patients with sports-related TBIs required subsequent transfer to a specialist facility or hospitalization. The most frequent causes of TBI were horse riding (11.7%), ice-skating (10.4%), riding all terrain vehicles (8.4%), tobogganing/sledding (8.3%) and bicycling (7.7%). American football accounted for 5.7% and combative sports including boxing, wrestling, martial arts and fencing made up 4.8%.[20]

Much work has been done on the epidemiology of American football-related head injuries. The annual rate of non-fatal head-related catastrophic injuries in American football has averaged around 0.3 per 100 000 for high school and college participants. The rate of fatal injuries has stabilised at 0.32 per 100 000 per year.[21]

The participant rate of acute head injury in amateur boxing is often less than in more popular sports such as horse riding and rugby union and absolute incidence is less. Fatalities in the ring are rare in amateur and professional boxing. There were 335 deaths between 1945 and 1979. The incidence of acute TBI has been reported in exposure terms, one study in the USA reporting a rate of 8.7 head injuries per 100 bouts in amateur boxing. In a study of amateur boxing in Denmark 5.7% to 7.8% of bouts were stopped because of a knockout.[22]

The cumulative effect of blows to the head and cerebral injury may result in chronic traumatic brain injury. A recent systematic review of observational studies has failed to find strong evidence to associate chronic traumatic brain injury with amateur boxing.[23] It is therefore important for the moral and philosophical arguments often cited against amateur and professional boxing to be informed by epidemiological data.

## Head injury requiring intensive care or neurosurgery

In a study from the UK, a rate of 40 per 100 000 was found for moderate to severe (10.9%) head injuries with a Glasgow Coma Scale of ≤12.[24] A figure of 4000 patients a year requiring neurosurgery in the UK has been reported.[25] In the paediatric population aged 0–14 years, an incidence of 5.6 per 100 000 per year has been quoted for admission to intensive care following a head injury.[19]

## Susceptibility to head injuries – apoE

There is evidence that genetic factors may predispose to a poorer outcome following head injury. The apolipoprotein E (apoE) is a protein that can influence the deposition of amyloid beta-protein in the cerebral cortex and is involved in neurodegeneration, brain injury and repair. Polymorphism of the apoE allele is associated with a worse outcome following head injury. Patients with the apoE epsilon 4 allele are more than twice as likely to have a poorer outcome at 6 months following head injury than those without.[26] Further studies have also shown that apoE epsilon 4 allele presence influences recovery from traumatic brain injury and this may be age dependent.[27]

## Prevention of head injury

Most TBI cases present with characteristic patterns of injury that are predictable and potentially preventable. Particular patterns may be caused by social, economic, behavioural or environmental factors. Identification of risk factors is therefore a prerequisite for devising preventive measures and public health policy. Attempts at reducing trauma from all mechanisms will also have the effect of reducing TBI to varying degrees. The prevention programmes for TBI focus on RTA prevention, cessation of drinking and driving, minimizing falls (particularly in the elderly), reducing sport injuries and decreasing violence and domestic abuse (particularly child abuse). Based on the standard principles of public health, William Haddon Jr, the first director of National Traffic Safety Bureau in the USA, proposed a conceptual model in the 1970s, the Haddon matrix, to address the problem of traffic safety.[28] The matrix illustrates the interaction of three factors – human, vehicle and environment – during three phases of an accident event – pre-accident, accident and post-accident. This concept has been successfully applied to the primary, secondary and tertiary prevention of RTAs and other types of accident (Table 1.4). In the USA, the remarkable reduction in mortality attributed to RTAs has been hailed as one of the main public health achievements of the twentieth century.[8] In the UK, primary prevention of accidents forms part of the government strategy for *Saving Lives: Our Healthier Nation*. This sets a public health target for reducing the incidence of serious injury from accidents by 10% and the mortality rate from accidents by 20% – saving 12 000 lives by the year 2010. A recent WHO report on road traffic injury prevention has summarized risk factors and interventions to reduce trauma from this common cause.[29]

Legislative policy and enforcement to control motor vehicle accidents by making wearing of helmets compulsory for cyclists and motorcyclists and reducing legal permissible alcohol levels for driving have been shown to be associated with a reduction in RTA associated head injuries.[29–31] Some countries have recently introduced a new regulation to prohibit the use of a handheld mobile phone while driving. Several studies have shown that the wearing of helmets by cyclists reduces the risk of head injury. In a recent Cochrane review of case-control studies, safety helmet use was associated with a 63%–88% reduction in the incidence of brain injury for all ages of cyclists. This protection was provided for crashes involving motor vehicles (69%) and all other causes (68%).[32] Evidence that wearing of helmets reduces injuries in skiers and snowboarders is also compelling.[33] Systematic reviews have shown that it is possible to reduce the incidence of falls by about 35% among older

**Table 1.4.** The Haddon matrix applied to prevention of road traffic accidents

| | Factors | | |
|---|---|---|---|
| Phase | People | Vehicle and equipment | Environment |
| Pre-accident (accident prevention) | Education Attitudes/behaviour Impairment (alcohol, drugs, fatigue) Police enforcement (traffic laws) Reflective clothing for pedestrians and cyclists | Roadworthiness Lighting (daytime lights on motorcycles) Braking and handling Speed limitation systems | Road design and layout (separation of car, cyclists, and pedestrians; better road marking and lighting) Speed limits Provision of transport alternatives |
| Accident (injury prevention/ limitation) | Use of seat belts Impairment (drink driving) | Crash-protective design and engineering Occupant restraints and safety devices (seat belts, air bags, child restraints) Use of helmets | Crash-protective roadside barriers/ objects (central reservation barrier, pedestrian crossing) |
| Post-accident (life sustaining and health improvement) | First aid and resuscitation Access to medical and rehabilitation services | Ease of access Fire risk | CCTV at danger points Access for rescue services (congestion) |

people.[34] Considering the wider determinants of public health, the role of health education and environmental engineering has been emphasized in the prevention of TBI. Examples of these efforts include education in schools about potential dangers around the home and road safety; education and examination of new motor vehicle drivers about risk factors for accidents; public health promotion campaigns to encourage use of helmets and seat belts and avoidance of alcohol and drugs when driving; better house designs to prevent falls and accidents; safer play areas for children and provision of cycle lanes.

## Summary

- TBI is an important global public health problem. Worldwide, around 10 million TBIs serious enough to result in hospitalization, long-term or lifelong disability, or death occur annually.
- About 5.3 million people in the USA and 6.2 million in the EU have some TBI-related disability, impairment, complaint or handicap.
- Average annual incidence rate of TBI in the EU is about 235 per 100 000 population.
- Average annual mortality rate of TBI in the EU is about 15 per 100 000 population.
- The risk of experiencing TBI is particularly high among children, young adults and the elderly.
- At all ages, males are about twice as likely as females to experience a TBI.
- The leading causes of TBI are RTAs, falls, struck by or against events, assault/violence and sports or recreation activities.

- Primary prevention of TBI includes prevention of RTAs, drinking and driving, falls, sport injuries and decreasing violence and domestic abuse.
- Legislation (e.g. seat belts, helmets, speed limits) and enforcement have been shown to reduce the incidence of TBI in the population.
- TBI is a public health problem that requires ongoing surveillance to monitor trends in the incidence and mortality, risk factors, causes and outcome (NCIPC has developed guidelines for surveillance of TBI http://www.cdc.gov/ncipc/). These data may help inform planning of services and identify individuals who are prone to suffering TBI and the situations where these accidents may occur.

# References

1. *International Statistical Classification of Diseases and Related Health Problems (Tenth Revision) 1992.* World Health Organization Geneva 1992. http://www.who.int/classifications/apps/icd/icd10online.
2. Bellner J, Jensen S-M, Lexell J, Romner B. Diagnostic criteria and the use of ICD-10 codes to define and classify minor head injury. *J Neurol Neurosurg Psychiatry* 2003; **74**: 351–2.
3. Murray G, Teasdale G, Braakman R, Cohadon F, Dearden M *et al.* The European Brain Injury Consortium Survey of Head Injuries. *Acta Neurochir* 1999; **141**: 223–36.
4. Murray CJ, Lopez AD. *Global Health Statistics.* Geneva: WHO, 1996.
5. Langlois J, Rutland-Brown W, Thomas K. Traumatic brain injury in the United States: emergency department visits, hospitalizations, and deaths. *Center for Disease Control and Prevention, National Center for Injury Prevention and Control.* Atlanta, Georgia, 2004.
6. Tagliaferri F, Compagnone C, Korsic M *et al.* A systematic review of brain injury epidemiology in Europe. *Acta Neurochir (Wien)* 2006; **148**: 255–68.
7. Tennant A. Admission to hospital following head injury in England: Incidence and socio-economic associations. *BMC Public Health* 2005; **5**: 21.
8. Centres for Disease Control and Prevention. Motor vehicle safety: a 20th century public health achievement. *Morbidity and Mortality Weekly Report* 1999; **48**: 369–74.
9. Bruns J, Hauser W. The epidemiology of traumatic brain injury: a review. *Epilepsia* 2003; **44 (Suppl 1)**: 2–10.
10. Hospital episodes statistics (2000/2001). Department of Health.
11. Foulkes M, Eisenberg H, Jane J, Marmarou A, Marshall L *et al.* The Traumatic Coma Data Bank: design, methods and baseline characteristics. *J Neurosurg* 1991; **75**: S8-14.
12. CRASH Trial Collaborators. Effect of intravenous corticosteroids on death within 14 days in 10 008 adults with clinically severe head injury (MRC CRASH Trial): randomised placebo controlled trial. *Lancet* 2004; **364**: 1321–8.
13. Kay A, Teasdale G. Head Injury in the United Kingdom. *World J Surg* 2001; **25**: 1210–20.
14. Tiret L, Hausherr E, Thicoipe M, Garros B, Maurette P, Castel J, Hatton F. The epidemiology of head trauma in Aquitaine (France), 1986: a community-based study of hospital admissions and deaths. *Int J Epidemiol* 1990; **19**(1): 133–40.
15. National Center for Injury Prevention and Control. Traumatic Brain Injury in the United States: a report to Congress 1999. Center for Disease Control and Prevention, US Department of Health and Health Services.
16. Cooper K, Tabbaddor K, Hauser W *et al.* The epidemiology of head injury in the Bronx. *Neuroepidemiology* 1983; **2**: 70–8.
17. Nell V, Brown D. Epidemiology of traumatic brain injury in Johannesburg – II. Morbidity, mortality and etiology. *Soc Sci Med* 1991; **33**(3): 289–96.
18. Thornhill S, Teasdale GM, Murray GD, McEwen J, Roy CW, Penny KI. Disability in young people and adults one year after head injury: prospective cohort study. *Br Med J* 2000; **320**: 1631–5.
19. Parslow R, Morris K, Tasker R, Forsyth R, Hawley C. Epidemiology of traumatic brain

injury in children receiving intensive care in the UK. *Arch Dis Child* 2005; **90**: 1182–7.

20. Gilchrist J, Thomas K, Wald M, Langlois J. Nonfatal traumatic brain injuries from sports and recreation activities – United States 2001–2005. *Morbidity and Mortality Weekly Report* 2007; **56**: 733–7.

21. Clarke K. The epidemiology of athletic head injuries. In: Canta RC, ed. *Neurologic Athletic Head and Spine Injuries*. USA, WB Saunders, 2000.

22. Jordan B. Head and spine injuries in boxing. In: Canta RC, ed. *Neurologic Athletic Head and Spine Injuries*. USA, WB Saunders, 2000.

23. Loosemore M, Knowles C, Whyte G. Amateur boxing and risk of chronic traumatic brain injury: systematic review of observational studies. *Br Med J* 2007; **335**: 809–12.

24. Yates P, Williams W, Harris A, Round A, Jenkins R. An epidemiological study of head injuries in a UK population attending an emergency department. *J Neurol Neurosurg Psychiatry* 2006; **77**: 699–701.

25. SBNS Working Party. Safe Neurosurgery 2000. *A report from the Society of British Neurological Surgeons. SBNS*, 35–43 Lincoln's Inn Fields, London.

26. Teasdale G, Murray G, Nicoll A. The association between apoE ε4, age and outcome after head injury: a prospective cohort study. *Brain* 2005; **128**: 2556–61.

27. Alexander S, Kerr M, Kim Y, Kamboh M, Beers S, Conley Y. Apoprotein E4 allele presence and functional outcome after severe traumatic brain injury. *J Neurotrauma* 2007; **24**: 790–7.

28. Haddon W Jr. A logical framework for categorizing highway safety phenomena and activity. *J Trauma* 1972; **12**: 193–207.

29. World report on road traffic injury prevention. Geneva, WHO, 2004.

30. W. Chiu, S. Huang, S. Tsai, J. Lin, M. Tsai, T. Lin, W. Huang. The impact of time, legislation and geography on the epidemiology of traumatic brain injury. *J Clin Neurosci* 2007; **14**: 930–5.

31. Sevadei F, Begliomini C, Gardini E, Giustini E, Giustini M, Taggi F, Kraus J. Effect of Italy's motorcycle helmet law on traumatic brain injuries. *Inj Prev* 2003; **9**: 257–60.

32. Thompson DC, Rivara FP, Thompson R. Helmets for preventing head and facial injuries in bicyclists. *Cochrane Database of Systematic Reviews* 1999, Issue 4. Art. No.: CD001855. DOI: 10.1002/14651858. CD001855.

33. Hagel BE, Pless IB, Goulet C, Platt RW, Robitaille Y. Effectiveness of helmets in skiers and snowboarders: case-control and case crossover study. *Br Med J* 2005; **330**: 281–3.

34. Gillespie L. Preventing falls in elderly people. *Br Med J* 2004; **328**: 653–4.

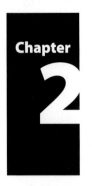

# Chapter 2

# The neuropathology of head injury

David A. Hilton

## Introduction

The neuropathological changes associated with head injuries are dependent on a number of factors, including both the type and severity of the injury, and the former can be divided into non-missile and missile types of injury. Non-missile injury (or blunt head injury) is usually due to rapid acceleration or deceleration of the head, with or without impact, or less commonly crushing of the head, and most often occur as the result of road traffic accidents or falls. Missile injuries are due to penetration of the skull by a rapidly moving external object, e.g. gunshot wounds, and result in a different pattern of brain injury. The neuropathology can be separated into focal (or localized) lesions such as contusions, haemorrhages, skull fractures or diffuse changes such as diffuse axonal injury, diffuse vascular injury, brain swelling and ischaemia. Although the lesions may develop at the time of the head injury (primary), many develop over a period of hours to days after the triggering event (secondary), and a significant minority of patients with severe head injury develop progressive neurological deterioration several years later. The pathological consequences of head injury are influenced by a number of factors including patient age, co-morbidity such as alcohol,[1] other injuries (particularly if they result in ischaemia or hypoxia), sepsis and medical treatment. In addition there is now clear evidence that genetic polymorphisms for the apolipoprotein gene have a significant effect on both the pathological changes[2] and clinical outcomes from head injury.[3]

## Focal injury

### Scalp injury

Focal injuries to the scalp such as abrasions and lacerations can be a useful indicator of the site of impact and may give some clues as to the type of object the brain came into contact with. Scalp lacerations may be an important route for infection and can result in excessive haemorrhage. Bruising may not always be a reliable indicator of impact location, for example, periorbital bruising is often associated with fractures of the orbital roofs following a contracoup injury to the occiput, and mastoid bruising ('battle sign') can be caused by blood tracking from a fracture of the petrous temporal bone.

### Skull fractures

These are not always of clinical importance, although they do indicate that significant force was involved in the head injury, and are associated with intracranial injury such as haemorrhage.[4,5] Linear fractures are the most common type, and extend from the point of impact along lines of least resistance, although their direction is also dependent upon the anatomy of the skull. A significant force exerted over a larger area of the skull may result in a

*Head Injury: A Multidisciplinary Approach*, ed. Peter C. Whitfield, Elfyn O. Thomas, Fiona Summers, Maggie Whyte and Peter J. Hutchinson. Published by Cambridge University Press. © Cambridge University Press 2009.

comminuted fracture with multiple fragments, whereas, if the force is exerted over a relatively small area of skull, a depressed fracture results, with a fragment of skull being protruded inwards indenting the brain. Diastatic fractures, which follow suture lines, are more common in children. Compound fractures increase the likelihood of intracranial infection via the laceration to the overlying skin. Skull-based fractures may result in cerebrospinal fluid (CSF) leakage and can extend into the air sinuses, causing aeroceles, and are also an important source of infection. Skull-based fractures extending along both petrous ridges and through the pituitary fossa result in a 'hinge' fracture, which indicates severe side to side impact of the head, and are usually associated with fatal head injuries. A 'ring' fracture encircling the foramen magnum usually results from severe hyperextension of the neck, or falls from a height, where the individual landed on their feet. A common type of skull-based fracture is that involving the orbital roofs due to contracoup injury when an individual falls backwards, hitting their occiput on a hard surface with the resulting shock-wave passing through the skull and fracturing these relatively thin bones.

## Brain contusions and lacerations

Tears to the pial membrane (lacerations) are often associated with underlying bruising (contusions). These may be of coup type, often associated with an overlying fracture (fracture contusion). More commonly contusions are due to contracoup injury and follow a stereo-typed pattern occurring at the frontal poles, orbital surfaces of the frontal lobes, temporal poles and lateral surfaces of the temporal lobes. These contracoup contusions are due to continued movement of the brain within the cranial cavity, particularly following rapid deceleration such as when the moving head hits a solid surface, and occur at sites where the skull has an irregular internal surface. Contusions are relatively uncommon in young infants where the floor of the skull has a smoother contour. Contusions may also occur following herniation of brain, either internally where brain is compressed against a dural edge, or externally via a craniectomy defect where brain is compressed against the skull edge. Contusions consist of areas of haemorrhage into brain parenchyma, often perpendicular to the cortical surface, and may continue to bleed over a period of hours after the initial injury, making a significant contribution to raised intracranial pressure. Haemorrhage may extend to the subcortical white matter, or through the leptomeninges into the subdural space, resulting in a 'burst lobe', most often in the frontal and temporal poles. After a period of days to weeks, the brain tissue will reabsorb, resulting in a wedge-shaped area of cavitation at the crests of the gyri, which has a brown color owing to the presence of blood breakdown products. Although contusions may be asymptomatic, they can be a cause of long-term epilepsy.

## Intracranial haemorrhage

### Extradural haemorrhage

Extradural haemorrhage results from direct impact and is uncommon at the extremes of age, but occurs in approximately 10% of severe head injury patients, most often in association with a fracture of the squamous temporal bone and tear in the underlying middle meningeal artery. However, particularly in children, where the bones are more flexible, a vascular tear may occur without a skull fracture. These are classically lens-shaped haematomas that accumulate over a period of hours as the dura is stripped from the skull, so that the patient may have an initial lucid interval. The volume of the haematoma is a predictor of outcome and most patients with more than 150 ml of blood have a poor prognosis.[6]

## Subdural haemorrhage

Subdural haemorrhage usually results from tearing of the bridging veins, particularly those adjacent to the superior sagittal sinus, in association with rapid acceleration or deceleration of the head, and does not require direct impact. It is more common in the elderly, as brain atrophy results in an increased capacity for the brain to move within the cranial cavity. Rarely, subdural haemorrhage may be due to other causes such as arterial bleeding, including ruptured arteriovenous malformations and berry aneurysms.[7] Subdural haemorrhage may present shortly after the head injury (acute subdural haemorrhage), 1–2 weeks later (subacute subdural haemorrhage) or more than 2 weeks later (chronic subdural haemorrhage). Chronic subdural haematomas are particularly common in the elderly, alcoholics and patients with a low intracranial pressure, such as those shunted following hydrocephalus. In some of these patients (particularly the elderly) the head injury may be relatively trivial and not remembered by the patient. Acute haematomas consist of soft clotted blood, often with a blackcurrant-jelly appearance. After several days, this breaks down into serous fluid, and after a period of 1–2 weeks a membrane of granulation tissue with proliferating fibroblasts and capillaries develops, initially on the dural aspect of the haematoma and later on the pial surface. Although the haematoma is usually eventually reabsorbed, re-bleeding is common, probably due to haemorrhage from the newly formed immature blood vessels,[8] although a number of other factors including excessive fibrinolysis may be involved.[9]

## Subarachnoid haemorrhage

Small collections of subarachnoid blood are fairly common after head injury, particularly in association with contusions and lacerations. Subarachnoid haemorrhage may also complicate intraventricular haemorrhage due to a leakage of blood through the exit-foraminae of the fourth ventricle. Occasionally, a massive subarachnoid haemorrhage may occur around the ventral aspect of the brainstem due to laceration of a vertebral artery, basilar artery or one of the smaller arteries.[10,11] This type of haemorrhage often results from an impact to the head or neck in an assault, and causes immediate collapse, and is often fatal. Patients who survive significant subarachnoid haemorrhage may develop hydrocephalus as a chronic complication.

## Intraventricular haemorrhage

In the context of head injury, intraventricular haemorrhage is usually secondary to either deep haemorrhages in the region of the basal ganglia or contusions.[12]

## Parenchymal haemorrhage

Parenchymal haemorrhage may occur secondary to contusions or in association with diffuse axonal injury, when they are usually deep seated in the region of the basal ganglia, thalamus and parasagittal white matter.

## Other types of focal injury
### Pituitary infarction

This may result from traumatic transection of the pituitary stalk or severe elevation of intracranial pressure.

### Brainstem avulsion

Severe hyperextension of the neck may result in brainstem avulsion, usually at the ponto-medullary junction or, less commonly, at the craniocervical junction, and unless incomplete, results in immediate death.

**Table 2.1.** Grading of traumatic axonal injury[19]

| Grade 1 | Axonal damage |
|---------|---------------|
| Grade 2 | Axonal damage and haemorrhagic lesions in corpus callosum |
| Grade 3 | Axonal damage and haemorrhagic lesions in corpus callosum and brainstem |

### Cranial nerve avulsion

Olfactory bulb injury, resulting in anosmia, is common after head injury, but other avulsions including the optic, facial and auditory nerves, also occur.

### Focal vascular injury

Carotid cavernous fistula, resulting in pulsating exophthalmos and carotid or vertebral artery dissections, also occur with head injuries.

## Diffuse injury

### Traumatic axonal injury

The term diffuse axonal injury (DAI) indicates widespread axonal damage within the brain, which may result from a number of insults including trauma, hypoxia, ischaemia and hypoglycaemia.[13,14] The neuropathological features of diffuse axonal injury following trauma differs from that seen after ischaemic injury.[15] Traumatic axonal injury (TAI) is caused by a rapid acceleration or deceleration of the head, particularly where there is rotational or coronal movement of the head.[16] TAI is particularly common following road traffic accidents, but may occur as a result of falls from a height and assaults[17] and is seen in the majority of patients with fatal head injury.[18] Patients with TAI are typically unconscious from the moment of injury and have a poor outcome, with death, severe disability and persistent vegetative state.[19] TAI is characterized by damage to axons, and in most cases, petechial haemorrhages. These haemorrhages, which are 3–5 mm across, occur instantaneously, and their presence determines the grade of TAI (see Table 2.1). They occur in the corpus callosum, often on either side of the midline, most extensively in the splenium, and in the dorso-lateral quadrant of the upper brain stem, usually in the superior cerebellar peduncle and predominantly unilateral (Fig. 2.1).

Axonal damage results in swollen, tortuous and transected fibres throughout the white matter, including the corpus callosum, parasagittal subcortical fibres, deep grey matter, cerebellar folia and brainstem tracts.[20] The axonal swellings can be seen with silver preparations after several hours survival and have been termed 'axon retraction balls'. However, axonal damage can be detected histologically by the accumulation of β-amyloid precursor protein as early as 35 minutes after head injury[21] (Fig. 2.2). After a period of several days to weeks, there is accumulation of microglia around damaged axons followed by Wallerian degeneration of axons resulting in shrinkage and grey discolouration of hemispheric white matter, atrophy of the brainstem and ventricular dilatation (Fig. 2.3). The axonal damage results from shearing forces exerted on long fibre tracts within the central nervous system causing damage to the axolemma, resulting in calcium influx and activation of calcium-dependent enzymes. Calpain activation results in damage to cytoskeletal proteins,[22,23] disrupting axonal transport mechanisms and resulting in accumulation of proteins at the site of injury and eventual axotomy.[24,25] Deep grey matter and parasagittal haemorrhages ('gliding contusions'), which are often bilateral, may be associated with TAI.

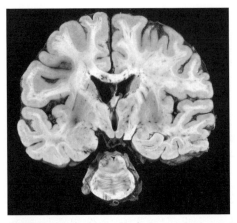

**Fig. 2.1.** Traumatic axonal injury resulting from a road traffic accident showing petechial haemorrhages within the corpus callosum and dorso-lateral quadrant of the brainstem. Also, note herniation contusion on parahippocampal gyrus, indicating previous brain swelling.

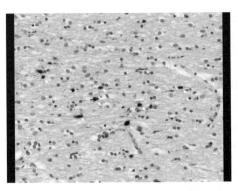

**Fig. 2.2.** Following immunocytochemistry for β-amyloid precursor protein, swollen darkly stained axons can be seen.

**Fig. 2.3.** Patient who survived in a persistent vegetative state for 4 years after traumatic axonal injury showing extensive loss and cavitation of hemispheric white matter, with atrophy of the corpus callosum and hydrocephalus ex vacuo.

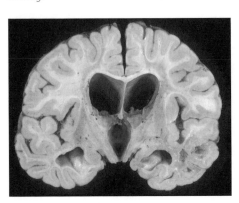

## Diffuse vascular injury

Some patients who die immediately following a severe acceleration or deceleration type of brain injury have widespread petechial haemorrhage throughout the brain due to shearing forces being exerted upon blood vessels. These patients do not survive long enough to develop any axonal changes.

## Brain swelling and cerebral ischaemia

Brain swelling is a common finding in patients with significant head injury, particularly in children and adolescents[26] and may be due to a number of factors including the primary brain injury, intracranial haematomas, epilepsy and systemic complications such as hypoxia, ischaemia and sepsis. Following brain injury, there may be an increase in cerebral blood volume due to vasodilation,[27] leakage of fluid due to incompetence of the blood–brain barrier (vasogenic oedema) and increased water content of cells within the central nervous system (cytotoxic oedema). Brain swelling results in raised intracranial pressure and a reduced cerebral perfusion pressure, causing ischaemic brain damage, which is most marked in susceptible regions such as the watershed areas, particularly at the borders of the anterior and middle cerebral artery territories, and within the Sommer's sector of the hippocampus.[28] Differential pressures between the intracranial compartments may result in herniation of brain and further more localized ischaemic injury; subfalcine herniation of the cingulate gyrus may result in compression of the anterior cerebral artery; transtentoral herniation (which is usually caudal, but may be rostral when there is a large posterior fossa haematoma) causes compression of the posterior cerebral artery, the parahippocampal gyrus and midbrain; transforaminal herniation of the brainstem (coning) causes ischaemia of vital brainstem functions and death.

## Fat embolism

Although not a direct result of head injury, fat embolism may be seen in patients with head injury who have long bone fractures. This syndrome classically causes dyspnoea, hypoxia and confusion 2–3 days after a traumatic incident with multiple petechial haemorrhages present in the white matter, and is due to lipid emboli released from the marrow lodging in lung and intracranial blood vessels.

## Inflicted head injury in childhood (non-accidental injury) – see also Chapter 4

The 'shaken baby syndrome' is important to recognize in young children and infants with unexplained head injuries. The relatively large head and weak neck, together with an immature brain, predispose infants and young children to brain injury resulting from shaking. Alertness to the syndrome should be raised by the presence of retinal haemorrhages, which are otherwise uncommon in infants more than a month after childbirth, and may be associated with other ocular injuries such as retinal tears, detachments, vitreous haemorrhage and retinal folds. These children often have a thin film of bilateral subdural haemorrhage, subarachnoid haemorrhage, haemorrhage into the optic nerve sheaths, cervical nerve roots and deep muscles of the neck. Traumatic axonal injury may be present, particularly in the lower medulla and upper cervical spinal cord.[29] There is usually marked brain swelling and, if an impact occurs, contusional tears within the white matter may occur in the orbital and temporal lobes. This constellation of injuries may occur as the result of severe shaking, with or without impact, although there is controversy as to the mechanisms causing these lesions.[30,31]

## Missile head injury

Impact of the head by an external object may result in a depressed skull fracture or penetration into the cranial cavity and focal brain damage. Penetrating injuries are common with gunshot wounds, but may also occur with knife stabs, particularly in the orbital and squamous temporal bones. Low velocity penetrating injuries of this type cause damage by direct injury to blood vessels, nerves and brain tissue and the complications caused by persisting haemorrhage and infection. High-velocity bullets (such as from rifles) often exit the skull (perforating injury) and may result in extensive brain damage from the massive shock wave caused.

## Progressive neurological degeneration

The pathological consequences of head injury may continue for a considerable time[32] and approximately 15% of patients who survive severe head injury undergo progressive neurological decline 10–20 years later, especially if the head injury is repetitive such as with boxers ('dementia pugilistica'). This neurological decline can result in a syndrome of incoordination, Parkinsonism, apathy and dementia and patients have a fenestrated septum pellucidum, degeneration of the substanta nigra and Alzheimer-type pathology in the cerebral cortex with neurofibrillary tangles and β-amyloid plaque deposition. β-amyloid deposition is seen in many head injury patients,[33] and the extent of deposition is determined by the apolipoprotein gene polymorphism.[34] Neurofibrillary tangle formation appears to be a relatively early event and has been seen in relatively young boxers.[35]

# Excitotoxicity and nitric oxide in head injury

The complex cascade of biochemical changes triggered by head injury is not fully understood, but some components may have a neuroprotective effect, whilst others may contribute to cell injury and death. Key factors in these processes are glutamate-mediated excitotoxicity and nitric oxide production, which will be briefly reviewed.

Widespread neuronal depolarization occurs with severe head injury and leads to massive release of several excitatory amino acids, including glutamate, which is elevated in extracellular fluid in models of head injury[36] and in the CSF of head injury patients.[37] Glutamate is widely distributed in the brain and acts on a number of receptors, including N-methyl-D-aspartate (NMDA) receptors, kainate receptors, α-amino-3-hydroxy-5-methyl-4-isoxazole proprionic acid (AMPA) receptors and metabotropic receptors. Over-stimulation of glutamate receptors causes massive calcium influx into neurons, which has been demonstrated in head injury,[38] and has a neurotoxic effect, particularly on dendrites.[39,40] A number of processes are triggered by calcium influx, including activation of calcium-dependent enzymes such as phospholipases, which cause cell membrane damage thus contributing to cerebral edema[41,42] and calpains, which degrade a range of cytoskeletal and other proteins,[22,23] disrupting axonal function. Excitatory amino acids also contribute to the release of reactive oxygen species ('free radicals'), which cause peroxidative damage to cell membranes, mitochondria, proteins and DNA.[43] Although the inflammatory response to head injury may contribute to tissue damage and release of reactive oxygen species,[44,45] inflammatory cytokines such as tumour necrosis factor, interleukin-1 and nerve growth factor also have neuroprotective properties.[46–49] Another product of inflammatory cells is nitric oxide (NO), which is also synthesized by neurons and endothelial cells by the actions of endothelial and neuronal nitric oxide synthases (eNOS and nNOS). In the first few hours after head injury, endothelial and neuronal NO production occurs, which have vasodilator[50,51] and neurotoxic effects,[52] respectively. NO produced by inflammatory cells, due to activation of inducible nitric oxide synthase (iNOS), occurs several hours after injury and may have an overall beneficial effect.[53] NO has a number of effects in the brain including increasing cerebral perfusion,[50] downregulating NMDA receptors thus attenuating excitotoxicity,[54] forming toxic peroxynitrite compounds with reactive oxygen species[55] and the inhibition of cell death mechanisms.[56] The location, timing and amount of NO production may alter the overall balance of these various actions, and determine whether there will be a neurotoxic or neuroprotective effect from NO.

Many of these processes contribute to cell injury, triggering apoptosis or 'programmed cell death', which occurs in both glia and neurons following head injury.[57] Cell death is associated with alterations in Bcl-2 gene expression, which is protective against apoptosis[58] and activation of caspases[59] which cleave cytoskeletal proteins,[60] and activate endonucleases which fragment DNA.[61] Many novel therapies are now being evaluated in animal and human trials, aimed at inhibiting the components of these processes that promote apoptosis, in order to improve outcome following head injury.

# References

1. Tien HC, Tremblay LN, Rizoli SB *et al.* Association between alcohol and mortality in patients with severe traumatic head injury. *Arch Surg* 2006; **141**: 1185–91.

2. Smith C, Graham DI, Murray LS, Stewart J, Nicoll JA. Association of apoE e4 and cerebrovascular pathology in traumatic brain injury. *J Neurol Neurosurg Psychiatry* 2006; 77: 363–6.

3. Sorbi S, Nacmias B, Piacentini S *et al.* ApoE as a prognostic factor for post-traumatic coma. *Nat Med* 1995; **1**: 852.

4. Servadei F, Ciucci G, Morichetti A *et al.* Skull fracture as a factor of increased risk in minor head injuries. Indication for a broader use of cerebral computed tomography scanning. *Surg Neurol* 1988; **30**: 364–9.

5. Mendelow AD, Teasdale G, Jennett B, Bryden J, Hessett C, Murray G. Risks of intracranial haematoma in head injured adults. *Br Med J (Clin Res Ed)* 1983; **287**: 1173–6.

6. Rivas JJ, Lobato RD, Sarabia R, Cordobes F, Cabrera A, Gomez P. Extradural hematoma: analysis of factors influencing the courses of 161 patients. *Neurosurgery* 1988; **23**: 44–51.

7. Tokoro K, Nakajima F, Yamataki A. Acute spontaneous subdural hematoma of arterial origin. *Surg Neurol* 1988; **29**: 159–63.

8. Yamashima T, Yamamoto S. How do vessels proliferate in the capsule of a chronic subdural hematoma? *Neurosurgery* 1984; **15**: 672–8.

9. Domenicucci M, Signorini P, Strzelecki J, Delfini R. Delayed post-traumatic epidural hematoma. A review. *Neurosurg Rev* 1995; **18**: 109–22.

10. Coast GC, Gee DJ. Traumatic subarachnoid haemorrhage: an alternative source. *J Clin Pathol* 1984; **37**: 1245–8.

11. Dolman CL. Rupture of posterior inferior cerebellar artery by single blow to head. *Arch Pathol Lab Med* 1986; **110**: 494–6.

12. Fujitsu K, Kuwabara T, Muramoto M, Hirata K, Mochimatsu Y. Traumatic intraventricular hemorrhage: report of twenty-six cases and consideration of the pathogenic mechanism. *Neurosurgery* 1988; **23**: 423–30.

13. Dolinak D, Smith C, Graham DI. Global hypoxia per se is an unusual cause of axonal injury. *Acta Neuropathol (Berl)* 2000; **100**: 553–60.

14. Dolinak D, Smith C, Graham DI. Hypoglycaemia is a cause of axonal injury. *Neuropathol Appl Neurobiol* 2000; **26**: 448–53.

15. Reichard RR, Smith C, Graham DI. The significance of beta-APP immunoreactivity in forensic practice. *Neuropathol Appl Neurobiol* 2005; **31**: 304–13.

16. Gennarelli TA, Thibault LE, Adams JH, Graham DI, Thompson CJ, Marcincin RP. Diffuse axonal injury and traumatic coma in the primate. *Ann Neurol* 1982; **12**: 564–74.

17. Graham DI, Clark JC, Adams JH, Gennarelli TA. Diffuse axonal injury caused by assault. *J Clin Pathol* 1992; **45**: 840–1.

18. Pilz P. Axonal injury in head injury. *Acta Neurochir Suppl (Wien)* 1983; **32**: 119–23.

19. Adams JH, Doyle D, Ford I, Gennarelli TA, Graham DI, McLellan DR. Diffuse axonal injury in head injury: definition, diagnosis and grading. *Histopathology* 1989; **15**: 49–59.

20. Strich SJ. Diffuse degeneration of the cerebral white matter in severe dementia following head injury. *J Neurol Neurosurg Psychiatry* 1956; **19**: 163–85.

21. Hortobagyi T, Wise S, Hunt N *et al.* Traumatic axonal damage in the brain can be detected using beta-APP immunohistochemistry within 35 min after head injury to human adults. *Neuropathol Appl Neurobiol* 2007; **33**: 226–37.

22. Johnson GV, Litersky JM, Jope RS. Degradation of microtubule-associated protein 2 and brain spectrin by calpain: a comparative study. *J Neurochem* 1991; **56**: 1630–8.

23. Kampfl A, Posmantur R, Nixon R *et al.* mu-calpain activation and calpain-mediated cytoskeletal proteolysis following traumatic brain injury. *J Neurochem* 1996; **67**: 1575–83.

24. Povlishock JT. Traumatically induced axonal injury: pathogenesis and pathobiological implications. *Brain Pathol* 1992; **2**: 1–12.

25. Maxwell WL, Graham DI. Loss of axonal microtubules and neurofilaments after stretch-injury to guinea pig optic nerve fibers. *J Neurotrauma* 1997; **14**: 603–14.

26. Graham DI, Ford I, Adams JH et al. Fatal head injury in children. *J Clin Pathol* 1989; **42**: 18–22.

27. Bouma GJ, Muizelaar JP, Fatouros P. Pathogenesis of traumatic brain swelling: role of cerebral blood volume. *Acta Neurochir Suppl* 1998; **71**: 272–5.

28. Graham DI, Ford I, Adams JH et al. Ischaemic brain damage is still common in fatal non-missile head injury. *J Neurol Neurosurg Psychiatry* 1989; **52**: 346–50.

29. Geddes JF, Hackshaw AK, Vowles GH, Nickols CD, Whitwell HL. Neuropathology of inflicted head injury in children. I. Patterns of brain damage. *Brain* 2001; **124**: 1290–8.

30. Geddes JF, Tasker RC, Hackshaw AK et al. Dural haemorrhage in non-traumatic infant deaths: does it explain the bleeding in 'shaken baby syndrome'? *Neuropathol Appl Neurobiol* 2003; **29**: 14–22.

31. Reece RM. The evidence base for shaken baby syndrome: response to editorial from 106 doctors. *Br Med J* 2004; **328**: 1316–17.

32. Smith DH, Chen XH, Pierce JE, Wolf JA, Trojanowski JQ, Graham DI et al. Progressive atrophy and neuron death for one year following brain trauma in the rat. *J Neurotrauma* 1997; **14**: 715–27.

33. Roberts GW, Gentleman SM, Lynch A, Graham DI. beta A4 amyloid protein deposition in brain after head trauma. *Lancet* 1991; **338**: 1422–3.

34. Nicoll JA, Roberts GW, Graham DI. Apolipoprotein E epsilon 4 allele is associated with deposition of amyloid beta-protein following head injury. *Nat Med* 1995; **1**: 135–7.

35. Geddes JF, Vowles GH, Robinson SF, Sutcliffe JC. Neurofibrillary tangles, but not Alzheimer-type pathology, in a young boxer. *Neuropathol Appl Neurobiol* 1996; **22**: 12–16.

36. Nilsson P, Hillered L, Ponten U, Ungerstedt U. Changes in cortical extracellular levels of energy-related metabolites and amino acids following concussive brain injury in rats. *J Cereb Blood Flow Metab* 1990; **10**: 631–7.

37. Zhang H, Zhang X, Zhang T, Chen L. Excitatory amino acids in cerebrospinal fluid of patients with acute head injuries. *Clin Chem* 2001; **47**: 1458–62.

38. Fineman I, Hovda DA, Smith M, Yoshino A, Becker DP. Concussive brain injury is associated with a prolonged accumulation of calcium: a $^{45}$Ca autoradiographic study. *Brain Res* 1993; **624**: 94–102.

39. Olney JW, Rhee V, Ho OL. Kainic acid: a powerful neurotoxic analogue of glutamate. *Brain Res* 1974; **77**: 507–12.

40. Olney JW, Ho OL, Rhee V. Cytotoxic effects of acidic and sulphur containing amino acids on the infant mouse central nervous system. *Exp Brain Res* 1971; **14**: 61–76.

41. Shohami E, Shapira Y, Yadid G, Reisfeld N, Yedgar S. Brain phospholipase A2 is activated after experimental closed head injury in the rat. *J Neurochem* 1989; **53**: 1541–6.

42. Dhillon HS, Donaldson D, Dempsey RJ, Prasad MR. Regional levels of free fatty acids and Evans blue extravasation after experimental brain injury. *J Neurotrauma* 1994; **11**: 405–15.

43. Dugan LL, Choi DW. Excitotoxicity, free radicals, and cell membrane changes. *Ann Neurol* 1994; **35** Suppl: S17–21.

44. Fee D, Crumbaugh A, Jacques T et al. Activated/effector CD4+ T cells exacerbate acute damage in the central nervous system following traumatic injury. *J Neuroimmunol* 2003; **136**: 54–66.

45. Feuerstein GZ, Wang X, Barone FC. Inflammatory gene expression in cerebral ischemia and trauma. Potential new therapeutic targets. *Ann NY Acad Sci* 1997; **825**: 179–93.

46. Bruce AJ, Boling W, Kindy MS et al. Altered neuronal and microglial responses to excitotoxic and ischemic brain injury in mice lacking TNF receptors. *Nat Med* 1996; **2**: 788–94.

47. Cheng B, Christakos S, Mattson MP. Tumor necrosis factors protect neurons against metabolic-excitotoxic insults and promote maintenance of calcium homeostasis. *Neuron* 1994; **12**: 139–53.

48. DeKosky ST, Styren SD, O'Malley ME et al. Interleukin-1 receptor antagonist suppresses neurotrophin response in injured rat brain. *Ann Neurol* 1996; **39**: 123–7.

49. Mattson MP, Goodman Y, Luo H, Fu W, Furukawa K. Activation of NF-kappaB protects hippocampal neurons against oxidative stress-induced apoptosis: evidence for induction of manganese superoxide dismutase and suppression of

peroxynitrite production and protein tyrosine nitration. *J Neurosci Res* 1997; **49**: 681–97.

50. Huang Z, Huang PL, Ma J *et al.* Enlarged infarcts in endothelial nitric oxide synthase knockout mice are attenuated by nitro-L-arginine. *J Cereb Blood Flow Metab* 1996; **16**: 981–7.

51. Dewitt DS, Smith TG, Deyo DJ, Miller KR, Uchida T, Prough DS. L-arginine and superoxide dismutase prevent or reverse cerebral hypoperfusion after fluid-percussion traumatic brain injury. *J Neurotrauma* 1997; **14**: 223–33.

52. Schulz JB, Matthews RT, Jenkins BG *et al.* Blockade of neuronal nitric oxide synthase protects against excitotoxicity in vivo. *J Neurosci* 1995; **15**: 8419–29.

53. Sinz EH, Kochanek PM, Dixon CE *et al.* Inducible nitric oxide synthase is an endogenous neuroprotectant after traumatic brain injury in rats and mice. *J Clin Invest* 1999; **104**: 647–56.

54. Lipton SA, Choi YB, Pan ZH *et al.* A redox-based mechanism for the neuroprotective and neurodestructive effects of nitric oxide and related nitroso-compounds. *Nature* 1993; **364**: 626–32.

55. Beckman JS, Beckman TW, Marshall PA, Freeman BA. Apparent hydroxyl radical production by peroxynitrite: implications for endothelial injury from nitric oxide and Superoxide. *Proc Natl Acad Sci USA* 1990; **87**(4): 1620–4.

56. Kim YM, Talanian RV, Billiar TR. Nitric oxide inhibits apoptosis by preventing increases in caspase-3-like activity via two distinct mechanisms. *J Biol Chem* 1997; **272**: 31138–48.

57. Newcomb JK, Zhao X, Pike BR, Hayes RL. Temporal profile of apoptotic-like changes in neurons and astrocytes following controlled cortical impact injury in the rat. *Exp Neurol* 1999; **158**: 76–88.

58. Nakamura M, Raghupathi R, Merry DE, Scherbel U, Saatman KE, McIntosh TK. Overexpression of Bcl-2 is neuroprotective after experimental brain injury in transgenic mice. *J Comp Neurol* 1999; **412**: 681–92.

59. Eldadah BA, Faden AI. Caspase pathways, neuronal apoptosis, and CNS injury. *J Neurotrauma* 2000; **17**: 811–29.

60. Aikman J, O'Steen B, Silver X *et al.* Alpha-II-spectrin after controlled cortical impact in the immature rat brain. *Dev Neurosci* 2006; **28**: 457–65.

61. Liu X, Zou H, Slaughter C, Wang X. DFF, a heterodimeric protein that functions downstream of caspase-3 to trigger DNA fragmentation during apoptosis. *Cell* 1997; **89**: 175–84.

# Chaper

# 3

# Experimental models of traumatic brain injury

H. C. Patel

## Introduction

The need for experimental traumatic brain injury (TBI) models comes from the drive to better understand TBI pathophysiology in order to improve outcome. Although there is no substitute for human studies, animal models offer unique advantages. There is uniformity of subjects, and the same injury can be repeated, enabling mechanistic and treatment effect studies. They allow for the creation of simple or complex injuries, whilst offering the ability to investigate global or focal change(s) from minutes to days following the insult. Experimental protocols can be pursued with attention to maintaining physiological stability minimizing secondary effects. Consistent injury requires uniformity of subject weight. The recruitment and follow-up issues that hamper clinical trials are eradicated. Animal studies permit multiple invasive tissue sampling procedures, trial of the widest dose range of candidate drug doses and full investigation at a histopathological level in fatal and non-fatal studies.

This chapter provides an overview of the methods and pathological features of experimental injury. Clinically relevant outcome measures employed following experimental brain injury are discussed. The studies described concentrate on rodent TBI models as these, for practical and financial reasons, are the most commonly used.

## Experimental TBI models

Denny-Brown and Russell pioneered early experimental head injury research. They classified injuries according to whether concussion was induced by acceleration or percussion injury, which essentially describes the creation of focal or diffuse injury.[1] The early characterization of forces implicated in generating injury has proved robust.[2] Large animal models also provided an early understanding of the pathophysiology of TBI including characterization of the pressure–volume curve.[3–5]

## Focal TBI models

### Weight drop model

This model involves a direct impact, using a free falling weight onto the head of a restrained anaesthetized animal to cause brain injury.[6] The weight and height of release are varied to create a spectrum of injury. The weight is directed down a fixed track or tube to allow for reproducibility. A craniotomy is normally performed (in the region overlying the right parietal lobe and hippocampus) before injury, although this method has also been described with an intact skull. Injury results in a contusion with focal neuronal, glial and vascular cell death immediately under the area of impact. With severe injury, a deep haemorrhagic contusion and contralateral injury has been reported.[6]

*Head Injury: A Multidisciplinary Approach*, ed. Peter C. Whitfield, Elfyn O. Thomas, Fiona Summers, Maggie Whyte and Peter J. Hutchinson. Published by Cambridge University Press. © Cambridge University Press 2009.

# Controlled cortical impact model

The controlled cortical impact model uses a pneumatic device to drive an impactor. This delivers a blow to the brain, thereby producing injury.[7] Again, this is performed following a craniotomy in an anaesthetized animal, and as with the weight drop method, injury severity and site of the lesion can be altered, with the advantage that there is no risk of rebound injury.[8] The changes in the brain following the insult are similar to those using the weight drop model, with evidence of contusional injury including neuronal and glial cell loss combined with a reactive microglial and astrocytic response. There is also some evidence of pericapillary haemorrhage within the lesion and petechial haemorrhage consistent with diffuse axonal injury in distant white matter tracts.

Overall, the weight drop and cortical impact models reliably induce cerebral contusions. Both are relatively simple, quick to perform and produce a wide spectrum of injury severity in a reproducible manner. The weight drop method has its critics mainly because there may be double injury caused by bouncing of the weight following initial impact.

# Acute subdural haematoma

Acute subdural haemorrhage may be induced by controlled cortical impact and impact acceleration injury (see below) models, but they are not seen consistently. Hence, subdural haematomas are induced by the direct placement of 300–400 µl of autologous blood into the rat subdural space following a small craniotomy.[9,10] This results in a zone of ischaemic brain damage underneath the subdural collection.[9] In order to mimic the brain swelling/diffuse injury that often accompanies acute subdural haemorrhage in man, autologous blood injection has been combined with the impact acceleration model (with or without a hypoxic insult).[10] This paradigm of injury has resulted in both ischaemic injury and cerebral oedema and is thought to be a more clinically relevant model.[10,11]

# Extradural haemorrhage models

In most extradural haemorrhage models, the compression is mimicked by inflating a balloon in the extradural compartment following a craniotomy.[11] Injury severity is controlled by changing either the volume of balloon inflation (0.1–0.4 ml), or the rate of inflation, and can be guided by intracranial pressure monitoring. Although the effect of blood in the extradural space is not replicated, this model does replicate radiological (midline shift, basal cistern effacement), and physiological (Cushing's response and anisocoria) disturbances associated with brainstem compression in the rat suggesting that this model may reproduce the common clinical scenario.[11]

# Diffuse TBI models

The focal models described above and the lateral fluid percussion model described below all have components of diffuse axonal injury, but contusional injury predominates. The inertial acceleration and impact acceleration models representing Denny–Brown and Russell's acceleration concussion injury, more consistently produce diffuse injury without a focal lesion.

## Diffuse axonal injury – inertial acceleration model

The inertial acceleration model was the first model of diffuse axonal injury and was described for non-human primates.[12] The injury is induced by the rapid deceleration of a moving frame that is rigidly fixed to the head. This results in a whiplash motion, initial coma and subcortical white matter injury consistent with diffuse axonal injury.[12] The forces needed to induce this injury are dependent on the weight of the brain, with lighter brains requiring exponentially high rotational/acceleration forces. Therefore, this method has mainly been restricted to studies in large animals.

Application of similar methodology to rodents using significantly higher rotational forces has been reported.[13] Fixation of a rotation device to the anaesthetised rodent using a head clip, a tooth hole and ear pins enabled a spring driven rapid rotation (2 ms) of the head in the range of 15° to 90°. Petechial haemorrhage in the temporal lobe and ventrolateral pons were the only observed macroscopic changes, with no evidence of contusional injury or subarachnoid haemorrhage. Axonal swelling and retraction balls characteristic of diffuse axonal injury were seen from 6 h and increased over time. These changes were initially only observed in the midbrain, medulla and upper cervical cord, although by 24 h these changes were also observed in the corpus callosum, internal capsule and optic tracts.

## Diffuse axonal injury – impact acceleration model

An impact acceleration model is commonly used to study diffuse injury in rats.[14] Injury is induced by dropping a weight onto a steel plate that is glued onto the skull, whilst the anaesthetized rat is supported on a foam bed of a known spring constant. Injury severity is altered by changing the height of release, weight and/or the spring constant of the foam.[14] The pathological changes are injury severity dependent and range from traumatic subarachnoid haemorrhage in the basal cisterns with mild injury, to extensive subarachnoid and intraventricular haemorrhage with frequent petechial haemorrhages in more severe injury. Axonal swelling is prominent, seen as early as 6 h after injury and reaching a maximum after 24 h. This is characterized by the accumulation of organelles in the peripheral axon and internalization of neurofilament at the core. Axonal injury is seen throughout the white matter with predominance in the optic tracts, cerebral peduncles and the pyramidal decussation. It is also observed to a lesser extent in the internal capsule and the corpus callosum without any evidence of focal contusion.[15] The addition of a laser to more precisely target the steel disc has been reported to produce a more consistent pattern of injury.[16]

## Focal axonal injury

The optic nerve stretch injury model representing diffuse axonal injury, first described in guinea pigs and then modified for mice, is the only pure experimental traumatic brain injury paradigm.[17,18] The injury is produced by the application of a transient (20 ms) traction force on the optic nerve exposed by detaching (a) the conjunctiva from the sclera and then (b) the extraocular muscles from the globe. The rapid elongation of the optic nerve by 20% results in an injury that leads to secondary axotomy. This is characterized by the hallmarks of axonal injury such as the presence of axonal swelling and axon retraction balls, neurofilament and microtubule disruption, disruption of fast axonal transport and accumulation of transported proteins within the first 24 h. There is also a progressive increase in axonal damage over time, ultimately leading to deafferentiation of the neuronal cell body.[17,18]

## Mixed focal and diffuse injury

The focal models of experimental injury described above, all result in a mixed focal and diffuse injury albeit with the focal injury component predominating. Changing the severity of injury or site of injury can, however, lead to more diffuse injury as typified by midline injury caused by controlled cortical impact of moderate or severe intensity. This results in axonal injury in the corpus callosum and internal capsule, in addition to distant hippocampal and thalamic degeneration and the contusion below the craniectomy site.[19] A better accepted model of combined injury is the lateral fluid percussion model in which injury is induced by releasing a pendulum from a known height onto a saline-filled reservoir that results in the impact of a fluid bolus against the dura on the side of the head of an anaesthetized experimental animal. The injury severity is controlled by the height from which the pendulum is released and the injury results in a focal contusion at the site of impact.[20] The presence of subdural haematoma, subarachnoid haemorrhage and white matter tears, as well as selective neuronal damage in the hippocampus and thalamus, have also been consistently noted. Lateral fluid percussion injury also consistently results in bilateral damage, with diffuse white matter damage distant from the site of injury. This mechanism of injury is therefore used to study 'mixed' brain injuries.[20]

## Outcome measurements in experimental TBI models

Most experimental studies concentrate on histopathological outcomes. Assessment of lesion volume alone is not a comprehensive outcome measure because it does not allow for the quantification of diffuse injury adequately, and the location of damage is of paramount importance. If experimental models are to be used as preclinical trials, clinically relevant outcome measures are required. Outcome assessment should therefore include a battery of outcome measures (e.g. cognitive, motor and sensory assessment), as well as specific surrogate measures that are implicated in influencing outcome in human head injury such as cerebral perfusion, cerebral blood flow, cerebral oedema, blood–brain barrier disruption and intracranial pressure monitoring.

## Behavioural assessment

Behavioural assessment encompasses a series of tests that have been designed to quantify motor and cognitive deficits. Motor assessments test strength (forelimb reflex, lateral pulsion, akinesia, bracing rigidity test), gait (beam walk, and balance tests, inclined plane test, rotarod test), reflex behaviours (Von Frey hair test, forelimb placing) and fine motor coordination (activity monitoring, grid walking tests).[21] They have been widely applied in experimental rodent TBI, with motor deficits observed following controlled cortical impact and lateral fluid percussion injury.[21]

Cognitive tests, which assess memory and learning, have been used as correlates of post-traumatic and retrograde amnesia.[22] The most commonly used paradigm is the Morris water maze comprising a circular water tank with a submerged platform.[23] To test memory, rats pre-injury are trained to find the submerged platform. Post-injury, the time taken and consistency with which the platform is found are taken as a marker for memory function. For the learning test paradigm, the time taken for the rats to find the platform from a fixed point is measured. Deficits of both short and long term in memory and learning have been reported following a variety of injury models in the rat.[21]

## Cerebral blood flow and cerebral oedema

Although temporally and spatially variable, cerebral ischaemia following TBI in humans is common and influences outcome.[24] For focal injury most studies in rats have also reported a reduction in the cerebral blood flow to up to 50% of baseline within 4 h of the injury.[25,26] The reduction in cerebral blood flow is observed up to 7 days post-injury in autoradiography studies in the rat and is related to injury severity.[25] A reduction in cerebral blood flow, reversible by early decompression, is also noted with the autologous blood injection model of acute subdural haemorrhage.[27] Cerebral oedema assessed using MRI-based techniques, wet dry methods and through the quantification of the extravasation of Evans blue dye (for vasogenic oedema), have all confirmed that brain water content increases following injury that is maximal at 24 hours, and persists for at least 1 week.[25,28] As in the clinical setting, blood–brain barrier opening is transient, and cerebral oedema is significantly worsened by secondary insults such as experimental hypoxia and hypotension in rodents.[28,29]

## Intracranial pressure monitoring/cerebral perfusion pressure

Currently, experimental measurement of ICP and CPP is largely limited to the period of anaesthetized immobilization. As with brain tissue, oxygen monitoring in the ambulant rodent, probe size and fixation for long-term use are currently being explored. Telemetry-based solutions with implantable probes offer a potential route for long-term monitoring, but these have not yet been fully characterized.

## Summary

Some critics have suggested that experimental TBI research will not translate into clinical gains, citing failings in experimental design, allied to the fundamental biological differences between species.[30,31] However, there are now well-characterized, histopathologically accurate, experimental TBI correlates of human TBI with robust methods of assessing clinically relevant acute pathophysiological events and cognitive outcomes. There has also been a realization that, in common with human head injury, there is a considerable heterogeneity in experimental TBI from differences in injuries between laboratories and lack of standardization of outcome measures and inappropriate experimental design. It is also increasingly accepted that outcome following brain injury cannot be based on a single, often histopathological, assessment. Hopefully, this increased understanding of the tools available will lead to their better application, which will lead to the translation of preclinical observations and hence to improvement in clinical outcome.

## References

1. Denny-Brown DR. Experimental cerebral concussion. *Brain* 1941; **64**: 93–164.

2. Holbourn AHS. Mechanics of head injury. *Lancet* 1943; **2**: 438–41.

3. Ommaya AK, Hirsch AE, Flamm ES, Mahone RH. Cerebral concussion in the monkey: an experimental model. *Science* 1966; **153**: 211–12.

4. Lofgren J, von Essen C, Zwetnow NN. The pressure–volume curve of the cerebrospinal fluid space in dogs. *Acta Neurol Scand* 1973; **49**: 557–74.

5. Lofgren J, Zwetnow NN. Cranial and spinal components of the cerebrospinal fluid pressure–volume curve. *Acta Neurol Scand* 1973; **49**: 574–85.

6. Feeney DM, Boyeson MG, Linn RT, Murray HM, Dail WG. Responses to cortical injury: I. Methodology and local effects of contusions in the rat. *Brain Res* 1981; **211**(1): 67–77.

7. Dixon CE, Clifton GL, Lighthall JW, Yaghmai AA, Hayes RL. A controlled cortical impact model of traumatic brain injury in the rat. *J Neurosci Methods* 1991; **39**(3): 253–62.

8. Morales DM, Marklund N, Lebold D et al. Experimental models of traumatic brain injury: do we really need to build a better mousetrap? *Neuroscience* 2005; **136**(4): 971–89.

9. Miller JD, Bullock R, Graham DI, Chen MH, Teasdale GM. Ischemic brain damage in a model of acute subdural hematoma. *Neurosurgery* 1990; **27**(3): 433–9.

10. Tomita Y, Sawauchi S, Beaumont A, Marmarou A. The synergistic effect of acute subdural hematoma combined with diffuse traumatic brain injury on brain edema. *Acta Neurochir Suppl* 2000; **76**: 213–16.

11. Burger R, Bendszus M, Vince GH, Roosen K, Marmarou A. A new reproducible model of an epidural mass lesion in rodents. Part I: Characterization by neurophysiological monitoring, magnetic resonance imaging, and histopathological analysis. *J Neurosurg* 2002; **97**(6): 1410–18.

12. Gennarelli TA, Thibault LE, Adams JH, Graham DI, Thompson CJ, Marcincin RP. Diffuse axonal injury and traumatic coma in the primate. *Ann Neurol* 1982; **12**(6): 564–74.

13. Xiao-Sheng H, Sheng-Yu Y, Xiang Z, Zhou F, Jian-ning Z. Diffuse axonal injury due to lateral head rotation in a rat model. *J Neurosurg* 2000; **93**(4): 626–33.

14. Marmarou A, Foda MA, van den Brink W, Campbell J, Kita H, Demetriadou K. A new model of diffuse brain injury in rats. Part I: Pathophysiology and biomechanics. *J Neurosurg* 1994; **80**(2): 291–300.

15. Foda MA, Marmarou A. A new model of diffuse brain injury in rats. Part II: Morphological characterization. *J Neurosurg* 1994; **80**(2): 301–13.

16. Cernak I, Vink R, Zapple DN *et al.* The pathobiology of moderate diffuse traumatic brain injury as identified using a new experimental model of injury in rats. *Neurobiol Dis* 2004; **17**(1): 29–43.

17. Gennarelli TA, Thibault LE, Tipperman R *et al.* Axonal injury in the optic nerve: a model simulating diffuse axonal injury in the brain. *J Neurosurg* 1989; **71**(2): 244–53.

18. Saatman KE, Abai B, Grosvenor A, Vorwerk CK, Smith DH, Meaney DF. Traumatic axonal injury results in biphasic calpain activation and retrograde transport impairment in mice. *J Cereb Blood Flow Metab* 2003; **23**(1): 34–42.

19. Hall ED, Sullivan PG, Gibson TR, Pavel KM, Thompson BM, Scheff SW. Spatial and temporal characteristics of neurodegeneration after controlled cortical impact in mice: more than a focal brain injury. *J Neurotrauma* 2005; **22**(2): 252–65.

20. Thompson HJ, Lifshitz J, Marklund N *et al.* Lateral fluid percussion brain injury: a 15-year review and evaluation. *J Neurotrauma* 2005; **22**(1): 42–75.

21. Fujimoto ST, Longhi L, Saatman KE, Conte V, Stocchetti N, McIntosh TK. Motor and cognitive function evaluation following experimental traumatic brain injury. *Neurosci Biobehav Rev* 2004; **28**(4): 365–78.

22. Povlishock JT, Hayes RL, Michel ME, McIntosh TK. Workshop on animal models of traumatic brain injury. *J Neurotrauma* 1994; **11**(6): 723–32.

23. Morris RG, Garrud P, Rawlins JN, O'Keefe J. Place navigation impaired in rats with hippocampal lesions. *Nature* 1982; **297** (5868): 681–3.

24. Graham DI, Ford I, Adams JH *et al.* Ischaemic brain damage is still common in fatal non-missile head injury. *J Neurol Neurosurg Psychiatry* 1989; **52**(3): 346–50.

25. Kochanek PM, Marion DW, Zhang W *et al.* Severe controlled cortical impact in rats: assessment of cerebral edema, blood flow, and contusion volume. *J Neurotrauma* 1995; **12**(6): 1015–25.

26. Shen Y, Kou Z, Kreipke CW, Petrov T, Hu J, Haacke EM. In vivo measurement of tissue damage, oxygen saturation changes and blood flow changes after experimental traumatic brain injury in rats using susceptibility weighted imaging. *Magn Reson Imaging* 2007; **25**(2): 219–27.

27. Sawauchi S, Marmarou A, Beaumont A, Signoretti S, Fukui S. Acute subdural hematoma associated with diffuse brain injury and hypoxemia in the rat: effect of surgical evacuation of the hematoma. *J Neurotrauma* 2004; **21**(5): 563–73.

28. Shapira Y, Setton D, Artru AA, Shohami E. Blood–brain barrier permeability, cerebral edema, and neurologic function after closed head injury in rats. *Anesth Analg* 1993; **77**(1): 141–8.

29. Unterberg AW, Stover J, Kress B, Kiening KL. Edema and brain trauma. *Neuroscience* 2004; **129**(4): 1021–9.

30. Croce P. *Vivisection or science? An investigation into testing drugs and safeguarding health*. London: Zed Books, 1999.

31. Perel P, Roberts I, Sena E *et al.* Comparison of treatment effects between animal experiments and clinical trials: systematic review. *Br Med J* 2007; **334**(7586): 197.

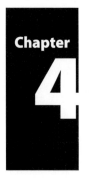

# Chapter 4

# Clinical assessment of the head-injured patient: an anatomical approach

Deva S. Jeyaretna and Peter C. Whitfield

## Introduction

The rapid and accurate clinical assessment of a head-injured patient is crucial. The initial management should be governed by attention to the airway, breathing and circulation according to the principles of the Advanced Trauma Life Support (ATLS) care system. This is vital not only to identify immediately life-threatening injuries but also to prevent secondary cerebral insults. The cervical spine should be immobilized, since patients with a head injury may also harbour a cervical spine injury.[1] The level of consciousness and pupil size and reaction should be determined early and at regular intervals when managing patients with TBI.

## History

The clinical history should be obtained from the patient, witnesses and paramedical staff as appropriate. History-taking should include details of the mechanism of the injury and status of the patient at the accident scene in addition to the following: past medical history, medications, allergies, smoking, alcohol or drug use and social circumstances. Symptoms depend upon the severity of the injury. In conscious patients, headache due to somatic pain from a scalp injury is common. The headache caused by raised ICP is exacerbated by coughing, straining or bending and is associated with nausea, vomiting and impaired consciousness. Deterioration can be extremely rapid, highlighting the low threshold required to undertake imaging investigations looking for intracranial mass lesions. Amnesia, repetitive speech and disorientation are very common early features, even after relatively minor trauma. Focal neurological deficits affecting any part of the brain and cranial nerves can occur. Anosmia due to disruption of the olfactory pathways is perhaps the most common focal symptom. CSF rhinorrhoea and otorrhoea occasionally may be reported by the patient at this early stage. Witnessed seizures should be noted.

## Examination

Neurological examination of the head-injured patient begins with an assessment of the level of consciousness and pupillary reactions. An external examination of the cranium and a tailored formal examination of cranial nerve and peripheral nerve function should their follow.

### Glasgow Coma Scale (GCS) assessment

The GCS is the most extensively used grading system for assessing the level of conscious-ness.[2] It is reproducible with high levels of interobserver agreement.[3] The scale is based on the best motor, verbal and eye-opening responses of the patient (Table 4.1) and is used to

*Head Injury: A Multidisciplinary Approach*, ed. Peter C. Whitfield, Elfyn O. Thomas, Fiona Summers, Maggie Whyte and Peter J. Hutchinson. Published by Cambridge University Press. © Cambridge University Press 2009.

**Table 4.1.** Glasgow Coma Scale

| | |
|---|---|
| *Eye opening* | |
| Eyes open spontaneously | 4 |
| Eyes opening to verbal stimuli | 3 |
| Eyes opening to painful stimuli | 2 |
| No eye opening | 1 |
| *Verbal response* | |
| Orientated | 5 |
| Confused | 4 |
| Inappropriate words | 3 |
| Incomprehensible sounds | 2 |
| No verbal response | 1 |
| *Motor response* | |
| Obeys commands | 6 |
| Localizing pain | 5 |
| Normal flexion to pain | 4 |
| Abnormal flexion to pain | 3 |
| Extension to pain | 2 |
| No motor response | 1 |

From Teasdale G, Jennett B (1974). Reproduced with permission from Elsevier. Copyright © 1974.

classify injury severity as minor (GCS 13–15), moderate (GCS 9–12) and severe (GCS 3–8). Repeated assessment of the GCS is of importance in monitoring the condition of the patient. Although other factors such as alcohol and iatrogenic administration of sedating drugs can affect the level of consciousness, they should not be assumed to be the cause of impaired consciousness. If the patient is unrousable, a central painful stimulus is applied. Supraorbital pressure is most commonly used. In clinical practice documentation of the motor score causes most difficulty. Localization to pain is noted if the patient raises the hand above the clavicle in response to central pain, or tries to remove the stimulus in response to a sternal rub. Flexion is characterized by flexion at the elbow with the forearm in a supinated position and the wrist held in a neutral or flexed position. Abnormal flexion is observed when flexion occurs at the elbow but the forearm is pronated with a flexed wrist posture. Extension occurs when the elbow extends and the arm rotates into a pronated position. Again, the wrist is usually flexed. A GCS of 3 represents no eye-opening to pain, no verbal response and no motor response to pain. This is usually annotated as E1,V1,M1 in the medical records. A GCS of 15 represents spontaneous eye opening, orientated (who they are, where they are, why they are where they are) and obeying commands; E4,V5,M6. If the patient is intubated or has a tracheostomy, the verbal response should be marked 'T'. This enables the eye opening and motor parameters to continue to be used to assess the level of consciousness. Sometimes severe periorbital swelling precludes accurate eye-opening responses. High spinal cord injury makes motor assessment difficult. However, the itemized GCS continues to provide useful information within these constraints. When recording the GCS, the scores of individual components should be noted rather than just the total, as patients with the same total GCS but with different component scores may have differing outcomes.[4] The motor component is generally regarded as the most accurate predictor of outcome.

## Pupillary reflexes

Examination of the pupillary reflexes provides critical information about the integrity of the optic and oculomotor pathways. Shining a light into one eye causes direct contraction of the ipsilateral pupil and consensual contraction of the contralateral pupil. Light-sensitive afferent fibres travel via the optic nerve into both optic tracts synapsing in the pretectal nuclei of the midbrain. These project bilaterally to the Edinger–Westphal nuclei, which supply parasympathetic fibres to the oculomotor nerves.[5,6] The oculomotor nerves emerge from the midbrain and travel anteriorly in the interpeduncular cistern and then along the ipsilateral free edge of the tentorium cerebelli before entering the cavernous sinus and orbit via the superior orbital fissure. The parasympathetic fibres cause contraction of the sphincter pupillae. In a patient with an expanding mass lesion, herniation of the medial temporal lobe (uncus) causes compression of the ipsilateral oculomotor nerve. The fibres to the ipsilateral sphincter pupillae cease to function, causing unopposed dilatation of the pupil, which fails to contract on direct or consensual testing.

When examining the eyes, pulsatile proptosis associated with orbital pain, ophthalmoplegia, reduced vision, chemosis and a bruit over the globe are the classical signs of a traumatic cavernous carotid fistula (CCF). Fundoscopy may reveal ocular injuries such as sub-retinal or vitreal haemorrhages.

## External examination

Inspect the scalp for signs of injury including bruising and lacerations; these are commonly found in cases of assault with direct impact injuries. Sometimes depressed skull fractures can be palpated. Subconjunctival haemorrhages and bleeding from the external auditory meatus may occur with skull base fractures. Otoscopy may reveal a haemotympanum. Other features associated with skull base fractures include periorbital and postauricular ecchymoses (Battle's sign), CSF rhinorrhoea and CSF otorrhoea.

The face should be examined for asymmetry, localized tenderness and fractures. Log-rolling enables a careful examination of the posterior aspect of the head and whole spine to be conducted.

## Cranial nerves

If the patient is conscious and cooperative, the cranial nerves should be examined systematically. In unconscious patients the brainstem reflexes (pupillary, corneal and gag) and gaze palsies should be noted. Oculocephalic and vestibulo-ocular reflexes are not normally conducted unless ascertaining the presence of any brainstem function when undertaking brainstem tests. Anosmia may occur due to tearing of the olfactory nerves at the cribiform plate. Patients with anosmia often report a change in the quality of taste sensation. Formal testing for sense of smell is performed using test bottles of peppermint solution and clove oil. Visual acuity, fields and pupillary reflexes are tested. Diplopia may be reported with impaired eye movements (Fig. 4.1). A complete oculomotor (III) nerve palsy results in a ptosis, ipsilateral pupillary dilatation unreactive to light directly or consensually, and the eye in the 'down and out' position. Trochlear (IV) and abducent (VI) nerve palsies result in vertical (a)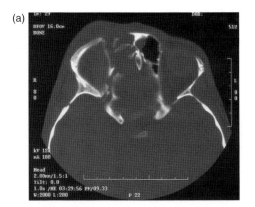

(b)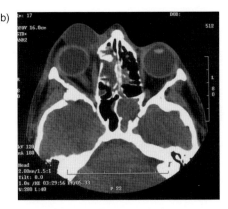

**Fig. 4.1(a) and (b).** Axial CT scans showing complex anterior fossa skull fractures. The patient had anosmia, no perception of light in the right eye and a visual field defect in the left eye. These injuries were consistent with trauma to the olfactory nerves and both optic nerves. The fractures were also complicated by a CSF rhinorrhoea.

and lateral gaze diplopia respectively. Superior orbital fissure fractures can result in cranial nerves III, IV, VI and the ophthalmic division of the trigeminal (V) nerve being injured. The trigeminal nerve is examined by testing sensation over the face and anterior scalp and the strength of the muscles of mastication. Branches can be injured distally by facial fractures or more proximal nerve injury can occur at the petroclinoid ridge near Meckel's cave.[7] The facial nerve (VII) supplies the muscles of facial expression and can be disrupted by fractures of the petrous temporal bone causing a complete lower motor neurone type of facial palsy. The corneal reflex, elicited by lightly touching the lateral aspect of each cornea and inspecting for bilateral blinking, tests the integrity of the trigeminal and facial nerve pathways. Hearing loss should be characterized as either sensorineural or conductive; both commonly occur after head trauma. The gag reflex is tested by touching the soft palate or pharynx with a stick or tongue depressor and observing elevation of the uvula. The afferent limb of the reflex tests the integrity of the glossopharyngeal (IX) nerve, whilst the vagus (X) causes contraction of the palatal musculature. Changes in the quality of voice are related to vagal injuries causing altered phonation. The spinal accessory nerve (XI) supplies the sternocleidomastoid and trapezius muscles. The hypoglossal nerve (XII) is rarely injured but does course through the anterior condylar canal and may be disrupted in fractures of the foramen magnum.

## Peripheral nervous system
A thorough examination of the peripheral nervous system may be impaired by a depressed level of consciousness and limb injuries. Furthermore, injuries of the brachial plexus, rarely the lumbosacral plexus and the peripheral nerves, can complicate the interpretation of abnormal findings. Observation of movement is important in assessing spinal cord function and corticospinal tract injury. Any asymmetry is documented. Unilateral motor signs (e.g. hemiplegia) may occur with an intracranial mass lesion and warrant further investigation.

## False localizing signs
The concept of false localizing signs was first described in 1904 by James Collier based on his examination and post-mortem study of 161 patients with intracranial tumours.[8] A false localizing sign occurs when the neurological signs elicited are a reflection of pathology distant from the expected anatomical locus.[9] The most common example is a VI nerve

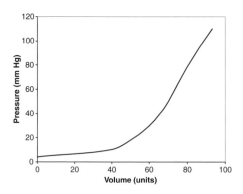

**Fig. 4.2.** Pressure–volume curve of the cerebrospinal fluid space based on work by Lofgren et al. in canine models.[11,12]

palsy presumably occurring due to traction of the nerve at the petroclinoid ligament, remote from the brainstem origin of the nerve. An intracranial mass lesion is usually associated with a contralateral hemiplegia due to either cortical dysfunction or compression of the ipsilateral cerebral peduncle. However, a supratentorial mass lesion can cause shift of the midbrain to the opposite side. The contralateral cerebral peduncle can then impinge on the tentorium cerebelli, causing the unexpected finding of an ipsilateral hemiplegia. At post-mortem this can be visualized as the Kernohan–Woltman notch indentating the midbrain.[10]

## Raised intracranial pressure

In 1783 Alexander Monro noted that the cranium was a rigid box containing a nearly incompressible brain. He observed that any increase in one of the component contents (brain, blood and CSF) required accommodation by displacement of the other elements. During the initial stages of rising intracranial pressure due to a mass lesion, cerebrospinal fluid and venous blood are displaced from the cranium buffering the change in pressure.[11,12] However, once the point of compensatory reserve has been reached, rapid elevation of the ICP occurs (Fig. 4.2). This may manifest as a fall in the level of consciousness and an oculomotor nerve palsy secondary to temporal lobe herniation.

## Intracranial herniation

Intracranial herniation is the pathological process of brain shifting from one compartment to another as a result of differential pressure gradients (Fig. 4.3). The dural folds normally minimize movement within the cranium. The falx cerebri is a sickle-shaped midline struc-ture that separates the cerebral hemispheres and decreases lateral movement. Anteriorly, it is attached to the crista galli and frontal crest. Posteriorly, it attaches to the internal occipital protuberance and the midline of the tentorium cerebelli suspending the latter structure. Supratentorial masses may cause displacement of the cingulate gyrus under the falx cerebri resulting in subfalcine herniation. This can cause compression of the anterior cerebral artery and subsequent ischaemia and infarction. The tentorium cerebelli supports the occipital lobes and separates them from the cerebellar hemispheres. The midbrain passes through the opening in the tentorium; the tentorial incisura. A supratentorial mass lesion commonly causes the uncus of the medial temporal lobe to herniate from the middle cranial fossa medially and downwards through the tentorial incisura compressing the oculomotor nerve and the midbrain. An oculomotor nerve palsy and contralateral hemiparesis usually occur and require urgent intervention. Compromise of the reticular activating system of the

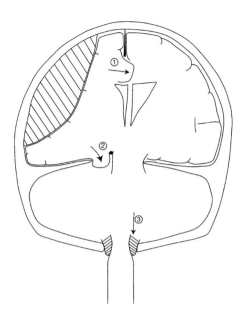

**Fig. 4.3.** Intracranial pressure gradients and brain herniation.

This coronal view shows an extradural haematoma causing (1) subfalcine herniation of the cingulate gyrus, (2) herniation of the uncus of the medial temporal lobe through the tentorial hiatus leading to compression of the ipsilateral oculomotor nerve, the posterior cerebral artery and the midbrain and (3) herniation of the cerebellar tonsils through the foramen magnum leading to compression of the cervicomedullary junction.

midbrain contributes to the impairment of consciousness. Uncal herniation can also compress the posterior cerebral artery leading to occipital lobe infarction and obstruction to the flow of cerebrospinal fluid through the aqueduct of Sylvius causing hydrocephalus.[13] Transtentorial herniation may also stretch perforating branches of the basilar artery causing secondary 'Duret' haemorrhages in the brainstem.[14]

Tonsillar herniation is the downward descent of the cerebellar tonsils through the foramen magnum. Mass lesions of the posterior fossa are more likely to cause tonsillar herniation, although any supratentorial mass can cause severe elevations of ICP throughout the cranial cavity leading to tonsil herniation. As the cerebellar tonsils descend, they compress the medulla and the fourth ventricle and efface the cisterna magna. Fourth ventricular compromise leads to obstructive hydrocephalus, compounding the situation. Direct compression of the medulla depresses the cardiac and respiratory centres leading to hypertension, bradycardia, ventilatory compromise and death.

## Non-accidental head injury

Non-accidental head injury is an important condition to consider when assessing a young child with a head injury. The neurosurgeon should engage in the management of the acute injury and enlist the assistance of an experienced paediatrician in determining the cause of the injury. Diagnostic errors are well recognized.[15] The terms 'battered baby' and 'shaken baby syndrome' imply specific mechanisms of injury and have been surpassed with the term 'non-accidental head injury'. The classical triad of features that strongly suggest a diagnosis of non-accidental head injury comprise subdural haematomas, retinal haemorrhages and brain injury (encephalopathy). In addition, the injuries are inflicted unwitnessed by a sole carer and the history is inconsistent with the clinical findings. Corroborative evidence includes features of previous trauma.

Mechanical experiments show that severe non-accidental head injury is most likely to be caused by the combination of shaking and impact rather than shaking alone. Scottish cases of suspected non-accidental head injury have identified four patterns of presentation.[16]

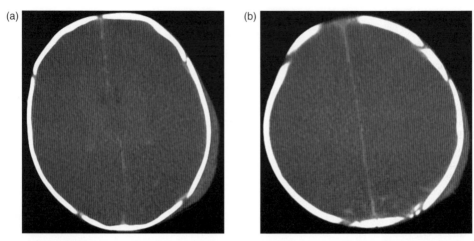

**Fig. 4.4(a) and (b).** CT scan of a probable case of non-accidental head injury.
The scan of this 1-month-old child showed a partly comminuted fracture of the left parietal bone with an overlying scalp swelling. This was consistent with extensive bruising on clinical examination. The brain appeared homogenous with a loss of grey–white differentiation, generalized brain swelling and ventricular effacement. Small subdural collections were present within the interhemispheric cleft and overlying the tentorium cerebelli. Some preservation of hyperdensity in the basal ganglia suggests diffuse hypoxic injury.

1. The cervicomedullary syndrome results from hyperflexion and hyperextension of the neck disrupting the integrity of the brainstem resulting in rapid death. At post-mortem, severe brain swelling due to hypoxia is evident with axonal disruption in the brainstem and trivial subdural haematomas.

2. Acute encephalopathy. This common mode of presentation is characterized by coma, seizures, apnoea and widespread retinopathy. There may be associated signs of impact trauma to the scalp (Fig. 4.4(a) and (b)).

3. Subacute non-encephalopathic presentation. The depression of conscious level is less severe without brain swelling and parenchymal hypodensities on CT scanning. Subdural haematomas and retinal haemorrhages may be seen.

4. Chronic subdural haematoma presentation. The child may present with features of an isolated chronic subdural haematoma. These include expanding head circumference, vomiting, failure to thrive, drowsiness and fits. Retinal haemorrhages are usually absent. The features develop a few weeks after primary trauma and an adequate explanation may not be found.

Geddes *et al.* postulated that hypoxia and ischaemia are important factors in causing the neuropathological changes of non-accidental head injury rather than the widespread traumatic axonal injury seen in adult head injury. They hypothesized that thin subdural haematomas may be consequential to venous or arterial hypertension rather than due to bridging vein disruption.[17,18] Others have emphasized the uncertainty of diagnostic accuracy if 'pathognomic' diagnostic criteria such as ocular haemorrhages and subdural haematomas are used in isolation.[19,20] In some cases other explanations of the trauma or insult (e.g. choking, vomiting, birth trauma) may be valid, although this is hotly contested by many paediatricians.[21] Corroborative evidence must be sought to identify the aetiology of the presentation in any individual case.

The management of the head-injured child is discussed in Chapter 21.

# References

1. Hadley MN, Walters BC, Grabb PA *et al.* Guidelines for the management of acute cervical spine and spinal cord injuries. *Clin Neurosurg* 2002; **49**: 407–98.
2. Teasdale G, Jennett B. Assessment of coma and impaired consciousness: a practical scale. *Lancet* 1974; **2**: 81–4.
3. Rowley G, Fielding K. Reliability and accuracy of the Glasgow Coma Scale with experienced and inexperienced users. *Lancet* 1991; **337**: 535–8.
4. Teoh LS, Gowardman JR, Larsen PD *et al.* Glasgow Coma Scale: variation in mortality among permutations of specific total scores. *Intens Care Med* 2000; **26**: 157–61.
5. Campbell WW. The ocular motor nerves. In DeJong's: *The Neurologic Examination*. 6th edn. Philadelphia, Lippincott Williams and Wilkins, 2005; 149–91.
6. Sinnatamby CS. Orbit and eye. In *Last's Anatomy: Regional and Applied*. 10th edn. Edinburgh, Churchill Livingstone, 1999; 389–402.
7. Katzen JT, Jarrahy R, Eby JB, Mathiasen RA, Margulies DR, Shahinian HK. Craniofacial and skull base trauma. *J Trauma* 2003; **54**(5): 1026–34.
8. Collier J. The false localising signs of intracranial tumour. *Brain* 1904; **27**: 490–508.
9. Larner AJ. False localising signs. *J Neurol Neurosurg Psychiatry* 2003; **74**: 415–18.
10. Kernohan JW, Woltman HW. Incisura of the crus due to contralateral brain tumor. *Arch Neurol Psychiatry* 1929; **21**: 274–87.
11. Lofgren J, von Essen C, Zwetnow NN. The pressure–volume curve of the cerebrospinal fluid space in dogs. *Acta Neurol Scand* 1973; **49**(5): 557–74.
12. Lofgren J. Zwetnow NN. Cranial and spinal components of the cerebrospinal fluid pressure-volume curve. *Acta Neurol Scand* 1973; **49**(5): 575–8.
13. Rhoton AL Jr. Tentorial incisura. *Neurosurgery* 2000; **47**(3 Suppl): S131–53.
14. Parizel PM, Makkat S, Jorens PG *et al.* Brainstem hemorrhage in descending transtentorial herniation (Duret hemorrhage). *Intens Care Med* 2002; **28**(1): 85–8.
15. Wheeler DM, Hobbs CJ. Mistakes in diagnosing non-accidental injury: 10 years' experience. *Br Med J* 1988; **296**: 1233–6.
16. Minns RA, Busuttil A. Four types of inflicted brain injury predominate. *Br Med J* 2004; **328**: 766.
17. Geddes JF, Vowles GH, Hackshaw AK, Nichols CD, Scott IS, Whitwell HL. Neuropathology of inflicted head injury in children I. Patterns of brain damage. *Brain* 2001; **124**: 1290–8.
18. Geddes JF, Vowles GH, Hackshaw AK, Nichols CD, Scott IS, Whitwell HL. Neuropathology of inflicted head injury in children II. Microscopic brain injury in infants. *Brain* 2001; **124**: 1299–306.
19. Lantz PE, Sinal SH, Stanton CA, Weaver RG Jr. Perimacular retinal folds from childhood head trauma. *Br Med J* 2004; **328**: 754–6.
20. Squier W. Shaken baby syndrome: the quest for evidence. *Dev Med Child Neurol* 2008; **50**: 10–14.
21. Reece RM. The evidence base for shaken baby syndrome: response to editorial from 106 doctors. *Br Med J* 2004; **328**: 1316–17.

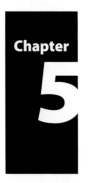

# Neuroimaging in trauma

Clare N. Gallagher and Jonathan Cole

## Introduction

Traumatic brain injury affects thousands of individuals every year worldwide. Injury severity is broad and can range from mild, with difficult to detect cognitive effects, to profound disturbances of consciousness with prolonged coma and persistent vegetative states. Imaging of brain injuries depends not only on the mechanism and severity of injury, but also the time since injury occurred. The purposes of imaging patients include immediate treatment decisions, attempts at prognosis and research into head injury pathophysiology. Both structural and ischaemic changes can be detected with recent advances in imaging techniques. This review will briefly outline the techniques available for traumatic brain injury and their usefulness in both the clinical and research settings.

## Acute imaging

The arrival of an injured patient in the emergency department often necessitates the decision whether or not to image the head and neck. This decision is, for the most part, clear when substantial neurological deficits are observed or if there is considerable suspicion of possible head injury. Acute imaging is directed at identifying lesions which need urgent surgical intervention or stabilization to prevent further injury. The full extent of the sustained injuries is determined after the patient has been resuscitated and stabilized.

## CT

CT scanning, which is now widely available in the emergency departments of most hospitals, has replaced the use of skull X-rays. Its ability to rapidly image trauma patients has made it invaluable for use in the acute phase following neurotrauma. An axial non-contrast CT can rapidly identify space-occupying haematomas requiring immediate removal. With examination of both the soft tissue and bony windows, fractures are also identified. CT has the advantage of being able to rapidly image the neck, chest, abdomen and pelvis. As time is important in evaluating the trauma patient, there is no other imaging technique that is more appropriate in the acute phase.[1] Indeed, the use of multidetector helical CT has reduced acquisition time to within 30 seconds, and image slices that are degraded by motion artefact can easily be repeated.[2] Development and validation of rules for evaluation of trauma patients with head CT guide the most efficient use of the technique.[3–5] The adoption of guidelines developed by The National Institute for Health and Clinical Excellence (NICE) in the UK has changed the way CT is used (Table 5.1).[6] These guidelines were based on the previously developed Canadian CT Head Rule (Table 5.2).[7] Overall, the guidelines have proved cost-effective with admission rates decreased from 9% to 4%. A decrease in skull X-ray use from 37% to 4% of patients with minor head injury and an increase in CT use from 3% of patients to 7% was shown.[6]

*Head Injury: A Multidisciplinary Approach*, ed. Peter C. Whitfield, Elfyn O. Thomas, Fiona Summers, Maggie Whyte and Peter J. Hutchinson. Published by Cambridge University Press. © Cambridge University Press 2009.

**Table 5.1.** NICE Guidelines for CT scanning in minor head injury

CT scan if any of the following are present:
- GCS less than 13 at any point since the injury
- GCS equal to 13 or 14 at 2 hours after the injury
- Suspected open or depressed skull fracture
- Any sign of basal skull fracture
- Post-traumatic seizure
- Focal neurological deficit
- More than one episode of vomiting
- Amnesia for greater than 30 minutes of events before impact

From National Institute for Health and Clinical Excellence (2007). CG56 *Head injury: Triage, assessment, investigation and early management of head injury in infants, children and adults. London*: NICE. Available from www.nice.org.uk/CG056 Reproduced with permission.

**Table 5.2.** Canadian CT head rule

CT scan for patients with minor head injury and any one of the following:

High risk
- GCS score <15 at 2 h after injury
- Suspected open or depressed skull fracture
- Any sign of basal skull fracture (haemotympanum, 'racoon eyes', cerebrospinal fluid otorrhoea/rhinorrhoea, Battle's sign)
- Vomiting ≥ two episodes
- Age ≥ 65 years

Medium risk
- Amnesia before impact >30 min
- Dangerous mechanism (pedestrian struck by motor vehicle, occupant ejected from motor vehicle, fall from height >3 feet or five stairs)

Reproduced from ref. 7. With permission from Elsevier. Copyright © 2001.

Primary head injury lesions seen on CT include acute extradural haematoma, acute subdural haematoma, subarachnoid haemorrhage, contusions, intracerebral haematoma and diffuse axonal injury (Fig. 5.1). However, initial CT scans with diffuse axonal injury (DAI) will be abnormal in only 20%–50% of cases.[1] Lesions that are visible are commonly located in the hemispheric subcortical lobar white matter, centrum semiovale, corpus callosum, basal ganglia, brainstem and cerebellum.[1] Due to the high percentage of normal scans, prognosis is difficult in patients with diffuse axonal injury. Some factors seen on initial scans do seem to correlate with outcome. Those that correlate with persistent vegetative state include: number of lesions, lesions in the supratentorial white matter, corpus callosum and corona radiata.[8] A recent study by Bigler *et al.* has indicated that there is poor correlation between acute CT and prognosis, apart from those patients with brainstem injury.[9]

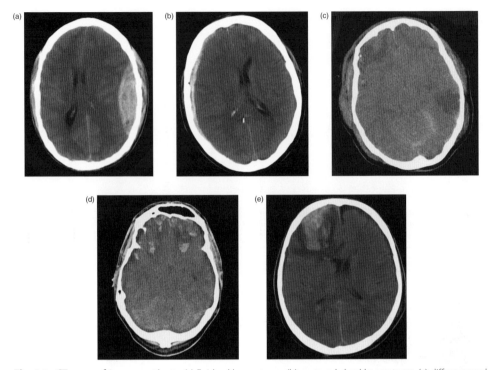

**Fig. 5.1. CT scans of trauma patients:** (a) Epidural haematoma, (b) acute subdural haematoma, (c) diffuse axonal injury, (d) bilateral frontal contusions, (e) haemorrhagic right frontal contusion with mass effect.

## Subacute imaging

### MRI

MRI is not routinely used in the acute phase of traumatic brain injury due to the technical difficulties of transporting critically ill patients and equipment compatibility. After the patient has been stabilized, MRI can be used to obtain a clearer picture of the extent of injury and information about prognosis while the patient is in an ICU setting. CT is superior to MRI in detecting haematoma, but in the acute phase MRI has a much higher sensitivity for detecting diffuse axonal injury (DAI).[10] DAI is characterized by acceleration–deceleration inertial forces.[11] Although regarded as a widespread injury, DAI is predominantly found in the parasagittal white matter, corpus callosum and pontine–mesencephalic junction. In the acute phase this is seen as punctate haemorrhages; however, DAI is often underestimated. In general, T1 and T2 sequences used for morphological studies have largely been replaced by FLAIR (fluid-attenuated inversion recovery). FLAIR sequences show T2 weighting but with hypointense CSF. These images show better resolution of cortical and periventricular lesions.[2] T2 and FLAIR produce hyperintense areas associated with non-haemorrhagic shear injury. T2* weighted gradient recalled echo (GRE) has been shown to be sensitive to blood breakdown products increasing the sensitivity for DAI. Local magnetic field inhomogeneities caused by the paramagnetic properties of haemosiderin result in lesions of low intensity following haemorrhage within the brain (Fig. 5.2). In addition to T2* GRE the use of ultra-fast sequences such as turbo Proton Echo Planar Spectroscopic Imaging

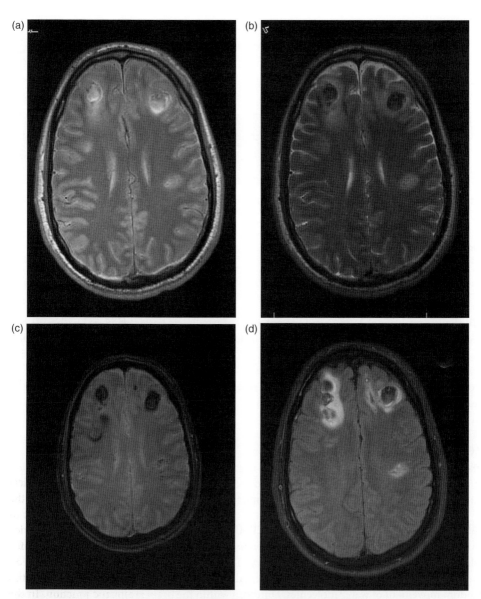

**Fig. 5.2.** MRI of trauma patient with DAI. (a) Proton density, (b) T2, (c) gradient echo, (d) FLAIR. Frontal contusions are apparent on all the sequences but differences in image contrast demonstrate different features of the lesions. The lesions appear more extensive on the T2 weighted sequence with regions of high signal surrounding the frontal contusions consistent with perilesional oedema. The FLAIR image shows T2 weighting but with attenuation of the CSF signal. This improves lesion detection particularly within cortical and periventricular regions. The frontal lesions appear hypodense on the gradient echo sequence which suggests haemorrhage within the lesion core. (Images courtesy of V. Newcombe, Wolfson Brain Imaging Centre, University of Cambridge.)

(t-PEPSI) has shown promise for assessment of DAI.[12] Newer gradient echo imaging methods have further improved the detection of haemorrhagic shearing injury. One such sequence, susceptibility weighted imaging (SWI), also utilizes the paramagnetic properties of haemorrhagic blood products.[13] SWI has also been shown to be more sensitive for evaluating

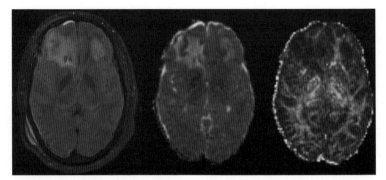

**Fig. 5.3.** MRI of trauma patient using diffusion-weighted imaging. The **FLAIR image (left panel)** demonstrates a large right frontal and smaller left frontal contusion. In the **ADC image (middle panel)** the region of the right frontal contusion is composed of tissue with mixed diffusion signal. There is a large region of bright signal (increased diffusion) mixed with areas of darker signal (restricted diffusion) consistent with vasogenic and cytotoxic oedema respectively. The **fractional anisotropy image (right panel)** demonstrates that white matter has diffusion which is less restricted and therefore has brighter signal. The frontal regions have reduced signal, particularly within the right frontal lobe, which is consistent with disruption of the white matter tracts. (The ADC and FA images are obtained as $2 \times 2 \times 2$ mm isotropic voxels, leading to a more 'pixelated' appearance when compared to other imaging data, which is acquired at higher resolution.) (Images courtesy of V. Newcombe, Wolfson Brain Imaging Centre, University of Cambridge.)

TBI than conventional MRI,[14] and the outcome of paediatric patients imaged with SWI has been shown to correlate with the number of lesions and numbers of locations affected.[15] Brainstem injuries are often not evident on CT scans. Mannion *et al.* used MRI to classify brainstem injury and determine outcome.[16] They classified injury into three types: I, secondary to supratentorial herniation, II, severe diffuse brain injury, III, isolated/remote brainstem injury. Outcome for types I and II was found to be poor, while outcome for type III was relatively good.

## Research techniques

The following techniques are not in general use for traumatic brain injury. They do provide information for use in research studies and for academic departments interested in brain injury and hold promise for more routine practice in the future.

## Diffusion-weighted and diffusion tensor imaging

Diffusion-weighted imaging (DWI) has been used extensively in the area of stroke and is a relative newcomer to traumatic brain injury. This technique relies upon the difference in isotropic diffusion of water molecules in normal and injured brain. Isotropic diffusion is the random movement of water molecules. Diffusion within the brain is affected by many factors and its measurement has been utilized following ischaemic stroke where a reduction in diffusion is an early sign of tissue injury consistent with cytotoxic oedema. It is thought that the increased intracellular concentration of water associated with cytotoxic oedema is more restricted in movement than the water that was initially extracellular. In addition, brain regions with vasogenic oedema and an increase in extra-cellular water demonstrate an increase in diffusion.[17] Images of such diffusion are generally displayed as maps of apparent diffusion coefficient (ADC), since signal on DWI images can be affected by T2 and T2* effects (Fig. 5.3). Using ADC maps, regions of restricted diffusion appear dark, while bright regions represent increased diffusion. Whilst not used as commonly as for the investigation of acute stroke, DWI has been used in trauma imaging.[17] DAI imaged by DWI does not have the same sensitivity for haemorrhagic lesions as T2* but does identify additional lesions to those found with T2* and FLAIR.[18–20] Schaefer *et al.* have shown that signal intensity on DWI correlates with modified Rankin score and that lesions in the corpus callosum also had a strong correlation with Rankin score, although a poor correlation with initial Glasgow Coma Scale.[21] This also applied to other MRI images. The combination of DWI with other MRI sequences may provide additional information about extent of injury and should be included in initial MRI imaging. Bradley and Menon have outlined in some detail the diffusion- and perfusion-weighted imaging associated with traumatic brain injury (TBI) and its complex interpretation.[22]

Measurements of water diffusion vary across the brain, depending upon the direction in which the tissue is examined. Owing to the structure of white matter tracts, water diffusion will appear less restricted along fibre tracts compared with perpendicular to the fibre tract. The directionality of diffusion is called anisotropy and is measured by diffusion tensor imaging (DTI).[23,24] DTI has found a role in the imaging of brain tumours and in anatomical studies with mapping of myelinated fibres as they are distorted by space occupying lesions or in the development of immature brain. Its use in trauma imaging is in its infancy and few papers have been published in this field. As with DWI and other MRI techniques its application in trauma is the study of diffuse axonal injury. It is hoped that DTI will be able to visualize changes that are not seen on conventional scans and give some information regarding prognosis both in severe and mild TBI. Many of the manuscripts published are case reports, but show some promising results.[25–28] Commonly, DTI is used to look at regions of interest in injured brain including the corpus callosum and fornix. While whole brain diffusion and fractional anisotropy may not detect changes, by using measurements from areas of interest in DAI, significant changes from control subjects can be found.[29] Secondary damage after traumatic brain injury may also be identified after injury in major white matter tracts and cortex. These changes were found to correlate with memory and learning.[30] Similarly, in the paediatric population DTI has also been correlated with deficits in cognitive processing after injury.[31,32] Nakayama *et al.* have been able to show disruption of the corpus callosum and fornix even without lesions identified by other radiological methods, in a severely injured patient with cognitive impairment.[28] DTI and other clinical markers such as GCS and Rankin score also show correlation.[33] Voss *et al.* have used DTI in combination with PET to examine two patients in a minimally conscious state.[34] Years after the initial traumatic brain injury, clinical improvement was noted with subsequent examination with both DTI and PET, suggesting axonal regrowth.

## Positron emission tomography

Positron emission tomography (PET) measures the accumulation of positron emitting radioisotopes within the brain.[35,36] These positron-emitting isotopes can be administered via the intravenous or inhalational route. 15-oxygen ($^{15}O_2$) is employed to measure cerebral blood flow, cerebral blood volume, oxygen metabolism ($CMRO_2$) and oxygen extraction fraction (OEF), while 18-fluorodeoxyglucose $^{18}FDG$) is used to measure cerebral glucose metabolism (CMRgluc). The emitted positrons are annihilated in a collision with an electron, resulting in release of energy in the form of two photons (gamma rays) released at an angle of 180º to each other. This annihilation energy can be detected externally using coincidence detectors, and the region of each reaction is localized within the object by computer algorithms. The images obtained are then generally co-registered with CT or MR to obtain anatomic relationships. Combining this information with other clinical parameters can be

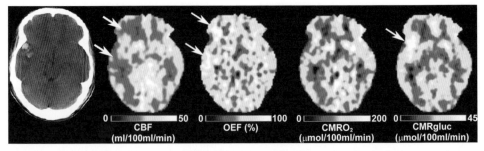

**Fig. 5.4.** PET scans of a patient with a right temporal contusion. The CBF is reduced in the frontotemporal regions with a corresponding increase in the oxygen extraction fraction and the cerebral metabolic rates for oxygen and glucose. (For colour version, see plate section.)

used to detect whether blood flow is sufficient to meet the needs of the injured brain. PET is very expensive, time consuming and requires extensive interventional expertise. PET in TBI is used mainly for research and its use is restricted to a few centres due to its dependence on a cyclotron to produce the short half-life radioisotopes required. The technique has been valuable in the identification of ischaemia after head injury. In response to a reduction in cerebral blood flow (CBF), the injured brain should increase oxygen extraction to meet energy requirements. Recent $^{15}O_2$ PET studies have shown regional pathophysiological derangements consistent with regional ischaemia, especially within the first day post-head injury (Fig. 5.4).[37,38] Indeed, using $^{15}O_2$ PET, the volume of ischaemic brain can be calculated based on the measurement of brain regions which demonstrate a critically high OEF.[37,38] This same group has shown that regions of ischaemia and hyperaemia can be found within the same patient, demonstrating the heterogeneous nature of derangements in flow metabolism coupling following TBI. In addition, brain regions that are unable to increase oxygen unloading through an increase in OEF may demonstrate tissue hypoxia due to microvascular collapse and perivascular oedema.[39,40] These data suggest that the injured brain may not be able to increase its oxygen extraction in response to a decrease in blood flow.[41] Numerous reports on cerebral ischaemia and abnormal metabolism following TBI have been published, indicating that significant interest remains in improving our understanding of head injury pathophysiology.[37,38,42–45]

## SPECT/Xenon-CT

Single photon emission computed tomography (SPECT) is a nuclear medicine imaging technique for the evaluation of blood flow. A radionucleotide is bound to a compound that crosses the blood–brain barrier and is trapped for at least the length of time required to image the patient. The uptake of the radiopharmaceutical is imaged by using a gamma camera. SPECT images are of a lower sensitivity than PET, are very sensitive to motion and require a longer imaging time than for MRI. In addition, in the clinical setting SPECT does not provide additional information to MRI for the management of severe traumatic brain-injured patients. In view of these limitations SPECT has largely been replaced by MRI and Xenon-CT. However, it has found application in the investigation of mild traumatic brain injury. Mild injury generally does not show structural abnormalities on conventional CT or MRI. In these cases it is sometimes hard to reconcile residual symptoms such as post-concussive syndrome with the lack of imaging abnormalities. Several studies have demonstrated the presence of SPECT abnormalities in mild injury even without CT

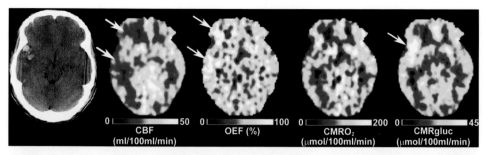

**Fig. 5.4.** PET scans of a patient with a right temporal contusion. The CBF is reduced in the frontotemporal regions with a corresponding increase in the oxygen extraction fraction and the cerebral metabolic rates for oxygen and glucose.

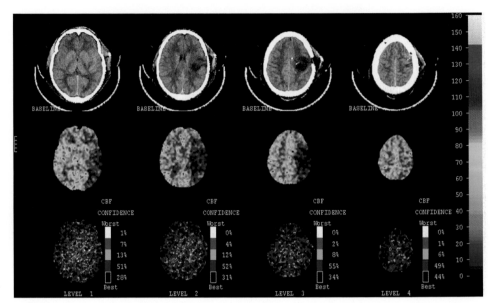

**Fig. 5.5.** Xenon CT of trauma patient. This scan was performed to evaluate regional perfusion in a patient with persistent elevated ICP. The patient shows reduced perfusion beneath a surgically elevated compound depressed skull fracture. The first row consists of CT images of various levels in the injured brain. Second row shows images of corresponding CBF values from 0–160 ml/100 g per min according to the colour scale at the right. The third row provides a visual display of the reliability of the imaging data across the different regions of the brain. The imaging data are reliant on several factors which include xenon delivery, uptake and patient movement. Data of the lowest quality will appear white and should be interpreted with caution, while the highest quality data will appear black. (Courtesy of P. Al-Rawi, University of Cambridge.)

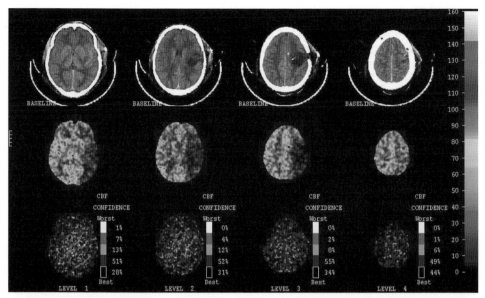

**Fig. 5.5.** Xenon-CT of trauma patient. This scan was performed to evaluate regional perfusion in a patient with persistent elevated ICP. The patient shows reduced perfusion beneath a surgically elevated compound depressed skull fracture. The first row consists of CT images of various levels in the injured brain. The second row shows images of corresponding CBF values from 0–160 ml/100 g per min according to the colour scale at the right. The third row provides a visual display of the reliability of the imaging data across the different regions of the brain. The imaging data are reliant on several factors which include xenon delivery, uptake and patient movement. Data of the lowest quality will appear white and should be interpreted with caution, while the highest quality data will appear black. (Courtesy of P. Al-Rawi, University of Cambridge.) (For colour version, see plate section.)

abnormality.[46] These abnormalities have been found to correlate with loss of consciousness, post-traumatic amnesia and post-concussive syndrome. New software (statistical parametric mapping) to analyse SPECT scans to increase objective evaluation may also lead to further development of this technique.[47]

Xenon-CT is a technique to quantify cerebral blood flow. Its usefulness in imaging traumatic brain injury is important in those cases where CBF is compromised. It does, however, have the advantage of being both simple and quick to perform (Fig. 5.5). Xenon-CT can be used with other techniques to determine the effect of loss of autoregulation during injury and its effect on cerebral perfusion and ICP.[48] This enables interventions to be taken to decrease hyperaemia leading to high ICP. Changes in cerebral blood flow have been correlated with outcome.[49] Patients who had lower cerebral blood flow at 3 weeks post-injury compared to normal controls had a worse neurological outcome than those who returned to normal.

## Summary

The field of neuroimaging is rapidly changing. For the clinical management of brain injury, CT and MRI are standards for both acute and subacute care. New techniques are giving us more information about the extent of injury, underlying physiological changes and anatomy. These are being developed to give us more information about prognosis, which even with our best efforts is still not predictable for many patients. Research tools are providing us with more information about the physiological changes leading to secondary injury, which will hopefully lead to better treatment of this devastating condition.

# Acknowledgements

The authors wish to acknowledge Dr V. Newcombe, Wolfson Brain Imaging Centre, University of Cambridge and Mrs P. Al-Rawi, University of Cambridge. CG is funded by Canadian Institute for Health Research.

# References

1. Toyama Y, Kobayashi T, Nishiyama Y *et al.* CT for acute stage of closed head injury. *Radiat Med* 2005; **23**: 309–16.

2. Teasdale E, Hadley DM. Imaging the head injury. In: Reilly P, Bullock R, eds. *Head Injury: Pathophysiology and Management*. 2nd edn. London, Hodder Educational. 2005; 169–214.

3. Stiell IG, Clement CM, Rowe BH *et al.* Comparison of the Canadian CT Head Rule and the New Orleans Criteria in patients with minor head injury. *J Am Med Assoc* 2005; **294**: 1511–18.

4. Smits M, Dippel DW, de Haan GG *et al.* External validation of the Canadian CT Head Rule and the New Orleans Criteria for CT scanning in patients with minor head injury. *J Am Med Assoc* 2005; **294**: 1519–25.

5. Sultan HY, Boyle A, Pereira M *et al.* Application of the Canadian CT head rules in managing minor head injuries in a UK emergency department: implications for the implementation of the NICE guidelines. *Emerg Med J* 2004; **21**: 420–5.

6. Hassan Z, Smith M, Littlewood S *et al.* Head injuries: a study evaluating the impact of the NICE head injury guidelines. *Emerg Med J* 2005; **22**: 845–9.

7. Stiell IG, Wells GA, Vandemheen K *et al.* The Canadian CT Head Rule for patients with minor head injury. *Lancet* 2001; **357**: 1391–6.

8. Lee B, Newberg A. Neuroimaging in traumatic brain imaging. *NeuroRx* 2005; **2**: 372–83.

9. Bigler ED, Ryser DK, Gandhi P *et al.* Day-of-injury computerized tomography, rehabilitation status, and development of cerebral atrophy in persons with traumatic brain injury. *Am J Phys Med Rehabil* 2006; **85**: 793–806.

10. Bradley WG, Jr. MR appearance of hemorrhage in the brain. *Radiology* 1993; **189**: 15–26.

11. Meythaler JM, Peduzzi JD, Eleftheriou E *et al.* Current concepts: diffuse axonal injury-associated traumatic brain injury. *Arch Phys Med Rehabil* 2001; **82**: 1461–71.

12. Giugni E, Sabatini U, Hagberg GE *et al.* Fast detection of diffuse axonal damage in severe traumatic brain injury: comparison of gradient-recalled echo and turbo proton echo-planar spectroscopic imaging MRI sequences. *Am J Neuroradiol* 2005; **26**: 1140–8.

13. Sehgal V, Delproposto Z, Haacke EM *et al.* Clinical applications of neuroimaging with susceptibility-weighted imaging. *J Magn Reson Imaging* 2005; **22**: 439–50.

14. Ashwal S, Holshouser BA, Tong KA. Use of advanced neuroimaging techniques in the evaluation of pediatric traumatic brain injury. *Dev Neurosci* 2006; **28**: 309–26.

15. Ashwal S, Babikian T, Gardner-Nichols J *et al.* Susceptibility-weighted imaging and proton magnetic resonance spectroscopy in assessment of outcome after pediatric traumatic brain injury. *Arch Phys Med Rehabil* 2006; **87**: 50–8.

16. Mannion RJ, Cross J, Bradley P *et al.* Mechanism-based MRI classification of traumatic brainstem injury and its relationship to outcome. *J Neurotrauma* 2007; **24**: 128–35.

17. Huisman TA. Diffusion-weighted imaging: basic concepts and application in cerebral stroke and head trauma. *Eur Radiol* 2003; **13**: 2283–97.

18. Huisman TA, Sorensen AG, Hergan K *et al.* Diffusion-weighted imaging for the evaluation of diffuse axonal injury in closed head injury. *J Comput Assist Tomogr* 2003; **27**: 5–11.

19. Kinoshita T, Moritani T, Hiwatashi A *et al.* Conspicuity of diffuse axonal injury lesions on diffusion-weighted MR imaging. *Eur J Radiol* 2005; **56**: 5–11.

20. Ezaki Y, Tsutsumi K, Morikawa M *et al.* Role of diffusion-weighted magnetic resonance imaging in diffuse axonal injury. *Acta Radiol* 2006; **47**: 733–40.

21. Schaefer PW, Huisman TA, Sorensen AG *et al.* Diffusion-weighted MR imaging in closed head injury: high correlation with

initial Glasgow Coma Scale score and score on modified Rankin scale at discharge. *Radiology* 2004; **233**: 58–66.

22. Bradley PG, Menon DK. Diffusion- and perfusion-weighted MR imaging in head injury. In: Gillard JH, Waldman AD, Barker PB, eds. *Clinical MR Neuroimaging Diffusion, Perfusion and Spectroscopy*. 1st edition. Cambridge, Cambridge University Press, 2005; 626–41.

23. Chan JH, Tsui EY, Peh WC *et al*. Diffuse axonal injury: detection of changes in anisotropy of water diffusion by diffusion-weighted imaging. *Neuroradiology* 2003; **45**: 34–8.

24. Lee JW, Choi CG, Chun MH *et al*. Usefulness of diffusion tensor imaging for evaluation of motor function in patients with traumatic brain injury: three case studies. *J Head Trauma Rehabil* 2006; **21**: 272–8.

25. Yen K, Weis J, Kreis R *et al*. Line-scan diffusion tensor imaging of the posttraumatic brain stem: changes with neuropathologic correlation. *Am J Neuroradiol* 2006; **27**: 70–3.

26. Ducreux D, Huynh I, Fillard P *et al*. Brain MR diffusion tensor imaging and fibre tracking to differentiate between two diffuse axonal injuries. *Neuroradiology* 2005; **47**: 604–8.

27. Naganawa S, Sato C, Ishihra S *et al*. Serial evaluation of diffusion tensor brain fiber tracking in a patient with severe diffuse axonal injury. *Am J Neuroradiol* 2004; **25**: 1553–6.

28. Nakayama N, Okumura A, Shinoda J *et al*. Evidence for white matter disruption in traumatic brain injury without macroscopic lesions. *J Neurol Neurosurg Psychiatry* 2006; **77**: 850–5.

29. Inglese M, Makani S, Johnson G *et al*. Diffuse axonal injury in mild traumatic brain injury: a diffusion tensor imaging study. *J Neurosurg* 2005; **103**: 298–303.

30. Salmond CH, Menon DK, Chatfield DA *et al*. Diffusion tensor imaging in chronic head injury survivors: correlations with learning and memory indices. *Neuroimage* 2006; **29**: 117–24.

31. Wilde EA, Chu Z, Bigler ED *et al*. Diffusion tensor imaging in the corpus callosum in children after moderate to severe traumatic brain injury. *J Neurotrauma* 2006; **23**: 1412–26.

32. Ewing-Cobbs L, Hasan KM, Prasad MR *et al*. Corpus callosum diffusion anisotropy correlates with neuropsychological outcomes in twins disconcordant for traumatic brain injury. *Am J Neuroradiol* 2006; **27**: 879–81.

33. Huisman TA, Schwamm LH, Schaefer PW *et al*. Diffusion tensor imaging as potential biomarker of white matter injury in diffuse axonal injury. *Am J Neuroradiol* 2004; **25**: 370–6.

34. Voss HU, Uluc AM, Dyke JP *et al*. Possible axonal regrowth in late recovery from the minimally conscious state. *J Clin Invest* 2006; **116**: 2005–11.

35. Baron JC, Frackowiak RS, Herholz K *et al*. Use of PET methods for measurement of cerebral energy metabolism and hemodynamics in cerebral vascular disease. *J Cereb Blood Flow Metab* 1989; **9**: 723–42.

36. Coles JP. Imaging after brain injury. *Br J Anaesth* 2007; **99**: 49–60.

37. Coles JP, Fryer TD, Smielewski P *et al*. Incidence and mechanisms of cerebral ischaemia in early clinical head injury. *J Cereb Blood Flow Metab* 2004; **24**: 202–11.

38. Coles JP, Fryer TD, Smielewski P *et al*. Defining ischemic burden after traumatic brain injury using $^{15}O_2$ PET imaging of cerebral physiology. *J Cereb Blood Flow Metab* 2004; **24**: 191–201.

39. Menon DK, Coles JP, Gupta AK *et al*. Diffusion limited oxygen delivery following head injury. *Crit Care Med* 2004; **32**: 1384–90.

40. Stein SC, Graham DI, Chen XH, Smith DH. Association between intravascular microthrombosis and cerebral ischemia in traumatic brain injury. *Neurosurgery* 2004; **54**: 687–91.

41. Pickard JD, Hutchinson PJ, Coles JP *et al*. Imaging of cerebral blood flow and metabolism in brain injury in the ICU. *Acta Neurochir Suppl* 2005; **95**: 459–64.

42. Cunningham AS, Salvador R, Coles JP *et al*. Physiological thresholds for irreversible tissue damage in contusional regions following traumatic brain injury. *Brain* 2005; **128**: 1931–42.

43. Wu HM, Huang SC, Hattori N *et al*. Selective metabolic reduction in gray matter acutely following human traumatic

brain injury. *J Neurotrauma* 2004; **21**: 149–61.

44. Vespa P, Bergsneider M, Hattori N *et al*. Metabolic crisis without brain ischaemia is common after traumatic brain injury: a combined microdialysis and positron emission tomography study. *J Cereb Blood Flow Metab* 2005; **25**: 763–74.

45. Menon DK. Brain ischaemia after traumatic brain injury: lessons from $^{15}O_2$ positron emission tomography. *Curr Opin Crit Care* 2006; **12**: 85–9.

46. Gowda NK, Agrawal D, Bal C *et al*. Technetium Tc-99 m ethyl cysteinate dimer brain single-photon emission CT in mild

traumatic brain injury: a prospective study. *Am J Neuroradiol* 2006; **27**: 447–51.

47. Shin YB, Kim SJ, Kim IJ *et al*. Voxel-based statistical analysis of cerebral blood flow using Tc-99 m ECD brain SPECT in patients with traumatic brain injury: group and individual analyses. *Brain Inj* 2006; **20**: 661–7.

48. Poon WS, Ng SC, Chan MT *et al*. Cerebral blood flow (CBF)-directed management of ventilated head-injured patients. *Acta Neurochir Suppl* 2005; **95**: 9–11.

49. Inoue Y, Shiozaki T, Tasaki O *et al*. Changes in cerebral blood flow from the acute to the chronic phase of severe head injury. *J Neurotrauma* 2005; **22**: 1411–18.

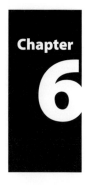

# Scoring systems for trauma and head injury

Maralyn Woodford and Fiona Lecky

Trauma care systems deal with patients who have an almost infinite variety of injuries requiring complex treatment. The assessment of such systems is a major challenge in clinical measurement and audit. Which systems are most effective in delivering best outcomes? Implementing recommendations for improved procedures will often incur additional costs – will the expense be worthwhile? Clearly, case-mix-adjusted outcome analysis must replace anecdote and dogma. Outcome prediction in trauma is a developing science that enables the assessment of trauma system effectiveness. This chapter will review some of the commonly used scoring systems and their particular applications in patients with traumatic brain injury.

The effects of injury can be defined in terms of **input** – an anatomical component and the physiological response – and **outcome** – mortality and morbidity. These must be coded numerically before we can comment with confidence on treatment or process of care. Elderly people survive trauma less well than others, therefore age must be taken into account and the association between gender and age is also considered to be important. Most recent work has been concerned with the measurement of injury severity and its relation to mortality. Assessment of morbidity has been less well studied, yet for every person who dies as a result of trauma there are two seriously disabled survivors.

## Input measures

Severity of injury is assessed through the anatomical component and the physiological response. These two elements are scored separately.

## Anatomical scoring system

The abbreviated injury scale (AIS), first published in 1969, is anatomically based. There is a single AIS severity score for each injury a patient may sustain. Scores range from 1 (minor) to 6 (incompatible with life)(Table 6.1).[1]

There are more than 2000 injuries listed in the 2005 dictionary, which is in its fifth edition. Intervals between the scores are not always consistent – for example, the difference between AIS3 and AIS4 is not necessarily the same as that between AIS1 and AIS2. (Copies of the booklet are available from www.carcrash.org.)

Patients with multiple injuries are scored by adding together the squares of the three highest AIS scores in three predetermined regions of the body. This is the injury severity score (ISS – Table 6.2). Scores of 7 and 15 are unattainable because these figures cannot be obtained from summing squares. The maximum score is 75 (25 + 25 + 25). By convention, a patient with an AIS6 in one body region is given an ISS of 75. The injury severity score is non-linear and there is pronounced variation in the frequency of different scores; 9 and 16 are common, 14 and 22 unusual.[2]

*Head Injury: A Multidisciplinary Approach*, ed. Peter C. Whitfield, Elfyn O. Thomas, Fiona Summers, Maggie Whyte and Peter J. Hutchinson. Published by Cambridge University Press. © Cambridge University Press 2009.

**Table 6.1.** Examples of injuries scored by the Abbreviated Injury Scale (AIS98 Update)

| Injury | Score |
|---|---|
| Shoulder pain (no injury specified) | 0 |
| Wrist sprain | 1 (Minor) |
| Closed undisplaced tibial fracture | 2 (Moderate) |
| Head injury – unconscious on admission but for less than 1 hr thereafter, no neurological deficit | 3 (Serious) |
| Incomplete transection of the thoracic aorta | 4 (Severe) |
| Complex liver laceration | 5 (Critical) |
| Laceration of the brainstem | 6 (Incompatible with life) |

**Table 6.2.** Injury severity score (ISS)

To obtain this:
- Use the AIS05 dictionary to score every injury
- Identify the highest AIS score in each of the following six areas of the body:
  1. head and neck
  2. face
  3. chest and thoracic spine
  4. abdomen, lumbar spine and pelvic contents
  5. bony pelvis and limbs
  6. body surface
- Add together the squares of the highest scores in three body areas

# Case study

A man is injured in a fall from a ladder while at work. He is disorientated on arrival; his mandible appears unstable and he has difficulty breathing. There is no external haemorrhage. There are abrasions around the left temple, left shoulder, left side of the chest and left knee. After a rapid sequence intubation, a CT brain scan shows a large subdural haematoma.

Radiographic examination of the cervical spine suggests no abnormality. There is a displaced fracture of the body of the mandible. There are also fractures of the left wrist, and left ribs (4–9) with a flail segment (Table 6.3).

For the purpose of the analysis described here, the ISS should be calculated only from injuries described by operative findings, imaging investigations or post-mortem reports. The ISS is an ordinal scale, therefore the overall score for a cohort of patients should be described by the median value and the interquartile range, rather than the mean. As 30% of patients with severe traumatic brain injury will have significant other injuries, a global anatomical scoring system needs to be used as extracranial injuries will have a significant bearing on outcome.

There are other ways of combining AIS values such as A Severity Characterization Of Trauma (ASCOT) and the New Injury Severity Score (NISS)[3,4] International Classification of Disease codes can be adapted to ISS scores but, in general, lack sufficient clinical detail, particularly for brain injury. ISS therefore remains the gold standard for scoring the anatomical severity of injury in multiply injured patients.

**Table 6.3.** Case study

| Injury | AIS score |
|---|---|
| Displaced fracture of body of mandible | 2 |
| Fracture of lower end of radius (not further specified) | 2 |
| Fracture of ribs 4–9 with flail segment | 4 |
| Abrasions (all sites) | 1 |
| Subdural haematoma (large) | 5 |

AIS05, Abbreviated injury scale ISS $= 5^2 + 4^2 + 2^2 = 45$.

## Physiological scoring systems

Historically, the physiological responses of an injured patient have been assessed by the revised trauma score (RTS). The physiological parameters that make up the RTS are respiratory rate, systolic blood pressure and Glasgow Coma Scale (GCS). The RTS was developed following statistical analysis of a large North American database to determine the most predictive independent outcome variables. Selection of variables was also influenced by their ease of measurement and clinical opinion. In practice the RTS is a complex calculation combining coded measurements of the three physiological values multiplied by a weighting factor, for each variable, derived from regression analysis of the database.

After injury, the patient's physiological response is constantly changing but for the purposes of injury scoring, and by convention, the first measurements, when the patient arrives at hospital, are used. If the patient is intubated before arrival, a RTS cannot be measured.

## Current practice

The latest European research has shown the GCS to be the most valuable physiological predictor at the time of Emergency Department presentation.[5] If the patient is intubated before arrival, a GCS measured at the scene of the incident can be used. Most trauma predictive models use the full GCS on arrival at the Emergency Department as physiological predictors.[6] TBI predictive models have been recently reviewed and used either the full GCS or the motor value of the GCS, however the timing of the latter is variable.[7–9] Various modifications of the scale have been suggested for use in small children. Some doctors reduce the maximum score to that which is consistent with neurological maturation. A more useful clinical device, which ensures more accurate communication and simplifies epidemiological research, is to retain the maximum score of 15 but redefine the descriptions (Table 6.4).[10]

## Trauma outcome prediction methodology

The degree of physiological derangement and the extent of anatomical injury are measures of the threat to life. Mortality will also be affected by the age and gender of the patient.

Traditionally, the 'TRISS methodology' combined four elements – the revised trauma score (RTS), the injury severity score (ISS), the patient's age, and whether the injury was blunt or penetrating – to provide a measure of the probability of survival.[11] From the database of the Trauma Audit & Research Network (TARN) the outcome prediction model has been updated to reflect the characteristics of the European trauma population and specifically includes:

**Table 6.4.** Modification of Glasgow Coma Scale for children

|  | Score |
|---|---|
| *Best verbal response* | |
| Appropriate words or social smiles, fixes on and follows objects | 5 |
| Cries but is consolable | 4 |
| Persistently irritable | 3 |
| Restless, agitated | 2 |
| Silent | 1 |
| *Eye and motor responses* | |
| Scored as in scale for adults | |

- outcome (survival or death) measured at 30 days reflecting outcomes from the injuries rather than any pre-existing diseases
- using the GCS as the only physiological marker. This improves the model and increases the number of cases that can be included in outcome predictions by 20%
- patients who are transferred to another hospital for further care, intubated at the scene and those with burn injuries
- injured children
- one model is now used for both blunt and penetrating injured patients
- as the age-related increases in mortality are more pronounced for males, the model incorporates an age/gender interaction

In order to achieve the best statistical model, there must be a balance between accurate prediction rates and clinical 'face validity'. The data used for the model's development must also reflect 'real world' data. The recent statistical modelling work at TARN reflects these concerns. Finally, the predictions of any model will only be valid if the dataset includes the great majority of index cases.

The probability of survival (**Ps**) of each injured patient is calculated using the following four factors:

· Age · Gender · Glasgow Coma Scale · Injury Severity Score

It is important to realize that **Ps** is a mathematical calculation; it is not an absolute measure of mortality but only an indication of the probability of survival. If a patient with a **Ps** of 80% dies, the outcome is unexpected because four out of five patients with such a **Ps** would be expected to survive. However, the fifth would be expected to die – and this could be the patient under study. The **Ps** is used as a filter for highlighting patients for study in multi-disciplinary trauma audit.

## Outcome prediction in traumatic brain injury (TBI)

It is clearly possible to use this approach to create a prognostic model for brain-injured patients. Guidelines for appraising the quality of prognostic models in healthcare are published elsewhere[12]. The anatomical, physiological and demographic variables used in a TBI model will depend on the setting and functional requirements of the model. For example, if a prognostic model is to be used for clinical audit and benchmarking then it is reasonable to include the ISS as the prognosis is calculated once all the specific injury details are known. The same model is more

**Table 6.5.** Common 'independent' prognostic variables in published head injury outcome prediction models (predicting outcome) – summarized from Perel *et al*.[7]

|  | Comments |
|---|---|
| Age | Present in more accurate models, predicting death or death and disability |
| GCS or motor GCS | Present in all accurate models |
| Blood pressure | Present in recent models |
| Hypoxaemia | Present in recent models |
| Pupillary reactivity | Present in all models |
| Pupillary size | Present in one European model |
| Oculocephalic reflex | Present infrequently |
| Mechanism of Injury | Present infrequently |
| ISS | Present in most models |
| CT classification | Present in models not using AIS / ISS |
| Intracranial haematoma | Present infrequently |
| Subarachnoid haemorrhage | Present as separate variable in models using CT classification |
| Midline shift | Present infrequently |

*Note:* Most models have studied only patients with moderate and severe TBI, lesser injuries are incorporated in general trauma models such as TARN.

difficult to use early in the patient's clinical course when the full injury descriptions from imaging and surgery, needed for ISS derivations, may not be available.

The utility of clinical variables will vary depending on the setting in which they are used, for example, the GCS provides good discrimination and outcome prediction when applied to the whole population of patients with head injury presenting to an emergency department.[13] The motor GCS is likely to be more useful and indeed more reliably measured if the subset of TBI patients to be studied is those ventilated on intensive care units. Table 6.5 summarizes the factors that have been found to have some prognostic ability for outcome after TBI in a recent systematic review of prognostic models.[7]

## Comparing systems of trauma care

Comparison of the probabilities of survival of all patients seen at a particular hospital with the observed outcome can be used as an index of overall performance. Probabilities of survival are combined in the 'standardized W statistic' (**Ws**) to assess a group of patients.[14] This provides a measure of the number of additional survivors, or deaths, for every 100 patients treated at each hospital accounting for different mixes of injury severity. The 'standardized Z statistic' (**Zs**) provides a measure of its statistical significance.

A high positive **Ws** is desirable as this indicates that more patients are surviving than would be predicted from the TRISS methodology. Conversely, a negative **Ws** signifies that the system of trauma care has fewer survivors than expected from the TRISS predictions. Consequently, poorly performing hospitals have the opportunity to evaluate their trauma care systems through comparative national audit and improve the care provided. Hospitals with outcomes better than those predicted should continue to monitor their healthcare system for injured patients to maintain clinical excellence.

51

# Applications of trauma outcome prediction

First developed in North America, the method used by TARN is now used in England and Wales, as well as throughout Europe and Australia, to audit the effectiveness of systems of trauma care and the management of individual patients.[15] The probability of survival methodology is applied in all patients with trauma who are admitted to hospital for more than 3 days, managed in an intensive care area, referred for specialist care or who die in hospital. Additional information is sought on the process and timing of care interventions and length of stay.

TARN provides a valuable method of comparing patterns of care in different parts of the country. It is reliant on careful collection of data in a consistent format to allow collation and comparison of results. Deaths caused by trauma are too varied, too complicated and too important to be discussed in isolation in individual hospitals.

The wider perspective of TARN is increasingly recognized as a valid approach to trauma audit and has been adopted by regional and national bodies. However, identification of deficiencies is valuable only if a mechanism exists to correct them. Local audit meetings and national comparisons must be used to stimulate appropriate changes in systems of trauma care.

The development of the TRISS and probability of survival methodologies has been a major advance in the benchmarking of trauma care. The detailed structure of the scales and the method of developing a single number to represent threat to life are under constant review.

European trauma registries are now collaborating through the EuroTARN initiative to compare crude outcomes (% mortality) in similar groups of patients. As there are large trauma system variations across Europe it is hoped this collaboration will help identify the true role and benefits of 'trauma centres' and other system characteristics that have yet to be determined.[16]

Recently, the outcome data from the 10 008 patients recruited into the CRASH trial (corticosteroid randomization after significant head injury) has been used to formulate prognostic models of head trauma.[17] Age, GCS, pupillary reactivity and the presence of major extracranial injury were prognostic indicators. CT scan findings that correlated with a poor outcome were petechial haemorrhages, obliteration of the third ventricle or basal cisterns, subarachnoid haemorrhage, midline shift and non-evacuated intracranial haematoma. A web-based prognostic calculator enables the 14-day mortality to be predicted from this large multinational pool of patients (www.crash2.lshtm.ac.uk/).

Measurement of outcome in terms of survival or death is, however, a crude yardstick. Further progress is required in measuring disability after injury. Most life-threatening visceral injuries leave the patient with little disability. Disability after musculoskeletal and brain injury are more common; however, many studies of disability suffer from losses to follow-up. Furthermore, it is uncertain whether the Glasgow Outcome Scale, commonly used in brain injury studies, adequately addresses the impact of extracranial injury on disability outcome.[18]

# Summary

Scoring systems for trauma have been developed which have facilitated the development of outcome prediction models, case mix adjustment and trauma system benchmarking. For trauma in general, which includes head injury, there is an international consensus that a TRISS or TRISS-like model should be used. These models contain measurement of host vulnerability (age, gender), anatomical severity of injury (ISS) and physiological derangement (GCS).

There are many head injury prognostic models in the literature that use varying combinations of variables. The gold standard is work in progress, but seems likely to include the types of scoring systems and variables used in general trauma models.

Further details of TARN can be obtained from www.tarn.ac.uk.

# References

1. Committee on Injury Scaling, Association for the Advancement of Automotive Medicine. The Abbreviated injury scale 1990 revision. Des Plaines, Illinois, 1990.
2. Baker SP, O'Neill B. The injury severity score: an update. *J Trauma* 1976; **16**: 882–5.
3. Champion HR, Copes WS, Sacco WJ *et al.* Improved predictions from A Severity Characterization of Trauma (ASCOT) over Trauma and Injury Severity Score (TRISS): results of an independent evaluation. *J Trauma* 1996; **40**: 42–9.
4. Osler TMD, Baker SPMPH, Long WMD. A modification of the Injury Severity Score that both improves accuracy and simplifies scoring. *J Trauma* 1997; **43**: 922–6.
5. Bouamara O, Wrotchford AS, Hollis S, Vail A, Woodford M, Lecky FE. A new approach to outcome prediction in trauma: a comparison with the TRISS model. *J Trauma* 2006; **61**: 701–10.
6. Champion HR, Sacco WJ, Copes WS, Gann DS, Gennarelli TA, Flanagan ME. A revision of the Trauma Score. *J Trauma* 1989; **29**: 623–9.
7. Perel P, Edwards P, Wentz R, Roberts I. Systematic review of prognostic models in traumatic brain injury. *BMC Med Inform Decision Making* 2006; **6**: 38.
8. Jennett B, Teasdale G. Aspects of coma after severe head injury. *Lancet.* 1977; **1**: 878–81.
9. Healey C, Osler T, Rogers F *et al.* Improving the Glasgow Coma Score scale: motor score alone is a better predictor. *J Trauma* 2003; **54**: 671–80.
10. The Child's Glasgow Coma Scale has evolved from adaptations to Jennett and Teasdale's Glasgow Coma Scale (Jennett, Teasdale. *Lancet* 1977; **1**: 878–81), by James and Trauner (James and Trauner. Brain insults in infants and children. Orlando: Grune & Stratton 1985; 179–82), Eyre and Sharples and by Tatman, Warren and Whitehouse (Tatman, Warren, Williams, Powell, Whitehouse. *Arch Dis Child* 1997; **77**: 519–21) and paediatric nurse colleagues, Kirkham and the British Paediatric Neurology Association GCS Audit Group.
11. Champion HC, Copes WS, Sacco WJ *et al.* The Major Trauma Outcome Study: establishing national norms for trauma care. *J Trauma* 1990; **30**: 1356–65.
12. Altman DG, Royston P. What do we mean by validating a prognostic model? *Stat Med* 2000; **19**: 453–73.
13. Stiell IG, Wells GA, Vandemheen K *et al.* The Canadian CT head rule for patients with minor head injury. *Lancet* 2001; **357**: 1391–6.
14. Hollis S, Yates DW, Woodford M, Foster P. Standardised comparison of performance indicators in trauma: a new approach to case-mix variation. *J Trauma* 1995; **38**: 763–6.
15. Lecky F, Woodford M, Yates DW. Trends in trauma care in England and Wales 1989–97. UK Trauma Audit and Research Network. *Lancet* 2000; **355**: 1771–5.
16. EuroTARN (2007) http://eurotarn.man.ac.uk/.
17. The MRC CRASH Trial Collaborators. Predicting outcome after traumatic brain injury: practical prognostic models based on large cohort of international patients. *Br Med J* 2008; **336**: 425–9.
18. Jennett B, Bond M. Assessment of outcome after severe brain damage: a practical scale. *Lancet* 1975; **1**: 480–4.

# Chapter 7

# Early phase care of patients with mild and minor head injury

Chris Maimaris

Mild head injuries (MHI) make substantial demands on health services all over the world. They consume time and resources including imaging and sometimes short stay hospital observation. A small proportion of patients may have persisting disabling symptoms, which preclude them from work for a long time, often needing support and costly rehabilitation.

## Definitions

Head injuries are classified into mild, moderate and severe according to severity at presentation. The use of the term **minor head injury** was commonly used interchangeably with **mild head injury** until the 1990s. In 1995 Teasdale suggested that the term minor should be used in a restrictive way for patients presenting with a GCS score of 15 versus those other mild head injured patients with GCS score of 13–14.[1] Other authors agreed with this classification.[2] Mild HI was originally defined as isolated head injury producing a GCS score of 13–15 at presentation. However, studies showed up to 40% of patients with an initial GCS of 13 had abnormal CT scans and 10% required neurosurgical treatment, with outcomes similar to moderate head injuries. The 1997 revision of the ATLS Manual recommended that patients with GCS of 13 should be classified as having moderate rather than mild head injury.[3] The definition of **mild** HI (MHI)is therefore accepted to be patients who on initial presentation have a GCS of 14–15 and **minor** HI describes the subset of patients with a GCS of 15 at presentation.

Traumatic brain injury (TBI) is used in the USA to refer to injury to the brain. The term head injury is used when there is clinically evident trauma above the clavicles such as scalp lacerations, periorbital ecchymoses, and forehead abrasions, whereas in TBI, the patient may have no signs of external injury. Mild traumatic brain injury is a term commonly used in the United States to describe mild head injury as defined above. "Concussion" is another loose term that is commonly used interchangeably with MHI.[4]

## Epidemiology

Head injuries comprise around 3%–5% of all Emergency Department attendances in the UK and 80%–90% of all head injuries are mild.[5] In the 1970s it was estimated that around one million patients with head injuries present to UK Emergency Departments per annum.[6] A study from Exeter estimated head injury incidence to be 450 per 100 000 population per year.[7] The National Institute of Clinical Excellence (NICE) recently estimated emergency department attendances with head injury to be around 700 000 per annum in England and Wales – a rate of more than 1200/100 000.[5] Studies from New Zealand estimate head injury attendances to be higher.[8] It is also known that many patients with mild head injury seek help at alternative health facilities such as minor injury units or GP surgeries and studies estimate that 40 cases of HI are medically treated outside hospital for every 100 seen in the emergency department.[9] Therefore, a more accurate estimate of the true incidence of head injury in the

*Head Injury: A Multidisciplinary Approach*, ed. Peter C. Whitfield, Elfyn O. Thomas, Fiona Summers, Maggie Whyte and Peter J. Hutchinson. Published by Cambridge University Press. © Cambridge University Press 2009.

population at large is close to 1500/100 000 and 95% of these are mild. Around 30% of all head injury attendances are children (defined as age <16) and an estimated 280 children/ 100 000 population require hospitalisation annually. The highest rates of attendances occur in the age group of 15 to 24-year-olds. The leading causes of mild head injury in the UK are falls, motor vehicle collisions, sporting injuries and assaults. Alcohol intake is present in up to 45% of head injured patients presenting to emergency departments.[5,9]

## Pathophysiology

Mild head injury can result from a direct blow to the head or from sudden deceleration or rotational forces that do not involve impact. The loss of consciousness, amnesia and other associated symptoms stem from direct injury to neurons and surrounding vasculature, with subsequent damage attributable to ischaemia and metabolic changes.

Early comparative studies demonstrated that patients without pathological findings on head CT scan may exhibit structural abnormalities on MRI, specifically in the cortex of the frontal and temporal lobes.[10] These findings correlated with behavioural and neuropsychological abnormalities. Diffuse axonal injury at the grey–white matter interface also has been demonstrated on MRI.[11] Functional neuro-imaging using PET and SPECT shows impaired cerebral glucose utilization and decreased cerebral blood flow after injury.[12,13]

Molecular modelling studies propose a state of excitatory neurotransmitter toxicity, whereby injury triggers a cascade of neuro-chemical and metabolic derangements resulting in anaerobic cellular metabolism and lactate production. These biochemical disturbances manifest as functional abnormalities and probably contribute significantly to the prolonged period of morbidity experienced by many patients in the absence of detectable structural lesions on CT/MRI scans.[14] Neuropsychological abnormalities that persist long after the initial injury, such as the 'post-concussive syndrome' are not identified with these anatomic imaging modalities. Future investigations that use more sensitive imaging tests and functional MRI may clarify the mechanisms and pathophysiology in patients with persistent symptoms.

## Clinical features and evaluation

The most common complaint after mild head injury is headache. However, many patients may not have any symptoms by the time they reach the emergency department. Other common symptoms are nausea and vomiting. Occasionally, patients may complain of disorientation, confusion or post-traumatic amnesia. Other important information to be sought during history-taking includes the mechanism of injury – ejection from vehicle, children struck by motor vehicles, falls from height – age (elderly patients are prone to sub-dural haematomas) and a history of bleeding diathesis or anticoagulation therapy.

The GCS should be monitored at presentation as a baseline reading and every 15–30 minutes thereafter. Scalp wounds or contusions should be examined thoroughly, assessing skin viability and the presence of foreign bodies. The wound should be palpated for any underlying bone fracture. Signs of skull base fractures should be sought. The ears should be examined with an auroscope to detect any CSF otorrhoea or haemotympanum – a dark red/blue appearance suggests blood behind the tympanic membrane. CSF rhinorrhoea – blood mixed with CSF from the nose – does not clot and forms tracks on blotting paper. Periorbital and retroauricular ecchymoses require careful inspection. A comprehensive neurological examination is essential to detect subtle neurological abnormalities such as unequal pupils, cranial nerve deficit or peripheral limb weakness/abnormalities. During evaluation of mild head injury patients, clinical evidence should be sought to identify the patients who are at risk of traumatic intra-cranial pathology and especially those that require neurosurgical intervention.

The neck should always be assessed for injury to the cervical spine. Patients who have neck symptoms suggestive of possible injury, patients who are confused or intoxicated and those with other distracting injuries require cervical spine imaging. A plain X-ray is per-formed and supplemented with further imaging (CT/MRI) as required. The ATLS and NICE Guidelines for imaging the C-Spine in the presence of head injury provide comprehensive recommendations and should be followed.[15,16]

## Imaging studies

The investigation of choice for adult and paediatric patients with mild head injury at presentation is CT scanning. This modality can detect underlying pathology and the presence of surgically significant lesions that require neurosurgical treatment or transfer of the patient from a District General Hospital (or Level II/III unit) to the neurosurgical centre.[17] Skull X-rays are indicated when there are no CT facilities and the patient is deemed to be at moderate or high risk of intracranial pathology. The presence of a linear, basal or depressed skull fracture, pneumocephalus or fluid in the sphenoid sinus raises the possibility of intra-cranial lesions and warrants urgent CT scanning.

Considerable debate about the indications for CT imaging of patients with mild head injury has occurred over the years. Prior to 2003 skull X-rays were widely used and only the most severe of mild head injury patients or those with a skull fracture were scanned due to shortage of CT scanning facilities or non-availability out of hours. With the increasing availability of CT facilities some centres adopted the Canadian CT scan rules before the National Institute for Clinical Excellence (NICE) Guidelines were published.[18,19] The 1999 Scottish Intercollegiate Guidelines (SIGN) advocated the use of skull X-rays, observation and selective use of CT imaging for mild head injury patients.[22] The UK adopted CT scanning as the investigation of choice in 2003 after the publication of the NICE Guidelines on the Management of Head injuries.[16] These are mainly based on the Canadian CT Head Rules and are updated regu-larly.[5,20,21] The ATLS course and some neurosurgical literature advocate CT scanning of all mild head injury patients and any patient with loss of consciousness.[3] However, because mild head injury is such a common condition, CT scanning of a large number of patients is impractical, expensive and exposes patients to high levels of irradiation. Therefore, further diagnostic workup hinges on risk stratification of mild head injury (Table 7.1).

Current medical opinion favours risk stratification for CT imaging supplemented when necessary with short stay hospital observation.[23] Patients with high risk features (Table 7.1) have a significantly increased incidence of brain injuries and haematomas and must undergo CT scanning and receive further treatment where necessary. CT scanning in the UK is sometimes not easily available for 24 hours a day and the NICE Guidelines make some recommendations as to which mild head injury cases should be scanned within one hour and those that can wait up to 8 hours.[5,16]

MRI is more sensitive than CT in detecting subtle brain injury such as diffuse axonal injury and some haemorrhagic lesions.[10] Studies have suggested that patients with long-term neuropsychological sequelae from mild head injury may have a normal initial CT scan. Such problems may be related to lesions that are seen initially only on MRI.[11] In the UK the availability of MRI is restricted and not used routinely for investigating MHI.

A urine toxicology screen and blood alcohol levels are useful laboratory investigations in the initial management of mild head injury. Alcohol usually affects the level of consciousness when

**Table 7.1.** Risk stratification of mild head injuries

| High-risk clinical features | Low-risk clinical features |
| --- | --- |
| GCS <13 when first documented by paramedic | No LOC |
| GCS <15 2-hours post-injury or after resusc | Currently asymptomatic or GCS 15 |
| Focal neurological deficit / unequal pupils | Initial GCS 14 but quickly improved to 15 |
| Any signs of Skull fracture – base/calvarium | No focal neurological abnormality and normal pupils |
| Post-traumatic seizures | Intact orientation or memory |
| Witnessed LOC >5 minutes | Trivial mechanism of injury |
| Post-traumatic confusion/amnesia >20 minutes | Injury >24hrs |
| Vomiting >2 times adults, or >3 times child | No evidence of intoxication |
| Coagulopathy-bleeding abnormality/warfarin | No serious distracting injury |
| Worsening headache not relieved by analgesia | Reliable home observation |
| Age >65 yr, <2 yr | |

Adapted from National Institute for Health and Clinical Excellence (NICE, 2007). Reproduced with permission.

the blood alcohol concentration is greater than 200 mg/dl. The combination of head injury and alcohol consumption is a very frequent presentation in the emergency department. An altered GCS cannot be assumed to be due to alcohol unless the alcohol level reaches that level and there are no external signs of any head injury or assault and the CT scan is unremarkable.[24]

# Initial care and observation

All trauma patients, including those with mild head injury, are resuscitated according to the ATLS principles. A full assessment of all the injuries determines the priorities for treatment. CT scanning is required for the mild head injury cases with high-risk features. Associated injuries and insults, especially hypoxia or hypovolaemia, need to be addressed promptly to avoid secondary brain injury. The patient should be stabilized before transfer to the imaging department. If CT imaging reveals evidence of intracranial pathology, the advice of the neurosurgical unit should be sought with the assistance of an image transfer system. Patients with mild head injury who require neurosurgical care should be transferred to using local protocols, to ensure optimal care. Mild head injury patients who have other associated injuries and do not require neurosurgical care are admitted to hospital for the treatment of these injuries but neurological observations should be carried out over at least 24 hours to ensure no neurological deterioration takes place.

Further management of the mild head injured patient is determined by the result of the CT scan and the condition of the patient (Fig. 7.1). Many of the patients with an isolated mild head injury and a normal or inconsequential CT scan require further hospital observation as determined by the various factors shown in the "Admission criteria" section of the management algorithm (Fig. 7.1). The objectives of hospital observation are to carry out regular neurological observations and allow time for the condition of the patient to improve and symptoms to resolve, especially in the presence of alcohol intoxication. The majority of patients usually improve over a period of 24 hours. Such patients are very suitably managed in short-stay observation wards or in Clinical Decision Units. On the rare occasion when the neurological observations deteriorate, rapid action in the form of further CT scanning and neurosurgical consultation should be conducted.

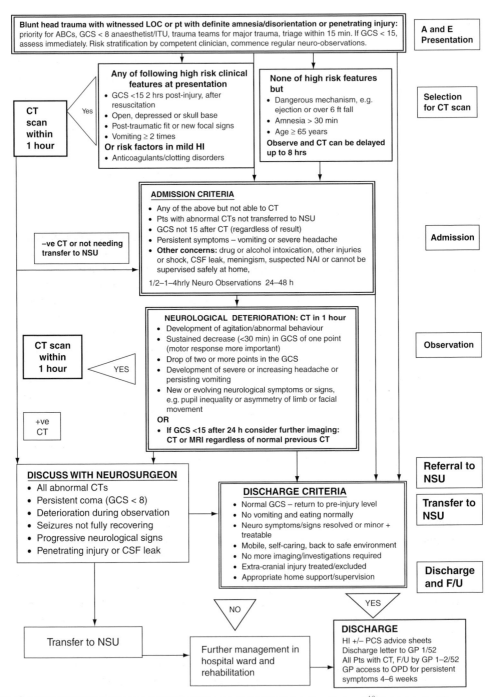

**Blunt head trauma with witnessed LOC or pt with definite amnesia/disorientation or penetrating injury:** priority for ABCs, GCS < 8 anaesthetist/ITU, trauma teams for major trauma, triage within 15 min. If GCS < 15, assess immediately. Risk stratification by competent clinician, commence regular neuro-observations.

**A and E Presentation**

**Any of following high risk clinical features at presentation**
- GCS <15 2 hrs post-injury, after resuscitation
- Open, depressed or skull base
- Post-traumatic fit or new focal signs
- Vomiting ≥ 2 times

**Or risk factors in mild HI**
- Anticoagulants/clotting disorders

**None of high risk features but**
- Dangerous mechanism, e.g. ejection or over 6 ft fall
- Amnesia > 30 min
- Age ≥ 65 years

**Observe and CT can be delayed up to 8 hrs**

**Selection for CT scan**

**CT scan within 1 hour** — Yes

**ADMISSION CRITERIA**
- Any of the above but not able to CT
- Pts with abnormal CTs not transferred to NSU
- GCS not 15 after CT (regardless of result)
- Persistent symptoms – vomiting or severe headache
- **Other concerns:** drug or alcohol intoxication, other injuries or shock, CSF leak, meningism, suspected NAI or cannot be supervised safely at home,

1/2–1–4hrly Neuro Observations 24–48 h

**Admission**

−ve CT or not needing transfer to NSU

**NEUROLOGICAL DETERIORATION: CT in 1 hour**
- Development of agitation/abnormal behaviour
- Sustained decrease (<30 min) in GCS of one point (motor response more important)
- Drop of two or more points in the GCS
- Development of severe or increasing headache or persisting vomiting
- New or evolving neurological symptoms or signs, e.g. pupil inequality or asymmetry of limb or facial movement

**OR**
- If GCS <15 after 24 h consider further imaging: CT or MRI regardless of normal previous CT

**Observation**

**CT scan within 1 hour** — YES

+ve CT

**DISCUSS WITH NEUROSURGEON**
- All abnormal CTs
- Persistent coma (GCS < 8)
- Deterioration during observation
- Seizures not fully recovering
- Progressive neurological signs
- Penetrating injury or CSF leak

**Referral to NSU**

**Transfer to NSU**

**DISCHARGE CRITERIA**
- Normal GCS – return to pre-injury level
- No vomiting and eating normally
- Neuro symptoms/signs resolved or minor + treatable
- Mobile, self-caring, back to safe environment
- No more imaging/investigations required
- Extra-cranial injury treated/excluded
- Appropriate home support/supervision

**Discharge and F/U**

Transfer to NSU

NO

Further management in hospital ward and rehabilitation

YES

**DISCHARGE**
HI +/− PCS advice sheets
Discharge letter to GP 1/52
All Pts with CT, F/U by GP 1–2/52
GP access to OPD for persistent symptoms 4–6 weeks

Fig. 7.1 Clinical pathway for managing mild head injuries. The Cambridge Protocol.[19] Reproduced with permission.

# Discharge and follow-up

Most patients with mild head injury and a normal neurological examination without indications for cerebral or cervical spine imaging may be discharged. Written instructions should be provided to the responsible, sober adult who will be monitoring the patient during the subsequent 24 hours. These describe the symptoms and signs of delayed complications of head injury. If there is doubt about the reliability of home observation, the patient should be kept in hospital for a short period, usually 12–24 hours. Indications for immediate medical attention include a new severe headache, vomiting, confusion, emotional lability, drowsiness, seizures or difficulty with coordination and balance. Patients should be encouraged to avoid alcohol for several days. Patients should also be advised that post-concussive symptoms lasting weeks to months may develop.

# Concussion

The term concussion refers to a temporary or brief interruption of neurological function after a minor head injury, which may involve loss of consciousness. It commonly occurs during contact sports (football, rugby, boxing) resulting from direct impact or rotational forces. The most common clinical features are amnesia for the traumatic event and confusion, the duration of which suggests the severity of injury sustained. Examination of the patient is usually normal and there may not be any external signs of injury. CT or MRI imaging does not reveal any abnormalities in the acute phase. In recent years there has been an upsurge of interest in the mechanisms of concussion due to its frequent occurrence in sports. A recent study has found 25% of concussed patients have abnormal cerebrovascular autoregulation for several days after the injury. During this period the brain may be vulnerable to additional minor head trauma.[25] A second mild head injury may result in severe consequences such as cerebral oedema and this has been labelled the 'second impact syndrome'. Therefore, patients who sustain concussion while playing sports should be advised to allow a period of rest before returning to sport activities. Sport organizations have developed guidelines. The International Rugby Board have ruled that an automatic 3-week suspension from all competitions and team practices must occur after a concussive injury.[26]

# Post-concussive syndrome (PCS)

Symptoms such as headache, dizziness, anxiety, impaired cognition and memory deficit may persist after mild head injury. In one study, this constellation of symptoms, known as post-concussive syndrome, affected more than 60% of patients 1 month after the injury.[27] Besides being distressing to the patient, family and the primary caregiver, PCS represents a significant economic burden. Patients miss an average of 4.7 work days after mild head injury as a result of post-concussive symptoms. Up to 20% of patients are unemployed at 1 year.[28] The cognitive impairment may have a profound impact on younger, high-achieving persons; deficits in memory and planning have been detected in amateur athletes as young as high school-age after mild head injury.[29]

It is difficult to predict which patients will progress to PCS. Most symptoms of uncomplicated mild head injury display a linear decline during the year after trauma. Whether the cause of these long-term impairments is structural or functional is unclear; there is a correlation with PCS symptoms and lesions in the hippocampus and temporal lobe detectable on PET or SPECT scans.[30] Regardless of the cause, the patient's complaints must be recognized as a clinical entity for which treatment options exist. It is very important to provide patients at risk with detailed information of post-concussive symptoms experienced after mild head injury.[9] Patients should be advised to seek help from their General Practitioner 4–6 weeks after injury if symptoms persist. If necessary, follow-up in a local head injury clinic or rehabilitation unit is recommended. A multidisciplinary team approach to follow-up involving the primary care physician, informed patient support groups (e.g. Headway in the UK) and the family is advisable.

# Children

The management of children with mild head injury is the same as for adults, bearing in mind some important distinctions. Overall, children have fewer mass lesions and more diffuse brain swelling than adults. Very young children (less than 1 year) are difficult to assess and may have suffered non-accidental injury (NAI). Children usually have more pronounced symptoms and signs: they look pale, are lethargic, vomit frequently and complain of headache and dizziness. Concussion in children may present as restlessness, irritability or confusion. Children may experience a brief 'impact seizure' at the time of relatively minor head trauma, but they recover fully and, by the time of assessment, are neurologically normal. This should be distinguished from a true post-traumatic seizure, which usually occurs sometime after recovery from the initial injury. Impact seizures do not predict post-traumatic seizures and may prompt more aggressive investigations than necessary. Occasionally, children with trauma to the back of the head may complain of transient 'post-concussive blindness' but recover fully within minutes to hours and with no permanent deficit.

The CT is the diagnostic imaging modality of choice for the evaluation of moderate and severe head injury in children. Younger children usually require sedation to carry out CT scanning and infants require a general anaesthetic. CT scanning is used in children with mild head injury who have high risk signs as in adults (see Table 7.1), including persisting vomiting, lethargy or increasing headache. The NICE Guidelines provide a sound method of deciding which children with MHI should be considered for scanning.[5,16] However, the risk of sedation should be weighed against the likelihood of an intracranial lesion. It is acceptable for young children with mild head injury to be observed initially for signs of deterioration before embarking on CT scanning. If after a period of 8–12 hours the symptoms do not improve, a scan should be organized. Skull X-rays may be a useful screening test in deciding whether to proceed to CT scanning in young children. In mild head injury, if the fontanelle is soft, neurological examination is normal and the skull X-rays show no fracture, a CT is not indicated. Complex stellate skull fractures or a tense fontanelle in an infant due to HI may be signs of NAI. These signs require further investigation by the paediatric team.

Children with minor head trauma, low-risk clinical features and normal examination can be discharged home, provided they receive competent observation by adults. Parents/guardians must be given advice sheets with warning signs and symptoms. If the home circumstances cannot guarantee this or the child is still symptomatic, admission to a hospital paediatric ward and regular observation must be arranged.

# References

1. Teasdale GM. Head injury. *J Neurol Neurosurg Psychiatry* 1995; **58**(5): 526–39.

2. Dubouri M, Ahmadi J, Farajbadgian M. Indications for brain CT scan in patients with minor head injury. *Clinical Neurology and Neurosurgery* 2007; **109**: 399–405.

3. American College of Surgeons Advanced Trauma Life Support (*ATLS*). *Student Manual*. 7th edition Chapter 6 Head injuries: 103, Chicago, 1997.

4. Cantu RC. An overview of concussion consensus statement since 2000. *Neurosurg Focus* 2006; **21**(4): E3.

5. NICE. Head injury: triage, assessment, investigation and early management of head injury in infants, children and adults. 2007 update. http://www.nice.org.uk/CGO56.

6. Jennett B. Epidemiology of head injury. *Arch Dis Child* 1998; **78**(5): 403–6.

7. Yates PJ, Williams WH, Harris A, Round A, Jenkins R. An epidemiological study of head injuries in a UK population attending an emergency department. *J Neurol Neurosurg Psych* 2006; **77**(5): 699–701.

8. Wrightson P, Gronwall D. Mild head injuries in NZ: incidence of injury and persisting symptoms: *NZ Med J* 1998; **111**: 99–101.

9. Wrightson P, Gronwall D. *Mild Head Injuries: A Guide to Management.* Definitions and epidemiology: 6–18. Oxford, Oxford University Press, 1999.

10. Levin HS, Amparo E, Eisenberg HM *et al.* Magnetic resonance imaging and computerized tomography in relation to the neurobehavioral sequelae of mild and moderate head injuries. *J Neurosurg* 1987; **665**: 706–13.

11. Mittl RL, Grossman RI, Hiehle JF *et al.* Prevalence of MR evidence of diffuse axonal injury in patients with mild head injury and normal head CT findings. *Am J Neuroradiol* 1994; **15**: 1583–9.

12. Bergsneider M, Hovda DA, Shalmon E *et al.* Cerebral hyperglycolysis following severe traumatic brain injury in humans: a positron emission tomography study. *J Neurosurg* 1997; **86**: 241–51.

13. Sakurada O, Kennedy C, Jehle J *et al.* Measurement of local cerebral blood flow with iodo [14C] antipyrine. *Am J Physiol* 1978; **234**: H59–66.

14. Hovda DA, Lee SM, Smith ML *et al.* The neurochemical and metabolic cascade following brain injury: moving from animal models to man. *J Neurotrauma* 1995; **12**: 903–6.

15. American College of Surgeons. *Advanced Trauma Life Support (ATLS) Instructor Manual.* 7th edition Chapter 7 C-Spine injuries. Chicago, 2004.

16. NICE 2003. Head injuries: triage, assessment, investigation and early management of head injuries in infants, children and adults. http://guidance.nice.org.uk/CG4/guidance/pdf/English.

17. Seeley HM, Maimaris C, Carroll G, Kellerman J, Pickard JD. Implementing the Galasko Report on the management of head injuries: the Eastern Region approach. *Emerg Med J* 2001; **18**: 358–65.

18. Boyle A, Santarius L, Maimaris C. Evaluation of the impact of the Canadian CT head rule on British practice. *Emerg Med J* 2004; **21**(4): 426–8.

19. Sultan HY, Boyle A, Pereira M, Antoun N, Maimaris C. Application of the Canadian CT head rules in managing minor head injuries in a UK emergency department: implications for the implementation of the NICE guidelines. *Emerg Med J.* 2004; **21**(4): 420–5.

20. Stiell IG, H. Lesiuk, G. A. Wells *et al.* The Canadian CT head rule study for patients with minor head injury: rationale, objectives, and methodology for phase I. *Ann Emerg Med* 2001; **38**: 160–9.

21. Stiell IG, Wells GA, Vandemheen K. The Canadian CT head rule study for patients with minor head injury. *Lancet* 2001; **357**: 1391–6.

22. Scottish Intercollegiate Guidelines Network. Early management of patients with a head injury. Edinburgh: Scottish Intercollegiate Guidelines(2000): http://www.sign.ac.uk/.

23. Haydel MJ, Preston CA, Mills TJ, Luber S, Blaudeau E, DeBlieux PM. Indications for computed tomography in patients with minor head injury. *N Engl J Med* 2000; **343**: 100–5.

24. Galbraith S, Murray WR, Patel AR, Knill-Jones R. The relationship between alcohol and head injury and its effect on the conscious level. *Br J Surg* 1976; **63**: 128–30.

25. Marx J, Hockburger R, Walls R (eds.) Head Injuries. In: *Rosen's Emergency Medicine.* 6th edition, Mosby, 2006.

26. Marshall SW, Spencer SJ. Concussion in Rugby: the hidden epidemic. *J Athletic Training* 2001; **36**(3): 334–8.

27. Rutherford WH, Merrett JD, McDonald JR. Symptoms at one year following concussion from minor head injuries. *Injury* 1979; **10**: 225–30.

28. Dikmen SS, Temkin NR, Machamer JE *et al.* Employment following traumatic head injuries. *Arch Neurol.* 1994; **51**: 177–86.

29. Alves WM, Macciocchi SN, Barth JT. Postconcussive symptoms after uncomplicated mild head injury. *J Head Trauma Rehabil* 1993; **8**: 48–59.

30. Umile EM, Sandel ME, Alavi A *et al.* Dynamic imaging in mild traumatic brain injury: support for the theory of medial temporal vulnerability. *Arch Phys Med Rehabil* 2002; **83**: 1506–13.

# Chapter

# 8

# Early phase care of patients with moderate and severe head injury

Duncan McAuley

## Introduction

Head injuries are classified into mild, moderate and severe according to their severity at presentation or after initial resuscitation.[1] In moderate head injuries (defined as Glasgow Coma Scale score 9–13) patients are typically lethargic, while in severe head injuries (GSC 3–8) patients are usually comatose. This chapter will discuss the early management of moderate and severe brain injury patients but, for convenience, use of the terms traumatic brain injury (TBI) and head injury will be used interchangeably.

In most countries road traffic collisions are the major cause of traumatic deaths and disability, although for the elderly falls are the leading cause. Despite an increased understanding of head injury pathophysiology, TBI remains a significant healthcare burden. Head injuries comprise about 5% of all emergency department (ED) attendances in the UK but only 10%–20% are moderate or severe.[2] The mortality rate is 6–10 per 100 000 per annum in the UK, making it a leading cause of death among young adults and children.[3] Mild head injuries have a mortality rate of about 0.1%, although up to 50% have significant disability as measured by the Glasgow Outcome Score.[4] For those with severe TBI, mortality may be 50% with a significant proportion dying in the first 6 hours.[5] Good long-term outcome, assessed by GOS, only occurs in 20% of these cases. Head injuries may become the most common global cause of death and disability by the year 2020.[6]

Traumatic brain injury has been traditionally divided into primary and secondary. Primary injury results from mechanical forces on the brain, while secondary injury is the consequence of further physiological insults, such as hypotension and hypoxia. Primary injury causes physical disruption of cell membranes and a disturbance in homeostasis leading to neuronal swelling, relative hypoperfusion and a cascade of neurotoxic events.[7] The distinction between primary and secondary periods of brain injury is not distinct with recent evidence that neuronal dysfunction may start hours after the injury.[8] Secondary brain injury is the main cause of in-hospital death after TBI and is principally due to brain swelling, with an increase in intracranial pressure (ICP) and subsequent cerebral hypoperfusion. Significant reduction of cerebral blood flow or elevated ICP causing cerebral herniation leads to further brain injury.

The early management of head injuries is aimed at reducing the progression of brain injury and secondary insults. There is evidence that prompt medical care and appropriate surgical intervention lead to improved outcomes, although very few interventions have been subjected to randomized, controlled trials.[9,10] Various groups have produced evidence-based or expert-derived guidelines for head injury management: European Brain Injury Consortium (EBIC, 1997: www.EBIC.nl), Scottish Intercollegiate Guidelines Network (SIGN, 2000: www.sign.ac. uk), Brain Trauma Foundation (BTF, 1995, 2000, 2007: www.braintrauma.org) and the National Institute for Clinical Excellence (2003, 2007: www.nice.org.uk).

*Head Injury: A Multidisciplinary Approach*, ed. Peter C. Whitfield, Elfyn O. Thomas, Fiona Summers, Maggie Whyte and Peter J. Hutchinson. Published by Cambridge University Press. © Cambridge University Press 2009.

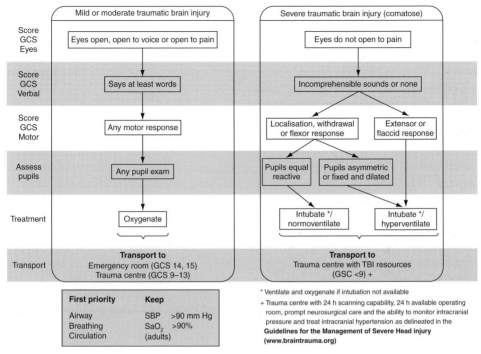

**Fig. 8.1.** Brain Trauma Foundation pre-hospital management algorithm. Reproduced with kind permission.

# Pre-hospital care

The role of advanced techniques in pre-hospital care has been debated for many years. A World Health Organization survey concluded there was insufficient evidence for many of the common pre-hospital interventions.[11] However, early identification of severe TBI at the scene with proper assessment, stabilization and transport destinations can reduce secondary injury. Specific guidelines for pre-hospital care of TBI have been produced by the Brain Trauma Foundation (Fig. 8.1).[12]

Failure to adequately maintain the airway is considered the leading cause of preventable deaths after trauma.[13] Few authorities would argue that many patients with TBI require early intubation but many debate whether this is best done at scene or in the emergency department. A retrospective study in San Diego demonstrated that intubation reduces the risk of death after isolated severe head injury from 50% to 23%.[14] Studies have shown the safety of using short-acting neuromuscular blockade to facilitate intubation by paramedics, although concerns have been raised that individual paramedics would have insufficient opportunities to maintain these skills. The use of neuromuscular blockade necessitates having appropriate rescue airway devices. Trials showing worsened outcomes when paramedics performed rapid sequence intubation (RSI) might be explained by the frequent use of hyperventilation rather than specific airway care.[15] Other, non-randomized, studies of pre-hospital intubation are limited because patients undergoing at scene intubation are likely to be more severely injured. In the UK paramedics are not trained to perform RSI but there are some pre-hospital doctors, trained in advanced airway techniques and use of end-tidal $CO_2$ monitoring to avoid hypo- or hyper-ventilation, working with paramedics within well-governed infrastructures.[16]

In most countries it is standard policy to maintain spinal immobilization for any patient with an appropriate mechanism of injury. The liberal use of spinal immobilisation has been questioned, claiming increased risk of respiratory problems and raised intracranial pressure.[17] Since spinal injuries are relatively rare (<6% of all multitrauma patients), very large trials would be required to properly investigate the role of spinal immobilization. Most guidelines encourage a conservative approach.[18]

Pre-hospital management of circulation aims to avoid shock by controlling haemorrhage and administering fluids. As well as application of pressure to control external bleeding, there are new products being investigated. The QuikClot® absorbent dressing is impregnated with the mineral zeolite, which promotes coagulation whilst absorption of fluids concentrates natural clotting factors. No product has, as yet, been shown to be superior to direct pressure.[19] Traditional fluid protocols involved infusion of a 2L crystalloid bolus. There is evidence for restricted use of fluids in patients with penetrating torso trauma.[20] However, TBI has a much worse outcome if associated with early hypotension. The Traumatic Coma Data Bank found hypotensive episodes (blood pressure <90 mm Hg) occurred at least once in 16% of patients with severe head injury by time of arrival to emergency department; hypotension was associated with doubling of mortality.[21] The choice of fluid may also be important; a meta-analysis found that hypertonic saline was associated with improved survival but other studies have not confirmed this.[22] Hypertonic saline/dextran may decrease intracranial pressure after TBI and offer a mortality benefit for those with severe head injuries but a definitive prospective trial is awaited.

In the USA coordinated systems of pre-hospital care, triage and transport to designated trauma centres have resulted in improved outcomes for TBI and it is common practice to bypass a local hospital to transport a patient to a trauma centre.[23] In the UK only 33% of major trauma patients were taken to trauma centres (major surgical specialties on site) in 1990 and nearly 75% of TBI patients underwent secondary transfer.[24] A survey in 1999 found only 30% of hospitals in England receiving trauma had on-site neurosurgery and only 79% had 24-hour availability of CT scans. There is evidence that individuals with TBI are more likely to survive if taken directly to a trauma centre rather than to a local hospital with secondary transfer.

There is little evidence that air-transport offers benefit over conventional land ambulance unless road journey times are excessive. Helicopter transport is limited by the need for suitable landing sites (at scene and hospital) and the difficulties of maintaining appropriate monitoring and patient access while in flight.

# Emergency department care

## General principles

Patients with severe head injuries should be received by a trauma team in the resuscitation room of the emergency department. It is important to gain information about mechanism of trauma as this can predict outcome. Pedestrians and cyclists fare worse than vehicle occupants, penetrating injuries fare worse than blunt and ejection from a vehicle carries a higher risk of TBI. ATLS protocols are the mainstay of early management for all trauma patients, including those with TBI. Pupillary responses in early severe head injury are more often due to brainstem hypoperfusion than to uncal herniation with third nerve compression.[16] Improving cerebral perfusion pressure will improve prognosis. However, an audit of 50 consecutive patients admitted to a regional neurosurgical centre suggested that ATLS protocols had given only modest improvements in patient care, relative to historical controls, at the expense of longer time spent in the emergency department.[26] This may be due to many ATLS violations including missed chest injuries, inadequate cervical immobilization and transfer before proper resuscitation.

## Airway

The airway should be secured in patients with severe head injury (GCS 3–8), those patients unable to maintain an adequate airway and those with hypoxia not corrected by supplemental oxygen. In children the benefits of endotracheal intubation need to be balanced against the difficulties inherent in intubating this population. Intubation should be confirmed by demonstration of $CO_2$ return. Many centres routinely intubate most moderate head injuries to allow controlled ventilation, avoid agitation and facilitate CT scanning. Care must be taken while intubating to avoid hyperextension of the cervical spine.

The choice of rapid sequence intubation (RSI) drugs must be considered in a patient with possible raised ICP. Many induction agents cause hypotension, while the insertion of laryngoscope and endotracheal tube may stimulate a reflex increase in ICP. Some authorities recommend the adjunctive use of an opioid to mitigate the sympathetic response to laryngoscopy and lidocaine to reduce the direct ICP response.[27] There is also debate whether suxamethonium causes an increase in ICP; small doses of non-depolarizing neuromuscular blocking agents can be used to mitigate this effect, although are not common practice in the UK.

## Breathing

Pre-hospital or in-hospital hypoxia ($PaO_2$ <7.9 kPa) is a strong predictor of outcome after TBI, although may be less important in children.[21] The exact target $PaO_2$ to aim for varies between guidelines. It is 13 kPa in the AAGBI guidelines.[28] Hyper- and hypocapnia can cause secondary brain injury and ventilation should be directed at the lower end of normocapnia ($PaCO_2$ 4.5–5.0 kPa). Hyperventilation lowers intracranial pressure (ICP) by causing cerebral vasoconstriction, which also leads to reduced cerebral blood flow (CBF). The reduction in CBF outweighs any benefit of reduced ICP and has been associated with adverse outcomes.[29] The use of prophylactic hyperventilation is no longer recommended before implantation of an ICP monitor and should only be used for brief periods when there are clinical signs of intracranial hypertension, such as motor posturing or pupil changes.[30]

## Circulation

Hypotension is an independent predictor of mortality in both adults and children after severe head injuries. Early (resuscitation) and late (definitive care) hypotension are separately and additively associated with increased mortality.[31] There is no evidence for the best fluid to use for TBI, but isotonic crystalloids are recommended by most guidelines. Hypotonic solutions may exacerbate cerebral oedema and should be avoided. The coexistence of other injuries, especially those likely to cause significant haemorrhage, such as vascular, intra-abdominal or pelvic, must be considered. Particular care is required if there is a spinal injury resulting in spinal shock with loss of sympathetic tone; excessive fluid administration to maintain blood pressure may lead to problems when the spinal shock recedes after 8–12 hours. Systolic blood pressure is easily measured but mean arterial pressure (MAP) is more relevant to calculate cerebral perfusion pressure (CPP). Optimal blood pressure remains undetermined; to maintain a CPP of 50 mmHg at the upper limit of normal ICP requires a MAP of 70 mmHg. The UK transfer guidelines suggest a MAP of >80 mmHg.[28] For children, age-related values should be used to define hypotension. There is insufficient evidence to support the routine use of pressor agents when fluids are unable to maintain blood pressure.

## Disability

The main aim of assessment is not to miss brain injury, especially among those presenting with a GCS of 9–13. This group of moderate brain injury patients includes cases who may 'talk and die'. Intoxication with alcohol or drugs can make examination difficult, but reduced consciousness should never be solely attributed to intoxicants without imaging.

GCS is the most universal scale of conscious level. Originally devised by Teasdale and Jennet in 1974 it is simple, quick, repeatable and has low inter-observer variation.[32] The GCS has been criticized for being inconsistent with the use of sedation or paralysis and not always performed correctly. No other scale is clearly superior and its use is recommended by the Brain Trauma Foundation and most other guidelines. The ATLS system advocates initial assessment using a simple four point scale: alert, responds to voice, responds to pain and unresponsive. This AVPU scale has not been validated as a predictor of outcome.

Many studies have looked at the prognostic power of post-resuscitation GCS and shown a steep decline in mortality as GCS increases from 3 to 8 and then a shallow decline from GCS 9–15. A drop in GCS is also significant, predicting the need for surgical evacuation of a subdural haematoma. It has been suggested that the motor component is as predictive as the global GCS score.[33] The adult GCS can also be used in children from age 5 onwards. A modified scale has been devised for pre-school children, although it is less sensitive to changes in conscious level.

Pupil size and reactivity can be affected through a number of mechanisms after head injury: eye and optic nerve trauma, third nerve injury, brainstem dysfunction and drug administration. TBI associated third nerve palsy typically occurs with ipsilateral compression of the nerve over the free edge of the tentorium. Unreactive pupils are associated with reduced consciousness level, hypotension and closed basal cisterns on CT brain scan. Bilateral unreactive pupils occur in 20%–30% of severe TBI patients and predict a 70%–90% chance of poor outcome. Asymmetrical pupils predict the presence of an operable mass lesion in about 30% of cases.[34]

## Imaging

Computed tomography (CT) is the mainstay of imaging in patients suffering head injuries. Although MRI is more sensitive, CT has the advantages of widespread availability, fast scan times and compatibility with monitoring and continued resuscitation.[35] MRI may be useful in the detection of brainstem lesions or diffuse axonal injury, particularly when there is an associated basal skull fracture. Use of CT has become much more widespread in the UK since the 2003 publication of the first NICE Guidelines on the Management of Head injuries.[36] Any patient with a GCS less than 13 on presentation or who fails to reach GCS 15 within 2 hours of injury warrants an urgent scan. Skull fractures can usually be identified on CT scan although a linear fracture may not be detectable if within the plane of the scan.[37] Depressed skull fractures with a fragment displaced more than 5 mm have a high probability of a dural tear and warrant surgical intervention. Skull X-rays also have a role in the detection of non-accidental injury in children.

In cases where CT scanning must be delayed by life-saving interventions, e.g. laparotomy or embolization, neurological assessment by insertion of an intraparenchymal ICP monitor or transcranial Doppler examination or exploratory burr holes should be considered. Recently, it was found that ultrasound measurement of the optic nerve sheath diameter may accurately predict the presence of raised ICP.[38] A finding suggestive of raised ICP will guide the surgeon in setting damage limitation priorities and prompt immediate neurosurgical consultation.

Due to the association between TBI and cervical spine trauma and the difficulty in clinical assessment when conscious level is decreased, CT imaging of the cervical spine is recommended. It is difficult to obtain a complete set of good-quality plain films in a comatose trauma patient, and many centres now perform only a lateral cervical spine radiograph followed by CT scanning. In a study of 437 intubated trauma patients, of whom 7% had an unstable cervical spine injury, CT scanning had a sensitivity of 98.1% and specificity of 98.8%.[39] In children CT scanning may be limited to C1-C3 after a lateral plain film in order to reduce radiation exposure. MRI is the modality of choice for detecting soft tissue injury or cord damage. Spinal cord injury without radiological abnormalities (SCIWORA) is rare, but reported in adults, although much more common in children. Spinal immobilization should continue until clinical assessment can be made.

## Pre ICU management

The use of mannitol is not supported by evidence, according to a recent Cochrane review.[40] Mannitol has been thought to reduce blood viscosity, thereby increasing cerebral blood flow leading to arteriolar vasoconstriction and so reducing ICP, in addition to its properties as an osmotic diuretic. Mannitol is still widely used, as 100 ml or 1 ml/kg of 20% solution both in the USA and UK. There is some evidence that hypertonic saline can be used as an alternative to mannitol, especially in children; infusions of 3% saline have been shown to reduce ICP.[41]

Anticonvulsants are not recommended routinely in TBI patients who are not fitting.[42] It is not uncommon, especially in children, for seizures to occur immediately or soon after head injury. In general, the risk of late seizures is not increased, although some types of head injury, such as penetrating injury and cortical contusions, are associated with an early risk of epilepsy. Phenytoin is the agent of choice for seizure prevention.[43]

Steroids were first used in head injuries in the 1960s, since they reduced cerebral oedema associated with tumours. More recently, recruitment into a large MRC study (CRASH) was terminated after recruitment of over 10 000 patients, when excess mortality was found in the steroid group.[44] The cause of the increased mortality is unclear. Other neuroprotective agents, such as magnesium and dexanabinol, have not shown a significant mortality or morbidity benefit in clinical trials.

## Injury priorities and patient transfer

Major extra-cranial injuries are found in about 50% of patients with TBI and the mortality of these can be very high, especially with associated pulmonary injuries requiring ventilation.[45] In head injury patients with blunt multiple trauma, it can be difficult to decide the priority of urgent laparotomy or craniotomy. Haemodynamically unstable patients need evaluation of their head, chest, abdomen and pelvis. They should have no unecessary investigations, control of haemorrhage by simple measures (and damage control surgery, if necessary) and then CT scan and treatment of the brain injury. Non-cranial injuries leading to haemorrhage and hypotension take priority. 'Damage control' surgery has developed from the knowledge that prolonged surgery can exacerbate hypothermia, coagulopathy and acidosis, all of which are associated with poor outcomes after trauma. The initial operation should aim to control haemorrhage with ligation of vessels and packing, removal of dead tissue, lavage of the abdominal cavity and then closure without tension, sometimes using a plastic sheet as temporary cover.

Bedside ultrasound scanning of the heart and abdomen (FAST scan) can be helpful in decision making. However, it may be necessary to consider treatment of the brain injury simultaneously with management of other injuries (laparotomy or thoracotomy), even without a CT scan to guide therapy. If there are signs of impending transtentorial herniation (unilateral posturing and/or unilateral dilated pupil), or if there is rapid progressive neurological deterioration (without extracranial cause), then measures to control ICP should be instituted. Blind burr holes to detect extra-axial collections may be appropriate as a last resort in some cases.

In haemodynamically stable patients with focal neurological signs, CT of the head with craniotomy should only be delayed long enough to allow rapid chest and pelvis X-rays and bedside FAST scan. Orthopaedic injuries are generally of secondary importance in multiple trauma, although fractures of the femur and pelvis can be life threatening. Femoral fractures can be managed with splinting and delay of definitive operation. Unstable pelvic fractures are associated with significant haemorrhage and often require laparotomy and early fixation. Fracture healing is known to be enhanced when there is a concomitant head injury, although the mechanism is unclear and the search for a responsible circulating factor continues.[47]

Most emergency departments in the UK have formal links with a regional neurosurgery centre, including electronic image transfer. However, transfer of patients can be limited by a lack of neuro-intensive care bed availability.[46] Transfer decisions may be aided by prognostic criteria such as age, initial GCS, severity of CT findings, pupillary response and time from injury. The presence of an acute subdural haematoma with bilateral fixed pupils is irretrievable unless the patient undergoes an emergent operation. Guidelines for the monitoring, escorts and organisation of TBI patient transfers have been published by the Anaesthetic Association of Great Britain and Ireland.[28]

# References

1. American College of Surgeons Advanced Trauma Life Support (*ATLS*) *Student Manual 7th Edition. Chapter 6: Head injuries*, Chicago, 1997.

2. NICE. Head injury: triage, assessment, investigation and early management of head injury in infants, children and adults. 2007 update. http://www.nice.org.uk/CG56.

3. Department of Health. *Hospital Episode Statistics* 2000/2001. www.hesonline.nhs.uk.

4. Thornhill S, Teasdale GM, Murray GD, McEwen J, Roy CW, Penny KI. Disability in young people and adults one year after head injury: prospective cohort study. *Br Med J* 2000; **320**: 1631–5.

5. Peek-Asa C, McArthur D, Hovda D, Kraus J. Early predictors of mortality in penetrating compared with closed brain injury. *Brain Inj* 2001; **15**: 801–10.

6. Murray CJ, Lopez AD. Global mortality disability and the contribution of the risk factors: global burden of disease study. *Lancet* 1997; **349**: 1436–42.

7. Werner C, Engelhard K. Pathophysiology of traumatic brain injury. *Br J Anaesth* 2007; **99**: 4–9.

8. Teasdale GM, Wasserberg J. The challenge of providing optimum care for the head injured. *Int Perspectives Traumatic Brain Injury* 1996; **5**: 10.

9. Mendelow AD, Gillingham FJ. Extradural haematoma: effect of delayed treatment (letter). *Br Med J* 1979; **2**(6182):134.

10. Patel HC, Menon DK, Tebbs S, Hawker R, Hutchinson PJ, Kirkpatrick PJ. Specialist neurocritical care and outcome from head injury. *Intens Care Med* 2002; **28**: 547–53.

11. Bunn F, Kwan I, Roberts I, Wentz R. Effectiveness of prehospital care. *Report to the World Health Organisation Pre-hospital Care Steering Committee*. Geneva: WHO, 2001.

12. Brain Trauma Foundation.*Guidelines for the prehospital management of traumatic brain injury*. New York: Brain Trauma Foundation, 2000. www.braintrauma.org.

13. Esposito TJ, Sanddal ND, Hansen *et al.* Analysis of preventable trauma deaths and

inappropriate care in a rural state. *J Trauma* 1995; **39**: 955–62.

14. Winchell RJ, Hoyt DB. Endotracheal intubation in the field improves survival in patients with severe head injury. *Arch Surg* 1997; **132**: 592–7.

15. Davis DP, Stern J, Sise MJ *et al*. A follow-up analysis of factors associated with head injury mortality after paramedic rapid sequence intubation. *J Trauma* 2005; **59**: 486–90.

16. MAGPAS guidelines. Mid Anglia General Practitioner Accident Service Guidelines. www.basics.org.uk.

17. Orledge JD, Pepe PE. Out of hospital spinal immobilisation: is it really necessary? *Acad Emerg Med* 1998; **5**: 203–4.

18. AANS/CNS Section on Disorders of the Spine and Peripheral Nerves. Guidelines for the management of acute cervical spine and spinal cord injuries. *Neurosurgery* 2002; **50** (Suppl): S7–S17.

19. Neuffer MC, McDivitt J, Rose D *et al*. Hemostatic dressings for the first responder: a review. *Mil Med* 2004; **169**: 716–20.

20. Bickell WH, Wall MJ, Pepe PE *et al*. Immediate versus delayed fluid resuscitation for hypotensive patients with penetrating torso injuries. *N Eng J Med* 1994; **331**: 1105–9.

21. Chesnut RM, Marshall LF, Klauber MR *et al*. The role of secondary brain injury in determining outcome from severe head injury. *J Trauma* 1993; **34**: 216–22.

22. Wade CE, Grady JJ, Kramer GC *et al*. Individual patient cohort analysis of the efficacy of hypertonic saline/dextran in patients with traumatic brain injury and hypotension. *J Trauma* 1997; **42** (5 Suppl): S61–5.

23. Mullins RJ, Veum-Stone J, Hedges JR *et al*. Influence of a statewise trauma system on the location of hospitalisation and outcome of injured patients. *J Trauma* 1996; **40**: 536–45.

24. Nicholl J, Turner J. Effectiveness of a regional trauma system in reducing mortality from major trauma: before and after study. *Br Med J* 1997; **315**: 1349–54.

25. Ritter A, Muizelaar JP, Barnes T *et al*. Brain stem blood flow, pupillary response and outcome in patients with severe head injuries. *Neurosurgery* 1999; **44**: 941–8.

26. Price SJ, Suttner NA, Aspoas R. Have ATLS and national transfer guidelines improved the quality of resuscitation and transfer of head-injured patients? A prospective survey from a regional neurosurgical unit. *Injury* 2003; **34**: 834–8.

27. Walls RM, Murphy MF. Increased Intracranial Pressure. In: Walls R, ed. *Manual of Emergency Airway Management*. Philadelphia, Lippincott, Williams & Wilkins, 2000.

28. Association of Anaesthetists of Great Britain and Ireland. *Recommendations for the transfer of patients with acute head injuries to neurosurgical units*. London: AAGBI, 2006.

29. Muizelaar JP, Marmarou A, Ward JD *et al*. Adverse effects of prolonged hyperventilation in patients with severe head injury: a randomized controlled trial. *J Neurosurg* 1991; **75**: 731–9.

30. Gabriel EJ, Ghajar J, Jagoda A *et al*. Guidelines for the pre-hospital management of traumatic brain injury. *J Neurotrauma* 2002; **19**: 111–74.

31. Fearnside MR, Cook RJ, McDougall P, McNeil RJ. The Westmead Head Injury Project outcome in severe head injury. A comparative analysis of pre-hospital, clinical and CT variables. *Br J Neurosurg* 1993; **7**: 267–79.

32. Teasdale G, Jennett B. Assessment of coma and impaired consciousness. A practical scale. *Lancet* 1974; **2**: 81–4.

33. Gill MR, Windemuth R, Steele R, Green SM. A comparison of the GCS score to simplified alternative scores for the prediction of traumatic brain injury outcome. *Ann Emerg Med* 2004; **45**: 37–42.

34. Chesnut RM, Gautille T, Blunt BA, Klauber MR, Marshall LE. The localizing value of asymmetry in pupillary size in severe head injury: relation to lesion type and location. *Neurosurgery* 1994; **34**: 840–5.

35. Cihangiroglu M, Ramsey RG, Dohrmann GJ. Brain injury: analysis of imaging modalities. *Neurol Res* 2002; **24**: 7–18.

36. NICE 2003. Head injury: triage assessment, investigation and early management of head injury in infants, children and adults. http://guidance.nice.org.uk/CG4/guidance/pdf/English.

37. RCR Working Party. *Making the Best Use of a Department of Clinical Radiology: Guidelines for Doctors*, 5th edition. London: The Royal College of Radiologists, 2003.

38. Blaivas M, Theodoro D, Sierzenski PR. Elevated intracranial pressure detected by

bedside emergency ultrasonography of the optic nerve sheath. *Acad Emerg Med* 2003; **10**(4): 376–81.

39. Brohi K, Healy M, Fotheringham T *et al.* Helical computed tomographic scanning for the evaluation of the cervical spine in the unconscious, intubated trauma patient. *J Trauma* 2005; **58**(5): 897–901.

40. Wakai A, Roberts I, Schierhout G. Mannitol for acute traumatic brain injury. *Cochrane Database of Systematlc Reviews* 2007, Issue 1. Art. No.: CD001049. DOI: 10.1002/14651858.CD001049.pub4.

41. Bayir H, Clark RS, Kochanek PM. Promising strategies to minimize secondary brain injury after head trauma. *Crit Care Med* 2003; **31**(1): S112–17.

42. Chadwick DW. Seizures and epilepsy after traumatic brain injury. *Lancet* 2000; **355** (9201): 334–6.

43. Tempkin NR. Antiepileptogenesis and seizure prevention trials with antiepileptic drugs: meta-analysis of controlled trials. *Epilepsia* 2001; **42**(4): 515–24.

44. Roberts I, Yates D, Sandercock P *et al.* Effect of intravenous corticosteroids on death within 14 days in 10 008 adults with clinically significant head injury (MRC CRASH trial): a randomised placebo-controlled trial. *Lancet* 2004; **364**: 1321–8.

45. Kotwica Z, Brzeziński J. Head injuries complicated by chest trauma a review of 50 consecutive patients. *Acta Neurochir* 1990; **103**: 109–11.

46. SBNS Working Party. Safe Neurosurgery 2000. *A report from the Society of British Neurosurgeons SBNS*, 35–43 Lincoln's Inn Fields, London.

47. Karuppal R. The effect of head injury on fracture healing. *J Orthop* 2007; **4**(1): e7 (www.jortho.org).

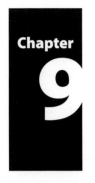

# Chapter 9

# Interhospital transfer of head-injured patients

Gareth Allen and Peter Farling

## Introduction

Neurosurgical services in the United Kingdom (UK) are organized regionally into 34 acute neuroscience centres. Traumatic brain injury is common and patients often present to local hospitals. Whilst it is difficult to calculate the overall need, in 1997 it was estimated that 11 000 interhospital transfers of critically ill patients occurred in the UK.[1] A high proportion of these was for traumatic brain injury and there is little doubt that the indications for transfer of acute brain injury have increased.[2] It has been demonstrated that the process of transfer may have adverse consequences in the general critically ill population, and it is widely accepted that the process of transferring any patient incurs inherent risks.[3] It is important therefore that, during the process of bringing the brain injured patient to a venue for definitive care, attention should be given to minimizing these risks at both individual patient and organizational levels. The need for standards for interhospital transfer was highlighted in 1994,[4] and since then guidelines have been produced by a number of organizations.[5–8]

Centrally based retrieval teams have become popular, particularly for transfer of paediatric patients, and this would solve the current manpower problem that occurs when the anaesthetist is absent from the referring hospital during a prolonged transfer. However mobilization of retrieval teams takes time and there is often a need to transfer patients with brain injury urgently. In situations where there is a time-critical lesion, such as an expanding intracranial haematoma, transfer by the referring team using the most appropriate members of staff available remains the preferred option.[9] All acute hospitals must retain the ability to resuscitate, stabilize and transfer critically ill patients.[6] This chapter will discuss the indications for transfer, the conduct of transfer and training implications.

## Indications for transfer

Accepting that transfer may have risks, it is important to have clear markers to identify patients who stand to benefit from being relocated.

Indications for transfer include:

(a) patients requiring neurosurgical intervention, e.g. evacuation of a haematoma, decompressive craniectomy, or drainage of cerebro-spinal fluid (CSF)

(b) patients requiring monitoring which cannot be provided at the referring hospital. In addition, some evidence indicates that there may be benefits to all patients with severe brain injuries, irrespective of plans for surgery, of receiving care in a dedicated neurosciences critical care unit,[2,10–13] particularly where this is headed by specialist neuro-critical care doctors.[14] However, given that demand may sometimes outstrip supply for these beds, first priority is usually given to patients who require surgery. As the

*Head Injury: A Multidisciplinary Approach*, ed. Peter C. Whitfield, Elfyn O. Thomas, Fiona Summers, Maggie Whyte and Peter J. Hutchinson. Published by Cambridge University Press. © Cambridge University Press 2009.

availability of computerised tomography (CT) has increased in district general hospitals so the need to transfer simply to facilitate imaging has decreased.

# Conduct of the transfer

The transfer should be agreed between the doctor in charge at the referring hospital and the receiving neurosurgical team. It is imperative to ensure that the receiving critical care and anaesthesia teams are also aware of the transfer of the patient. The precise destination of the patient, whether operating theatre, intensive care unit (ICU), or emergency department should be ascertained, as well as the urgency of the journey. It has been shown that 1 to 2 hours may commonly elapse between arriving in a neurosurgical hospital and surgery commencing.[15]

Information passed to the neurosurgical team must include the patient's age and medical history, mechanism and time of injury, initial and current neurological status, presence of drugs or alcohol, extracranial injuries, physiological status, details of patient management and findings of imaging. The use of a standardized neurosurgical referral letter has been shown to more consistently provide all relevant information than non-standardized *ad hoc* documents.[7,16]

The transfer of CT images between hospitals using image linking is now somewhat taken for granted and has greatly improved communication between doctors. Prior to the introduction of this technology inappropriate patient transfers were more common than today,[17] including many for which the transfer would have been particularly hazardous.[18] Today the capacity exists to obtain all radiological images digitally. These digital images can then be made available over local area networks, and with the advent of higher bandwidths, and the use of compression algorithms, even very large files can be sent rapidly over distances without loss of image quality.[19] It is vital that all hospitals receiving trauma patients have the ability to both obtain and transfer images to the neurosurgical department.

Various problems may occur during transfer, some being unique to the interhospital environment. During movement into and out of the vehicle, inadvertent decannulations or extubations may occur. Vehicles used, whether land or air based, often lack space. This, coupled with the motion of the vehicle and potential for poor lighting, makes patient observation and the performance of procedures more challenging than in the hospital environment. Monitoring alarms and inadvertent disconnections may also take longer to be noticed. The climate within the transport vehicle may be more variable than in a hospital, with patients potentially being exposed to excessive heat or cold depending on the location and the season. The motion of the vehicle may affect the patient's physiology. Hypoxaemia may be precipitated by vibrations loosening secretions and possibly provoking bronchospasm as well as by head-down tilt whilst ascending hills. Haemodynamic changes during transport, hypotension and occasionally hypertension, are common and thought to be precipitated by changes in preload and afterload.[20] This is caused by the mass movement of blood volume during acceleration and deceleration as well as by tilt induced by hills. Intracranial pressure (ICP) may be increased by vibration, noise, head down tilt or by worsening of intracranial pathology. Previously undiagnosed conditions may present or treated conditions may deteriorate; all in a location where physical help is usually unavailable. The patient is totally reliant on portable equipment during the transfer. Since 2002 all transfer equipment and vehicles are subject to regulations published by the European Committee for Standardisation (CEN).[21] In addition, although unlikely, road accidents with patient and staff injury have occurred during transfers. It is vital that appropriate medical indemnity and personal injury assurance be provided for the staff undertaking the transfer.

Unsurprisingly, therefore, problems during transfer have been found to occur in up to 34% of transfers of the critically ill with up to 37% having worse observations after the journey.[22,23] Audit data obtained by a dedicated critical care transfer team revealed that hypoxaemia was the commonest adverse event (15%), hypotension occurring in 10%, cardiac arrhythmia in 7% and equipment failure in 9%.[20] The need for emergency re-intubation was rare (0.4%). Data from the 1970s and 1980s showed that hypotension and hypoxaemia were very common on arrival at neurosurgical centres – up to 30% of patients in one series.[24] Improvement in these figures has occurred with time, and data from the 1990s show hypotension occurring in 12% and hypoxaemia in 6% of transfers.[25] More attention to stabilization of the patient prior to transfer is a key component in this improvement.[26]

Allowing for the fact that time to evacuation of an intracranial haematoma inversely correlates with the chance of a good outcome,[27,28] it is accepted that transfer must be accomplished as rapidly as possible allowing for patient safety. However, this must not occur at the expense of adequate assessment and resuscitation. There is little merit in decreasing the time to surgery at the expense of increasing the degree of systemically originated secondary brain injury. For these reasons, the direct involvement of experienced senior staff in patient management and in the decision making process is vital. For the reasons outlined above, all life threatening injuries must be attended to at the referring hospital. In one study untreated life-threatening extracranial injuries were present in almost one in ten patients arriving at neurosurgical centres.[29] Scalp injuries are probably the most frequently overlooked injury, and the potential for significant haemorrhage from these must be appreciated.[30] Immobilization of any fractures should be performed and the cervical spine stabilized appropriately. The use of spinal boards during the secondary transfer of patients does not have a firm evidence base, and the risk of precipitation of severe pressure damage must be appreciated. Unsurprisingly, formal guidelines are lacking regarding their use in a transfer setting and the decision currently rests with the staff directly involved with each transfer.

## Primary transfer to tertiary referral centres

Common sense would dictate, and limited medical evidence indicate, that any injured patient is best served by travelling directly to a centre where definitive care can be provided.[31] This is supported by the fact that as few as 33% of patients undergoing a secondary transfer may arrive within 4 hours of injury at a neurosurgical operating theatre, the median time in one study being over 6 hours.[15] To apply this principle to the head-injured patient requires a number of criteria to be satisfied. Firstly, the patient should be correctly diagnosed as having sustained a head injury. To fail in this respect exposes a patient with unconsciousness due to systemic cardiorespiratory insufficiency or drug overdose to risks of a longer transfer whilst unstable, and places further pressure on neurosurgical centre intensive care services. Secondly, facilities must exist to stabilize the patient and then rapidly undertake the longer journey to the neurosurgical centre. These requirements can be met using helicopter-based ambulance services, with a suitably experienced, equipped and assisted doctor on board. Where systems such as this are in place, delays would appear to be consistently less than those cited above, however several hours may still elapse from injury to surgical intervention.[32] It is noteworthy that examination of outcome data from similar air transport teams has shown no benefit to either mortality or functional outcome.[33] It must be borne in mind that helicopter transport presents its own unique set of problems, particularly concerning management of complications occurring *en route*, and the experience and training of the teams involved must be rigorous.[34,35]

**Table 9.1.** Recommendations for the safe transfer of patients with brain injury

High-quality transfer of patients with brain injury improves outcome.

1. There should be designated consultants in the referring hospitals and the neuroscience units with overall responsibility for the transfer of patients with brain injuries.

2. Local guidelines on the transfer of patients with brain injuries should be drawn up with the referring hospital trusts, the neurosciences unit and the local ambulance service. These should be consistent with established national guidelines. Details of the transfer of responsibility for patient care should also be agreed.

3. While it is understood that transfer is often urgent, thorough resuscitation and stabilization of the patient must be completed before transfer to avoid complications during the journey.

4. All patients with a Glasgow Coma Scale less than or equal to 8 requiring transfer to a neuroscience unit should be intubated and ventilated.

5. Patients with brain injuries should be accompanied by a doctor with appropriate training and experience in the transfer of patients with acute brain injury. They must have a dedicated and adequately trained assistant. Arrangements for medical indemnity and personal accident insurance should be in place.

6. The standard of monitoring during transport should adhere to previously published standards.

7. The transfer team must be provided with a means of communication. A mobile telephone is suitable.

8. Education, training and audit are crucial to improving standards of transfer.

Reproduced with permission from the Association of Anaesthetists of Great Britain and Ireland.[8]

# Management of 'non-surgical' patients in district general hospitals

Evidence citing improvement in outcome for brain-injured patients by medical management in specialized units has attracted some controversy. Large scale retrospective data suggest a 26% mortality increment with management in non-neurosurgical centres.[2] Attention must be paid to the content of the care as well as the location. Previously, some centres had demonstrated trends towards improved outcome using multi-modal monitoring and protocols for investigation and management of detected abnormalities.[11–13] Available evidence suggests that the average district hospital receiving trauma will care for 15 severe head injuries per year, making hospital volume a potential factor in outcome.[36] District hospitals are less likely to have access to ICP monitoring, and unlikely to have capacity to drain CSF if required. However where adequate facilities exist, and in conjunction with general surgical support, some non-neurosurgical centres have shown comparable results.[37] Caring for such patients at a distance from full neurosurgical support means that controlled expedient transfer may be needed in the event of a deterioration, for instance, if decompressive craniectomy is required.

## Maintaining standards for interhospital transfers

Given the large number of transfers occurring and the associated risks, maintenance of quality is paramount. To this end, several guidance documents have been published, including those published by the Neuroanaesthesia Society of Great Britain and Ireland in conjunction with the Association of Anaesthetists of Great Britain and Ireland.[5,8] A summary of their recommendations is given in Table 9.1 and several of the points noted bear further examination.

The role of the designated consultant should be one of quality control and include organization of audit, incident collation, education, and liaison with appropriate staff – medical and non-medical. Recent audits show that up to 50% of UK hospitals have not formally identified a staff member for this role.[38] Transfer of these patients should be a subject for audit.

In addition to those patients with a Glasgow Coma Scale (GCS) of less than or equal to eight, other patients may require pre-emptive intubation in order to preclude the need for this procedure *en route*. They include those with a downward trend in the GCS, those with airway injuries, bilateral mandibular fractures often being cited as an example, or those with suboptimal respiratory function.

A 'doctor with appropriate experience' is usually taken to mean one capable of performing any necessary procedures during the transfer, and with knowledge of the pathophysiology of brain injury. An anaesthetist with 2 years' experience is often cited as appropriate;[7] however, changes in medical training in the UK may necessitate review of this level of experience.

The standard of monitoring should not be less than that in the hospital from which the patient is leaving, and as a minimum should include ECG, invasive blood pressure, pulse oximetry, capnography, and temperature.[6] Although central venous pressure monitoring is usually not essential, the line itself is a reliable port of access and invaluable should the need for vasoactive drugs for maintenance of perfusion pressure be required during transfer. Line placement, however, should not delay transfer; particularly for surgical intervention. The pupillary reflexes must be monitored for signs of neurological deterioration. Airway pressure, inspired oxygen concentration and ventilator settings must be observed. It is essential that all observations and interventions are recorded; an anaesthetic chart is usually well suited to this purpose and specifically designed transfer charts are used in certain regions.

## Checklists

It is recommended that checklists be used when preparing a patient for transfer.[8] As a general rule, there should be a suitable doctor, with functioning equipment and a suitable assistant to transfer a suitable patient in a suitable vehicle, to a clear pre-arranged destination. Examples of checklists are shown in Table 9.2.

Available functioning equipment must include a portable ventilator, adequate oxygen supply, monitors as detailed above, full range of airway management equipment, infusion pumps, equipment for intercostal drain insertion, full range of vascular access equipment, equipment for ALS management of cardiac arrest and warming equipment. A supply of sedatives, neuromuscular blocking drugs, analgesics, anticonvulsants, vasoactive drugs and intravenous fluids should be available, as well as osmotic agents for the management of intracranial hypertension.

## Training

Medical training in general and anaesthesia training in particular is undergoing change. The development of competency-based training provides an opportunity to include transfer skills in a structured training programme. Furthermore, formal assessment by a supervising consultant during an accompanied transfer has been introduced in some areas.[39] Safe Transfer and Retrieval (StaR) courses are organized by the Advanced Life Support Group at venues throughout the UK,[40] and some local hospitals provide 'Training for Transfer'.[41] These courses provide a multidisciplinary 'hands-on' approach promoting best practice and awareness of legislation relating to equipment.

**Table 9.2.** Transfer checklist

*Respiratory checklist*
Airway secure
$PaO_2$ >13.0 kPa, $PaCO_2$ 4.5 – 5.0 kPa
Chest X-ray reviewed after placement of ETT/central access /gastric tubes
Life threatening thoracic injuries ruled out/treated

*Circulatory checklist*
Appropriate reliable i.v. access
Volume repletion
MAP>80 mmHg, HR<100/min (or age appropriate value for children)
No signs of systemic hypoperfusion
Cross-matched blood to travel with patient where possible

*Trauma checklist*
Cervical spine stabilized
External haemorrhage (e.g. scalp lacerations) controlled
Rib fractures/pneumothoraces excluded/treated
Intrathoracic/abdominal bleeding adequately excluded
Pelvic/long bone fractures stabilized

*Brain checklist*
Signs of critically raised ICP sought and acted on as needed
Seizures controlled
All appropriate imaging and clinical details with patient/electronically transferred where available

# Summary

Inter-hospital transfer of the head injured patient is common and demanding. Hospitals that receive patients with severe head injuries should retain the capability for their resuscitation, stabilization and transfer. The goal is the delivery of a patient to the neuroscience unit in a timely fashion, with a safe airway, mean arterial pressure > 80 mmHg, ICP < 20 mmHg, $PaO_2$ >13 kPa, $PaCO_2$ 4.5 – 5.0 kPa, normothermic and normoglycaemic, and with no untreated life-threatening extracranial injuries. Extensive high quality guidelines are available from a number of sources and checklists should be used during preparation for the transfer. Involvement of senior staff in both administration, clinical decision making and training is vital in maintaining quality.

# References

1. Mackenzie PA, Smith EA, Wallace PGM. Transfer of adults between intensive care units in the UK. *Br Med J* 1997; **314**: 1455–6.
2. Patel HC, Bouamra O, Woodford M *et al.* Trauma Audit and Research Network. Trends in head injury outcome from 1989 to 2003 and the effect of neurosurgical care: an observational study. *Lancet* 2005; **366**(9496): 1538–44.
3. Duke G, Green JV. Outcome of critically ill patients undergoing interhospital transfer. *Med J Aust* 2001; **174**(3): 122–5.
4. Oakley P. The need for standards for interhospital transfer. *Anaesthesia* 1994; **49**: 565–6.
5. Association of Anaesthetists of Great Britain and Ireland. *Recommendations for the transfer of patients with acute head injuries to neurosurgical units.* London: The Neuroanaesthesia Society of Great Britain and Ireland and the Association of Anaesthetists of Great Britain and Ireland, 1996.
6. Intensive Care Society. *Guidelines for the transport of the critically ill adult.* Intensive

Care Society 2002. http://www.ics.ac.uk/downloads/icstransport2002mem.pdf.

7. NICE Guidelines. Head injury: triage, assessment, investigation and early management of head injury in infants, children and adults. HMSO 2003. http://www.nice.org.uk.

8. The Neuroanaesthesia Society of Great Britain and Ireland and the Association of Anaesthetists of Great Britain and Ireland. *Recommendations for the safe transfer of patients with brain injury*. London: NASGBI and AAGBI, 2006.

9. Farling P, Smith M. Transfer of brain injured patients – time for a change? *Anaesthesia* 2006; **61**: 1–2.

10. Seeley HM, Hutchinson P, Maimaris C *et al.* A decade of change in regional head injury care: a retrospective review. *Br J Neurosurg* 2006; **20**(1): 9–21.

11. Elf K, Nilsson P, Enblad P. Outcome after traumatic brain injury improved by an organized secondary insult program and standardized neurointensive care. *Crit Care Med* 2002; **30**(9): 2129–34.

12. Clayton TJ, Nelson RJ, Manara AR. Reduction in mortality from severe head injury following introduction of a protocol for intensive care management. *Br J Anaesth* 2004; **93**(6): 761–7.

13. Patel HC, Menon DK, Tebbs S *et al.* Specialist neurocritical care and outcome from head injury. *Intens Care Med* 2002; **28**: 547–53.

14. Varelas PN, Conti MM, Spanaki MV *et al.* The impact of a neurointensivist-led team on a semiclosed neurosciences intensive care unit. *Crit Care Med* 2004; **32**(11): 2191–8.

15. Lind CR. Transfer of intubated patients with traumatic brain injury to Auckland City Hospital. *ANZ J Surg* 2005; **75**(10): 858–62.

16. Keaney J, Fitzpatrick MO, Beard D *et al.* A standardised neurosurgical referral letter for the interhospital transfer of head injured patients. *J Accid Emerg Med* 2000; **17**(4): 257–60.

17. Eljamel MS, Nixon T. The use of a computer-based image link system to assist interhospital referrals. *Br J Neurosurg* 1992; **6**(6): 559–62.

18. Lee T, Latham J, Kerr RS *et al.* Effect of a new computed tomographic image transfer system on management of referrals to a regional neurosurgical service. *Lancet* 1990; **336**(8707): 101–3.

19. Hawnaur J. Recent advances: Diagnostic Radiology *Br Med J* 1999; **319**: 1168–71.

20. Ridley S, Carter R. The effects of secondary transport on critically ill patients. *Anaesthesia* 1989; **44**: 822–7.

21. Medical vehicles and their equipment – Road ambulances EN 1789:1999. http://www.cenorm.be.

22. Ligtenberg JJ, Arnold LG, Stienstra Y *et al.* Quality of interhospital transport of critically ill patients: a prospective audit. *Crit Care* 2005; **9**(4): 446–51.

23. Rohan D, Dwyer R, Costello J *et al.* Audit of Mobile Intensive Care Ambulance Service. *Irish Med J* 2006; **99**(3): 76–8.

24. Gentleman D, Jennett B. Hazards of interhospital transfer of comatose head-injured patients. *Lancet* 1981; **2**(8251): 853–4.

25. Dunn LT. Secondary insults during the interhospital transfer of head-injured patients: an audit of transfers in the Mersey Region. *Injury* 1997; **28**(7): 427–31.

26. Andrews PJD, Piper IR, Dearden NM. Secondary insults during intrahospital transport of head-injured patients. *Lancet* 1990; **335**: 327–30.

27. Mendelow AD, Karmi MZ, Paul KS *et al.* Extradural haematoma: effect of delayed treatment. *Br Med J* 1979; **1**(6173): 1240–2.

28. Seelig JM, Becker DP, Miller JD *et al.* Traumatic acute subdural hematoma: major mortality reduction in comatose patients treated within four hours. *N Engl J Med* 1981; **304**(25): 1511–18.

29. Henderson A, Coyne T, Wall D *et al.* A survey of interhospital transfer of head-injured patients with inadequately treated life-threatening extracranial injuries. *ANZ J Surg* 1992; **62**(10): 759–62.

30. Fitzpatrick MO, Seex K. Scalp lacerations demand careful attention before interhospital transfer of head injured patients. *J Accid Emerg Med* 1996; **13**(3): 207–8.

31. Young JS, Bassam D, Cephas GA *et al.* Interhospital versus direct scene transfer of major trauma patients in a rural trauma system. *Am Surg* 1998; **64**(1): 88–91.

32. Wright KD, Knowles CH, Coats TJ *et al.* 'Efficient' timely evacuation of intracranial haematoma – the effect of transport direct to a specialist centre. *Injury* 1996; **27**(10): 719–21.

33. Di Bartolomeo S, Sanson G, Nardi G *et al.* Effects of 2 patterns of prehospital care on the outcome of patients with severe head injury. *Arch Surg* 2001; **136**(11): 1293–300.

34. Bernard SA. Paramedic intubation of patients with severe head injury: a review of current Australian practice and recommendations for change. *Emerg Med Austr* 2006; **18**(3): 221–8.

35. Davis DP, Stern J, Sise MJ *et al.* A follow-up analysis of factors associated with head-injury mortality after paramedic rapid sequence intubation. *J Trauma-Injury Infect Crit Care* 2005; **59**(2): 486–90.

36. McKeating EG, Andrews PJ, Tocher JI *et al.* The intensive care of severe head injury: a survey of non-neurosurgical centres in the United Kingdom. *Br J Neurosurg* 1998; **12**(1): 7–14.

37. Havill JH, Sleigh J. Management and outcomes of patients with brain trauma in a tertiary referral trauma hospital without neurosurgeons on site. *Anaesth Intens Care* 1998; **26**(6): 642–7.

38. Allen G, Farling P, Mullan B. Designated consultants for the interhospital transfer of patients with brain injury. *J Intens Care Soc* 2006; **7**(2): 13–15.

39. Spencer C, Watkinson P, McCluskey A. Training and assessment of competency of trainees in the transfer of critically ill patients. *Anaesthesia* 2004; **59**: 1242–55.

40. Safe Transfer and Retrieval (STaR) Advanced Life Support Group. http://www.alsg.org.

41. Mark J. Transfer of the critically ill patient. *Anaesthesia News* July 2004; 2–4. ISSN 0959-2962.

# Chapter 10

# Principles of head injury intensive care management

Martin Smith

The intensive care management of traumatic brain injury (TBI) is complex and requires a coordinated and stepwise approach. The aim is to provide general intensive care support and interventions targeted to the injured brain. Cerebral ischaemia is the dominant factor determining secondary brain injury and recent studies characterizing its incidence and mechanisms have demonstrated that the ischaemic burden is correlated with outcome after TBI.[1] Prevention and treatment of cerebral ischaemia is the major goal of the intensive care management of TBI and is associated with improved outcome.[2]

## Monitoring

The monitoring of critically ill head-injured patients has become increasingly complex. Besides the close monitoring and assessment of cardiac and respiratory functions common to all critically ill patients, several techniques are now available for global and regional brain monitoring.[3,4] Cerebral monitors allow measurement of intracranial and cerebral perfusion pressures and estimation of cerebral blood flow, assessment of cerebral oxygenation and measurement of brain tissue biochemistry.[5-7] Although elevated intracranial pressure (ICP) correlates with higher risk of mortality and morbidity after TBI, not all patients with intracranial hypertension have poor outcome.[8] This is not surprising because monitoring of ICP and cerebral perfusion pressure (CPP) cannot confirm in an individual patient whether the CPP target is sufficient to meet the brain's metabolic demands at a particular moment in time. A recent study has demonstrated that brain resuscitation after TBI, based on control of ICP and CPP alone, does not prevent cerebral hypoxia in some patients.[9] Measurement of ICP and CPP in association with monitors of the *adequacy* of cerebral perfusion, such as cerebral oxygenation and brain tissue biochemistry, provide a more complete picture of the injured brain and its response to treatment.[3] There is preliminary evidence to suggest that therapy directed to maintain brain tissue oxygenation as well as ICP and CPP is associated with reduced mortality after severe TBI.[10] Multimodality intracranial monitoring is now widely employed during neurointensive care to provide early warning of impending brain ischaemia and guide targeted therapy in order to optimize cerebral perfusion and oxygenation (see Chapters 11 and 12).

## Treatment

Consensus guidance for the management of TBI has been available for many years and the most comprehensive, from the Brain Trauma Foundation, has recently been revised.[11-13] Due to the lack of class I data from randomized controlled trials, the majority of the recommendations are at level II or III based on data from small prospective or retrospective studies, observational studies or case series. Despite this, rigorous and continuous monitoring and management on the intensive care unit is associated with improved outcome after TBI.[14-16]

*Head Injury: A Multidisciplinary Approach*, ed. Peter C. Whitfield, Elfyn O. Thomas, Fiona Summers, Maggie Whyte and Peter J. Hutchinson. Published by Cambridge University Press. © Cambridge University Press 2009.

# General aspects of treatment

The intensive care management of severe TBI has undergone extensive revision as evidence accumulates that longstanding and established practices are not as efficacious or innocuous as previously believed.[17,18] Traditional therapies such as fluid restriction and hyperventilation have been called into question and are no longer recommended and newer therapies, such as therapeutic hypothermia, remain controversial. The sole goal of identifying and treating intracranial hypertension has been superseded by a focus on the prevention of secondary ischaemic insults by a multi-faceted neuroprotective strategy incorporating a systematic, stepwise approach to control of raised ICP and maintenance of adequate CPP and cerebral oxygen delivery.[14–16]

Secondary systemic physiological insults, particularly hypotension and hypoxaemia, have adverse effects on outcome, and their anticipation, prevention and treatment are key aspects of the intensive care management of TBI.[2,14,16] Mechanical ventilation is mandatory to ensure adequate oxygenation and normal arterial carbon dioxide tension.[16,19] Even short periods of hypotension are associated with adverse neurological outcome and should be meticulously avoided.[2,19,20] Euvolaemia is the primary cardiovascular goal and intravascular volume should initially be maintained with isotonic crystalloids and colloids to achieve a central venous pressure of 5–10 mmHg.[14,16] A vasoactive agent, such as dopamine or norepinephrine, should be added if adequate blood pressure is not achieved with fluid resuscitation. General intensive care principles should be applied in all cases and tight glycaemic control, aggressive management of pyrexia, early enteral nutrition and seizure management are of particular importance.[15,16] The best outcomes are achieved when care is provided by a multidisciplinary team whose collective goal is to minimize secondary brain injury. Meticulous management of mechanical ventilation and cardiovascular variables may be just as important in determining outcome as the intervention of a neurosurgeon! The details of the intensive care management of TBI are summarized in Table 10.1. and discussed in detail in Chapters 13 and 14.

# Neurosurgical intervention

In the acute phase, evacuation of an expanding haematoma is the primary goal of neuro-surgical treatment. Life-saving surgery should be available within 4 hours of injury and immediately during management on the intensive care unit. Delay in surgical treatment continues to be a major preventable cause of morbidity and mortality.[21] In severe TBI, when patients are unconscious or sedated as part of their treatment, clinical signs, such as pupil changes, may occur late when irreversible tissue damage or shift of brain substance may already have occurred. Despite the absence of class I evidence demonstrating the outcome benefit of ICP monitoring, there is a large body of clinical evidence supporting its use to detect intracranial mass lesions early as well as to guide therapeutic interventions.[5,22] In patients with severe TBI, ICP monitoring should therefore be established on admission to the intensive care unit at the latest. Neurosurgical techniques, such as external ventricular drainage or decompressive craniectomy, are increasingly being used to control intracranial hypertension refractory to medical therapy (see Chapter 17).

### Physiological neuroprotection

High ICP and low CPP may result in cerebral ischaemia and are associated with increased mortality and worse outcome in survivors.[23] Conventional approaches to the management of TBI have therefore concentrated on a reduction in ICP to prevent secondary ischaemic

**Table 10.1.** Summary of intensive care management of patients with severe head injury

| | |
|---|---|
| Ventilation | • $PaO_2$ >13 kPa & $PaCO_2$ 4.5–5.0 kPa |
| | • PEEP ($\leq$10 cm $H_2O$) to maintain oxygenation |
| | • Strategies to minimize risk of pneumonia |
| Cardiovascular | • MAP >90 mmHg |
| | • Normovolaemia |
| | • Dopamine or norepinephrine |
| ICP and CPP targets | • Maintain CPP 50–70 mmHg |
| | • ICP <20 mmHg |
| ICP and CPP management | • Sedation/analgesia |
| | • Volume expansion plus norepinephrine to maintain CPP |
| | • Osmotic therapy (mannitol or hypertonic saline) |
| Options for resistant intracranial hypertension | • Moderate hyperventilation |
| | • Moderate hypothermia |
| | • CSF drainage |
| | • Barbiturates |
| | • Decompressive craniectomy |
| Miscellaneous | • Normoglycaemia |
| | • Enteral nutrition |
| | • Thromboembolic prophylaxis |
| | • Seizure control |

injury. However, there has been a shift of emphasis from primary control of ICP to a multi-faceted approach of maintenance of CPP and brain protection following evidence in the 1990s that induced hypertension using fluid resuscitation and vasoactive agents to maintain CPP > 70 mmHg is associated with improved outcome.[24] Therapies to maintain high CPP, however, are controversial because of the high incidence of complications. In one study, there was a five-fold increase in the occurrence of acute lung injury (ALI) in a group of head injured patients managed with a CPP threshold of 70 mmHg vs. 50 mmHg.[25] In another, outcome was as good in patients treated with a modest CPP target (60 mmHg vs. 70 mmHg) and systemic complications occurred less frequently.[26]

An alternative approach utilises a lower CPP target of > 50 mmHg (the Lund concept) with volume-targeted therapy. This aims to minimize increases in intracapillary hydrostatic pressure and intracerebral water content thereby avoiding secondary rises in ICP.[27] Whilst the Lund concept is not universally accepted, recent evidence indicates that excessive CPP is associated with a lower likelihood of favourable outcome after TBI.[23]

The Brain Trauma Foundation now recommends that the CPP target after severe TBI should lie between 50–70 mmHg and that aggressive attempts to maintain CPP > 70 mmHg should be avoided because of the risk of ALI.[28] It is also now clear that a CPP threshold exists on an individual basis in a time dependent manner and that optimal CPP should be defined for each patient individually and frequently.[29]

# Systemic complications

Systemic complications are common after TBI and are independent contributors to morbidity and mortality.[30] They represent risk factors that are potentially amenable to treatment and early recognition and prompt intervention may improve outcome.[31] Respiratory complications are most frequent, occurring in up to 80% of patients, with those sustaining the severest injury being most at risk.[30] Ventilator acquired pneumonia is a particular problem and occurs in 45%–60% of patients.[30,32] The intensive care management of head injury-associated non-neurological organ dysfunction and failure presents a significant challenge because optimum treatment for the failing systemic organ system may have potentially adverse effects on the injured brain and vice versa.[31] These challenges are discussed in Chapter 14.

### Protocol-driven treatment

Many studies have shown that protocol-driven strategies for head injury management are effective in reducing mortality and improving outcome.[33–36] These usually incorporate stepwise introduction of higher intensity treatment, moving from one step to the next if ICP and CPP targets remain unachieved.[16,33] Patel et al. demonstrated, in head injured patients with raised ICP in the absence of intracranial mass lesions, that the establishment of an evidence-based management protocol resulted in a significant reduction in mortality (from 59.6% to 40.4%), with a high proportion of favourable outcome in survivors, compared to historic controls.[35] In a similar study that included all categories of severe head injury admitted to the ICU, Elf et al. described a standardised treatment protocol and compared recent mortality rates to two previous periods – one before the availability of a neurointensive care unit and the other after the establishment of a basic neurointensive care unit without protocolized treatment strategies.[34] Each time period showed a decrease in mortality from 40% to 27% to 2.8%, in association with an increase in the incidence of good functional outcome in survivors from 40% to 68% to 84%. The striking improvements noted in these studies suggest that high quality intensive care, with the delivery of targeted therapeutic interventions, impacts not only on survival but also on the *quality* of survival after head injury.

The majority of studies examining the introduction of protocolized management strategies for head injury have used historic control groups and it is therefore impossible to be certain that other factors have not contributed to the demonstrated outcome benefits. Clayton et al. attempted to deal with this issue in a study in which the introduction of an evidence-based management protocol resulted in a reduction in ICU mortality from around 20% to 13.5% and in hospital mortality from 24.5% to 20.8% in patients with severe head injury.[33] This occurred despite an increase in the median age and APACHE II score of the patient population after implementation of the protocol. Although historic controls were used in this study, the ICU in which the patients were managed also admitted patients with other disease processes. The ICU mortality for those without head injury did not change significantly over the same period, strongly suggesting that the benefits to the head-injured patients derived from the introduction of the protocol-driven management paradigm.

### Specialized neurointensive care vs. general intensive care

There is also evidence that the management of head injured patients in a specialised neurointensive care unit might bring additional outcome benefits compared to management in a general ICU.[37–39] The reasons for this are likely to be multifactorial and the potential outcome benefits have recently been reviewed.[36]

Neurointensive care teams, incorporating a dedicated neurointensivist, reduce hospital mortality and length of stay and are associated with fewer significant medical complications in critically ill brain injured patients.[40–42] In a large prospective study of 42 ICUs, Diringer *et al.* investigated outcome of patients with intracerebral haemorrhage admitted to a general ICU compared to those admitted to a specialized neurointensive care unit.[43] Being admitted to a specialized unit was associated with decreased hospital mortality but, in contrast to other studies, also with increased length of stay. The benefits of specialized neurointensive care units are likely to occur because neurointensivists and their teams focus on the interplay between the brain and other systems and integrate all aspects of neurological and medical management into a single care plan.[39] Members of a neurointensive care team are familiar with the unique aspects of the disease processes and the effects of interventions in head injured patients. For example, blood pressure control is more aggressive in neurointensive care units compared to general ICUs, resulting in a lower incidence of systemic, often iatrogenic, hypotension.[44] Furthermore, other physiological derangements, such as fever, hyperglycaemia and sodium disturbances, are likely to be managed more aggressively in a neurointensive care unit compared to a general ICU.[37] Acute rehabilitation is also important in securing improved long-term neurological outcomes after TBI and intervention from neurophysiotherapists is likely to occur earlier and more reliably in a specialist unit than in a general ICU.

In summary, the provision of a dedicated cohort of medical, nursing and other healthcare professionals, supervision of care by a dedicated neurointensivist and involvement of senior neurosurgeons with rapid access to surgical intervention, is likely to have a positive impact on patient management and outcome.[37,38,43]

## Variations in practice

Despite available evidence and guidance, there are considerable variations in the implementation of established intensive care management and monitoring strategies between head injury centres.[45]

In 1996 only 50% of neurosurgical centres in the UK routinely monitored ICP in comatose head-injured patients and ICP monitoring was never used in 8% of centres.[46] By 2001, 75% of UK centres were monitoring ICP in the majority of patients with severe head injury and it seems likely that this change was driven by awareness and implementation of published guidelines.[45] In a study from the USA, ICP monitors were placed in only 58% of patients who fulfilled established criteria for monitoring, and therapies to reduce raised ICP were routinely applied in patients with no monitoring.[47] Although ICP monitoring was almost universal in a Canadian study of severe TBI, only 20% of neurosurgeons believed that outcome was affected by ICP monitoring.[48]

Bulger *et al.* examined variations in care on outcome in patients with severe head injury and found that centres that aggressively monitor, and therefore presumably manage, ICP have better outcomes.[47] The unanswered question is whether aggressive ICP monitoring and management *per se* improve outcome or whether they are simply a proxy marker for units that provide higher standards of overall care and an integrated approach to management. Whatever the reason, adherence to a protocol for head injury management based on the Brain Trauma Foundation guidance is associated with reduced mortality and significantly improved functional outcome in survivors.[49] Invasive monitoring and management of systemic and cerebral variables results in increased resource usage, but the improvements in outcome are likely to justify the increased cost of the treatment episode.[50]

There is also evidence to suggest that aggressive and targeted intensive care after head injury might result in increased levels of therapy intensity without improving outcome. A UK study demonstrated only weak evidence of an association between intensive head injury monitoring and management and outcome compared to supportive intensive care management strategies.[51] Cremer *et al.* recently investigated the effect of ICP and CPP targeted therapy on outcome and therapy intensity in 333 patients with severe TBI.[52] Patients managed in two head injury centres were compared. In centre A, ICP was not monitored but supportive intensive care was provided to maintain MAP > 90 mmHg, with other therapeutic interventions directed by clinical observations and CT findings. In centre B, ICP was monitored and treatment provided to maintain ICP < 20 mmHg and CPP > 70 mmHg. Intensity of treatment, measured by use of sedatives, vasoactive drugs, mannitol and barbiturates, was greater in centre B and the median time on mechanical ventilation was also greater in centre B (12 days vs. 5 days, $P < 0.001$). Hospital mortality was similar between the two centres (34% vs. 33%, $P = 0.87$) and the odds ratio for a more favourable outcome following ICP and CPP-targeted therapy was 0.95 (95% confidence interval, 0.62–1.44).

These conflicting data suggest that a prospective, randomized, controlled trial of the intensive care management of severe TBI, including ICP and CPP-targeted therapy, is more necessary than ever. Furthermore, the recent evidence suggesting that targeting brain tissue oxygenation in addition to ICP and CPP might bring additional outcome benefits suggests that any trial should be extended to include treatment targeted to all aspects of multimodal monitoring.[10] However, the practical and ethical issues of such a study are considerable.

## Summary

The intensive care management of head injury is complex and requires a coordinated and stepwise approach, including clinical assessment, imaging, monitoring and optimization of ICP and CPP. With improved understanding of the pathophysiology of the injured brain, new diagnostic, prognostic and treatment modalities will become available and these should be incorporated into established management strategies. The complex treatment modalities applied after TBI call for interdisciplinary collaboration between neurosurgeons, neuro-intensivists, specialist nurses and therapists. Specialized neuromonitoring and neuroimaging techniques must also be available and the neurointensive care unit serves as the focal point for these combined efforts.

## References

1. Coles JP, Fryer TD, Smielewski P *et al.* Defining ischemic burden after traumatic brain injury using 15O PET imaging of cerebral physiology. *J Cereb Blood Flow Metab* 2004; **24**: 191–201.

2. Chesnut RM, Marshall LF, Klauber MR *et al.* The role of secondary brain injury in determining outcome from severe head injury. *J Trauma* 1993; **34**: 216–22.

3. Tisdall MM, Smith M. Multimodal monitoring in traumatic brain injury: current status and future directions. *Br J Anaesth* 2007; **99**: 61–7.

4. Timofeev I, Gupta A. Monitoring of head injured patients. *Curr Opin Anaesthesiol* 2005; **18**: 477–83.

5. Steiner LA, Andrews PJ. Monitoring the injured brain: ICP and CBF. *Br J Anaesth* 2006; **97**: 26–38.

6. Nortje J, Gupta AK. The role of tissue oxygen monitoring in patients with acute brain injury. *Br J Anaesth* 2006; **97**: 95–106.

7. Tisdall MM, Smith M. Cerebral microdialysis: research technique or clinical tool. *Br J Anaesth* 2006; **97**: 18–25.

8. Resnick DK, Marion DW, Carlier P. Outcome analysis of patients with severe head injuries and prolonged intracranial hypertension. *J Trauma* 1997; **42**: 1108–11.

9. Stiefel MF, Udoetuk JD, Spiotta AM *et al*. Conventional neurocritical care and cerebral oxygenation after traumatic brain injury. *J Neurosurg* 2006; **105**: 568–75.

10. Stiefel MF, Spiotta A, Gracias VH *et al*. Reduced mortality rate in patients with severe traumatic brain injury treated with brain tissue oxygen monitoring. *J Neurosurg* 2005; **103**: 805–11.

11. Maas AI, Dearden M, Teasdale GM *et al*. EBIC-guidelines for management of severe head injury in adults. European Brain Injury Consortium. *Acta Neurochir (Wien)* 1997; **139**: 286–94.

12. Maas AI, Dearden M, Servadei F, Stocchetti N, Unterberg A. Current recommendations for neurotrauma. *Curr Opin Crit Care* 2000; **6**: 281–92.

13. The Brain Trauma Foundation. The American Association of Neurological Surgeons. The Joint Section on Neurotrauma and Critical Care. *J Neurotrauma* 2007; **24**: S1–S106.

14. Dutton RP, McCunn M. Traumatic brain injury. *Curr Opin Crit Care* 2003; **9**: 503–9.

15. Vincent JL, Berre J. Primer on medical management of severe brain injury.*Crit Care Med* 2005; **33**: 1392–9.

16. Helmy A, Vizcaychipi M, Gupta AK. Traumatic brain injury: intensive care management. *Br J Anaesth* 2007; **99**: 32–42.

17. Coles JP, Fryer TD, Coleman MR *et al*. Hyperventilation following head injury: effect on ischemic burden and cerebral oxidative metabolism. *Crit Care Med* 2007; **35**: 568–78.

18. Roberts I, Schierhout G, Alderson P. Absence of evidence for the effectiveness of five interventions routinely used in the intensive care management of severe head injury: a systematic review. *J Neurol Neurosurg Psychiatry* 1998; **65**: 729–33.

19. The Brain Trauma Foundation. The American Association of Neurological Surgeons. The Joint Section on Neurotrauma and Critical Care. Blood pressure and Oxygenation. *J Neurotrauma* 2007; **24**: S7–S13.

20. Chesnut RM. Avoidance of hypotension: *conditio sine qua non* of successful severe head-injury management. *J Trauma* 1997; **42**: S4–S9.

21. Leach P, Childs C, Evans J, Johnston N, Protheroe R, King A. Transfer times for patients with extradural and subdural haematomas to neurosurgery in Greater Manchester. *Br J Neurosurg* 2007; **21**: 11–15.

22. The Brain Trauma Foundation. The American Association of Neurological Surgeons. The Joint Section on Neurotrauma and Critical Care. Indications for intracranial pressure monitoring. *J Neurotrauma* 2007; **24**: S37–S44.

23. Balestreri M, Czosnyka M, Hutchinson P *et al*. Impact of intracranial pressure and cerebral perfusion pressure on severe disability and mortality after head injury. *Neurocrit Care* 2006; **4**: 8–13.

24. Rosner MJ, Rosner SD, Johnson AH. Cerebral perfusion pressure: management protocol and clinical results. *J Neurosurg* 1995; **83**: 949–62.

25. Robertson CS, Valadka AB, Hannay HJ *et al*. Prevention of secondary ischemic insults after severe head injury. *Crit Care Med* 1999; **27**: 2086–95.

26. Huang SJ, Hong WC, Han YY *et al*. Clinical outcome of severe head injury in different protocol-driven therapies. *J Clin Neurosci* 2007; **14**: 449–54.

27. Nordstrom CH. Physiological and biochemical principles underlying volume-targeted therapy – the "Lund concept". *Neurocrit Care* 2005; **2**: 83–95.

28. The Brain Trauma Foundation. The American Association of Neurological Surgeons. The Joint Section on Neurotrauma and Critical Care. Cerebral perfusion pressure thresholds. *J Neurotrauma* 2007; **24**: S59–64.

29. Vespa P. What is the optimal threshold for cerebral perfusion pressure following traumatic brain injury? *Neurosurg Focus* 2003; **15**: E4.

30. Zygun DA, Kortbeek JB, Fick GH, Laupland KB, Doig CJ. Non-neurologic organ dysfunction in severe traumatic brain injury. *Crit Care Med* 2005; **33**: 654–60.

31. Lim HB, Smith M. Systemic complications after head injury: a clinical review. *Anaesthesia* 2007; **62**: 474–82.

32. Zygun DA, Zuege DJ, Boiteau PJ et al. Ventilator-associated pneumonia in severe traumatic brain injury. *Neurocrit Care* 2006; **5**: 108–14.

33. Clayton TJ, Nelson RJ, Manara AR. Reduction in mortality from severe head injury following introduction of a protocol for intensive care management. *Br J Anaesth* 2004; **93**: 761–7.

34. Elf K, Nilsson P, Enblad P. Outcome after traumatic brain injury improved by an organized secondary insult program and standardized neurointensive care. *Crit Care Med* 2002; **30**: 2129–34.

35. Patel HC, Menon DK, Tebbs S, Hawker R, Hutchinson PJ, Kirkpatrick PJ. Specialist neurocritical care and outcome from head injury. *Intens Care Med* 2002; **28**: 547–53.

36. Suarez JI. Outcome in neurocritical care: advances in monitoring and treatment and effect of a specialized neurocritical care team. *Crit Care Med* 2006; **34**: S232–8.

37. Smith M. Neurocritical care: has it come of age? *Br J Anaesth* 2004; **93**: 753–5.

38. Menon D. Neurocritical care: turf label, organizational construct, or clinical asset? *Curr Opin Crit Care* 2004; **10**: 91–3.

39. Rincon F, Mayer SA. Neurocritical care: a distinct discipline? *Curr Opin Crit Care* 2007; **13**: 115–21.

40. Suarez JI, Zaidat OO, Suri MF et al. Length of stay and mortality in neurocritically ill patients: impact of a specialized neurocritical care team. *Crit Care Med* 2004; **32**: 2311–17.

41. Varelas PN, Conti MM, Spanaki MV et al. The impact of a neurointensivist-led team on a semiclosed neurosciences intensive care unit. *Crit Care Med* 2004; **32**: 2191–8.

42. Mirski MA, Chang CW, Cowan R. Impact of a neuroscience intensive care unit on neurosurgical patient outcomes and cost of care: evidence-based support for an intensivist-directed specialty ICU model of care. *J Neurosurg Anesthesiol* 2001; **13**: 83–92.

43. Diringer MN, Edwards DF. Admission to a neurologic/neurosurgical intensive care unit is associated with reduced mortality rate after intracerebral hemorrhage. *Crit Care Med* 2001; **29**: 635–40.

44. Qureshi AI, Bliwise DL, Bliwise NG, Akbar MS, Uzen G, Frankel MR. Rate of 24-hour blood pressure decline and mortality after spontaneous intracerebral hemorrhage: a retrospective analysis with a random effects regression model. *Crit Care Med* 1999; **27**: 480–5.

45. Wilkins IA, Menon DK, Matta BF. Management of comatose head-injured patients: are we getting any better? *Anaesthesia* 2001; **56**: 350–2.

46. Jeevaratnam DR, Menon DK. Survey of intensive care of severely head injured patients in the United Kingdom. *Br Med J* 1996; **312**: 944–7.

47. Bulger EM, Nathens AB, Rivara FP, Moore M, MacKenzie EJ, Jurkovich GJ. Management of severe head injury: institutional variations in care and effect on outcome. *Crit Care Med* 2002; **30**: 1870–6.

48. Sahjpaul R, Girotti M. Intracranial pressure monitoring in severe traumatic brain injury – results of a Canadian survey. *Can J Neurol Sci*. 2000; **27**: 143–7.

49. Fakhry SM, Trask AL, Waller MA, Watts DD. Management of brain-injured patients by an evidence-based medicine protocol improves outcomes and decreases hospital charges. *J Trauma* 2004; **56**: 492–9.

50. Palmer S, Bader MK, Qureshi A et al. The impact on outcomes in a community hospital setting of using the AANS traumatic brain injury guidelines. Americans Associations for Neurologic Surgeons. *J Trauma* 2001; **50**: 657–64.

51. Murray LS, Teasdale GM, Murray GD, Miller DJ, Pickard JD, Shaw MD. Head injuries in four British neurosurgical centres. *Br J Neurosurg* 1999; **13**: 564–9.

52. Cremer OL, van Dijk GW, van Wensen E et al. Effect of intracranial pressure monitoring and targeted intensive care on functional outcome after severe head injury. *Crit Care Med* 2005; **33**: 2207–13.

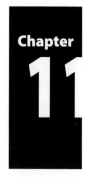

# Intracranial pressure monitoring in head injury

Ruwan Alwis Weerakkody, Marek Czosnyka, Rikin A. Trivedi and Peter J. Hutchinson

## Introduction

### Background

Intracranial pressure (ICP) has long been recognized as a vital variable able to affect cerebral function in the acute phase following head injury. Since the work of Lundberg, ICP has become a major part of brain monitoring in head injury and also in a number of other clinical scenarios.[1] As well as providing direct insight into the pathophysiology of the damaged brain, information and parameters derived from ICP and its waveform provide valuable information about impending trends and events as well as end-prognosis in brain-injured patients.

### Definitions and physiology

ICP can be interpreted as the environmental pressure acting within the cranial vault. Three main elements contribute to it: the brain parenchyma, blood and cerebrospinal fluid (CSF). These three elements are contained within a space of fixed volume that is enclosed by a relatively rigid and inextensible skull; they are themselves relatively incompressible. Any changes in volume in one of these elements, are compensated by the others, and lead to changes in ICP.

These describe the terms of the Monro–Kellie doctrine, which underlies the fundamental relationship between cerebral volume and ICP. In recent years its absolute doctrinal validity has been challenged in view of the fact that distension of the dural space within the lumbar canal allows limited changes in the net volume of the craniospinal system to take place. Nevertheless, the underlying concept generally holds true in describing the mechanism behind pathological changes in ICP.

## Importance of ICP monitoring in head injury

The physiological significance of raised ICP lies in its effect on cerebral blood flow (CBF). ICP acts as an additional opposing influence to the intrinsic driving force of arterial pressure and therefore has a direct impact on cerebral perfusion pressure (CPP=MAP-ICP). Maintaining cerebral perfusion pressure is important in order to maintain adequate and stable cerebral blood flow (Fig. 11.1).

Since both MAP and ICP can vary a great deal under normal conditions, mechanisms exist to maintain an adequate and stable cerebral blood flow by means of changing vascular resistance in response to cerebral perfusion pressure and local biochemical changes (autoregulation). Autoregulation acts over a limited range of CPP, with low CPP marking loss of autoregulatory reserve (Fig. 11.2). Therefore, maintaining CPP within its limits is vital to ensure stable cerebral blood flow. Following head injury, the limits of cerebral autoregulation may become narrowed, shifted up (along the axis of CPP) or may be impaired altogether.

*Head Injury: A Multidisciplinary Approach*, ed. Peter C. Whitfield, Elfyn O. Thomas, Fiona Summers, Maggie Whyte and Peter J. Hutchinson. Published by Cambridge University Press. © Cambridge University Press 2009.

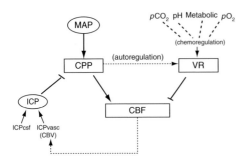

**Fig. 11.1.** Intracranial pressure and cerebral blood flow. MAP, mean arterial pressure; ICP, intracranial pressure (composed of distinct contributions from cerebrospinal fluid (ICPcsf) and the vascular compartment (ICPvasc)); CBV, cerebral blood volume; CPP, cerebral perfusion pressure; VR, cerebral vascular resistance; CBF, cerebral blood flow. '→' excitatory; '--|' inhibitory; ---> variable influences.

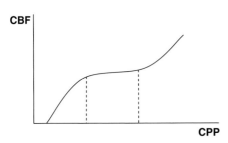

**Fig. 11.2.** Autoregulation of cerebral blood flow (CBF). Stable CBF is maintained over a limited range of cerebral perfusion pressure (CPP) [dotted lines].

Therefore, restoration of cerebral autoregulation as an important intrinsic mechanism preventing cerebral ischaemia or hyperaemia becomes an important target in various intensive care management protocols.

### Technology

A number of methods for measuring ICP exist. These employ one of two modalities: fluid-filled catheters or pressure micro-transducers, in various forms (Table 11.1). Sites for ICP measurement are shown in Fig. 11.3.

The 'gold standard' for measuring ICP is widely recognized as the intraventricular catheter connected to an external pressure transducer, (intraventricular pressure at the foramen of Monro where there is unobstructed flow to CSF is generally considered the reference point for ICP).[2,3] Such a system also allows CSF withdrawal in response to raised ICP. The practical limitations to intraventricular pressure measurements include infection and difficulty of insertion in advanced brain swelling. The risk of infection increases over time and is in the range of 6%–8% overall.[4,5]

Technological advances have allowed pressure microtransducers to evolve as reliable alternatives to the intraventricular system. These are based on strain-gauge pressure or fibre-optic sensors. The best of these are thought to be the intraparenchymal probes.[6] These have the advantage of very low infection rate and in vitro testing of modern probes has shown them to be accurate, with minimal zero-drift.[7] The main disadvantage of the latter lies with the caveat that intraparenchymal pressures may not reflect true ICP, in view of the considerable pressure gradients that can occur in the presence of focal lesions.[8] Since these probes cannot be re-zeroed after insertion, the added effect of zero drift also ought to be considered. Automatically re-zeroing devices are still in the process of development.[9]

Less invasive pressure transducers, such as subarachnoid, subdural and extradural devices, although increasingly accurate, are questionable in terms of providing true measures

**Table 11.1.** Intracranial pressure measurement – methods and their properties

|  | Advantages | Disadvantages |
|---|---|---|
| Intraventricular catheter | Measure of 'true' intracranial pressure<br>Treatment of raised ICP possible by drainage of CSF<br>Re-zeroing possible | Most invasive<br>High Infection risk<br>Can be difficult to insert |
| Intraparenchymal probe | Lower infection rate<br>Probably most accurate of the microtransducer devices | Only measures local pressure (not entirely accurate in presence of intracranial pressure gradients)<br>Zero-drift (cannot re-zero) |
| Subarachnoid probe | Lower infection rate<br>Less invasive | Limited accuracy<br>High failure rate |
| Epidural probe | Lower infection rate<br>Less invasive<br>Easy insertion | Limited accuracy |
| Lumbar CSF pressure | Usually simple procedure<br>Extracranial | Unreliable as indicator of ICP<br>Can be dangerous in presence of mass lesions |
| Non-invasive methods | Non-invasive; none of the above complications | Still in development (limited or insufficient precision) |

ICP, intracranial pressure; CSF, cerebrospinal fluid

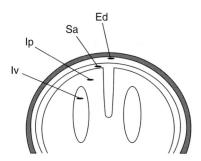

**Fig. 11.3.** Sites for ICP measurement. Iv, intraventricular; Ip, intraparenchymal; Sa, subarachnoid space; Ed, extradural.

of ICP.[3] Measurement of lumbar CSF pressure is not reliable in the context of head trauma and may be dangerous in the presence of intracranial mass lesions.[2,3]

Non-invasive methods of ICP measurement, which would eliminate the risk of haemorrhage that accompanies all current methods, are still in the process of research and development. Proposed methods include those based on transcranial ultrasonography or measurement of tympanic membrane displacement.[10,11]

## Process

When measuring ICP in the head-injured patient with intraparenchymal microsensors one ought to bear in mind that pressures may not be evenly distributed. In terms of obtaining the most reliable measures of ICP, averaging over at least 30 minutes with the patient lying still in the horizontal position is required. Ideally, continuous measures of pressure and pulse amplitude with description of pressure dynamics overnight, during natural sleep should be made.

### Normal values

Normal ICP is often quoted as being 'less than 15 mmHg', but in reality there is no universally attributable 'normal' value for ICP; it varies between and within individuals, depending on age, body posture and clinical condition. In the horizontal position, it is thought to be in the range of 7–15 mmHg in normal healthy adults,[12] in the vertical position it has been found to be slightly negative (but not lower than –15 mm Hg).[13]

Values for raised ICP also vary, depending on the clinical context. In head injury, pressures above 20 mmHg are considered abnormal, with aggressive treatment initiated above 25 mm Hg. In children, treatment thresholds for ICP are again different, varying with age.[14]

## Common patterns of ICP in head injury

ICP varies with time, taking the form of a wave. In acute states, continuous monitoring of ICP reveals a few patterns,[3] which may be classified as follows (Fig. 11.4):

1. Low and stable ICP (<20 mmHg), typically seen following uncomplicated head injury or in the early stages post trauma

2. High and stable ICP (>20 mmHg), the most common following head trauma

3. Vasogenic waves: Plateau 'A' waves (steep increases in ICP remaining at a high level for 5–20 minutes) and 'B' waves (oscillations at 0.5–2 Hz).

4. ICP waves related to changes in cerebral blood flow (transient hyperaemic events)

5. Refractory intracranial hypertension – refers to a large and rapid rise in ICP that is often fatal unless drastic aggressive measures such as decompressive craniectomy are instigated.

## Analysis of ICP waveform

The waveform obtained from continuous monitoring can itself be analysed in two main ways:

(a) Frequency analysis

(b) Derivations obtained from the wave

### Frequency analysis

The ICP waveform has been found to comprise three distinct components; that is, it can be thought of as a composite of overlapping waveforms of different periodicities or 'fundamental frequencies'. These waveforms, like any wave, can be isolated and analysed using spectral analysis, which displays the relative intensities of the different frequency components, contributing to the overall waveform (Fig. 11.5).[15] (Note that any wave can be thought of as a complex of a number of different pure sinusoidal waves of different frequencies, with the 'fundamental frequency' usually determining the overall periodicity of the wave.)

The periodicities of these components, termed pulse waves, respiratory waves and slow waves, have been found to correspond with the heart rate (at 50–180 bpm), the respiratory

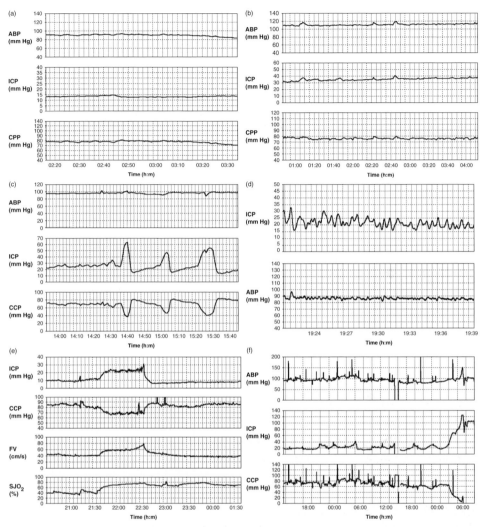

**Fig. 11.4.** ICP Patterns. (a) Low and stable ICP; (b) high and stable ICP; (c) plateau waves; (d) B waves (e) hyperaemia; (f) development of refractory intracranial hypertension

cycle (at 8–20 cycles per minute) and changes in the vascular bed (0.3–3 cycles per minute), respectively.[3,15]

## Pulse wave

The pulse waveform reflects the contribution of arterial pulsations to ICP. Spectral analysis of the pulse waveform reveals a fundamental frequency equal to the heart rate.[15] The amplitude of the fundamental component of the pulse wave can provide useful information about homeostatic mechanisms regulating cerebral blood flow.[15,16] An equivalent means of evaluating the pulse waveform is by time-domain analysis, where the averaged peak-to-peak amplitude of ICP caused by arterial pulsation during a single heartbeat is calculated.

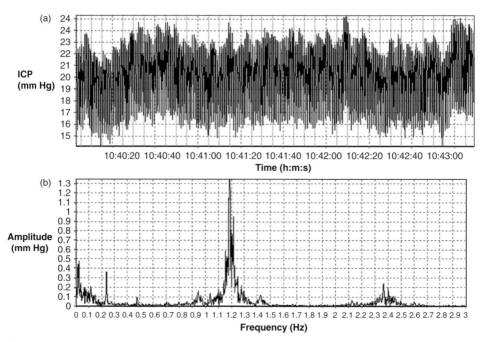

**Fig. 11.5.** Frequency components of ICP waveform. (a) ICP waveform in time; (b) spectral representation of ICP waveform. Reproduced from ref. 13 with permission.

Good correlation has been found between the amplitude of the fundamental component (derived by spectral analysis) and that of peak-to-peak amplitude (derived from time-domain analysis). The former has the advantage of being less influenced by noise from other frequency components, whereas, it may be affected by irregularities in heart rate [15]

The amplitude of the fundamental component (AMP) has been found to relate to a number of important physiological parameters. Firstly, there is a positive correlation of AMP with mean ICP. This relationship holds up to an upper 'breakpoint', corresponding to a state of maximal vasodilatation of the cerebral arterial bed (Fig. 11.6). This can hypothetically be said to delimit the upper limit of properly working vasodilation, occurring when CPP decreases. It can usually be observed beyond the lower limit of autoregulation of CBF. At lower pressures another breakpoint is observed, indicating transition between the flat and exponential part of the pressure volume curve, distinguishing between good and exhausted compensatory reserve, respectively (see below and Fig. 11.7).

Secondly, AMP correlates with the pulse amplitude of CBF velocity and the systemic arterial pulse wave (Fig. 11.8). Finally, AMP has, in itself, shown to relate to outcome (with the highest AMP seen in patients who died). However, this is likely to be related to the relationship between AMP and mean ICP, demonstrated by the fact that in head injury fatal outcome is strongly associated with greater average ICP (>20 mmHg).[17]

### Respiratory waves and slow waves

The respiratory waveform is related to the frequency of the respiratory cycle (8–20 cycles per minute). All those components showing periodicities between 0.3 and 3 minutes are

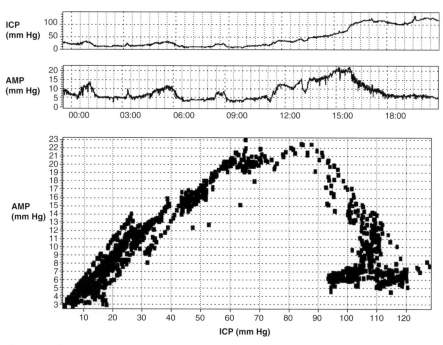

**Fig. 11.6.** The AMP pressure curve. Top panel: simultaneous tracings of AMP and ICP. Bottom panel: the linear relationship in the AMP pressure graph holds up to an upper breakpoint, corresponding to maximum vasodilation. AMP, amplitude of fundamental component (first harmonic) of ICP pulse wave. Reproduced from ref. 15 with permission.

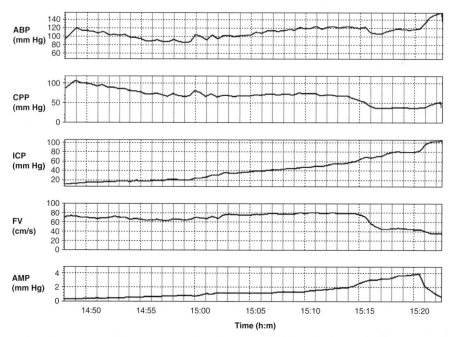

**Fig. 11.7.** Relationship between AMP and other variables. Simultaneous tracings over time. ABP, mean arterial blood pressure; CPP, cerebral perfusion pressure; ICP, intracranial pressure; FV, cerebral blood flow velocity; AMP, amplitude of fundamental component (first harmonic) of ICP pulse wave.

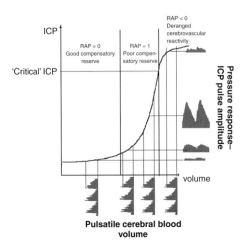

**Fig. 11.8.** RAP, pressure–volume curve and model of dependent changes in the response of ICP pulse-wave to pulsatile cerebral blood flow. The transformation of pulsatile changes in cerebral blood flow to changes in the ICP pulse-wave depends on the pressure–volume curve. The first, relatively flat part of the curve represents good compensatory reserve. The second steep part indicates an escalation in ICP secondary to vasodilatation (poor compensatory reserve). The terminal portion indicates exhaustion of compensatory reserve (collapse of arterial bed as ICP overcomes ABP, with a corresponding late increase in compliance). RAP, indicator of compensatory reserve. Reproduced from ref. 15 with permission.

classified as slow waves.[15] It is thought that the latter reflect changes in cerebral blood volume (CBV) that result from changes in vasomotor tone and have provided the substrate for calculation of other derived indices of autoregulatory reserve (see later).[18] Recent evidence has also demonstrated that a lower magnitude of slow waves correlates with unfavourable outcome in patients with intracranial hypertension.[19]

## Derivations
Certain secondary parameters can be used to derive more specific information about the state of intracranial homeostatic mechanisms.

### RAP index and compliance
Since the experiments of Lofgren *et al.* in the early 1970s the relationship between intra-cerebral volume (and more specifically CBV) and ICP has been well studied (Fig. 11.8).[20–25] This relationship is fundamental to cerebral perfusion. It directly reflects the limited compensatory reserve that exists before further vasodilatation gives rise to a rather dramatic increase in ICP to a level that threatens and eventually occludes cerebral blood flow.

The relationship between the pulse amplitude (AMP) and mean ICP can be considered a reflection of intracranial compensatory reserve. This is based on the principle, first investigated by Avezaat and Eijndhoven that the pulsatile component of cerebral blood volume associated with each heartbeat is accompanied by a variable increase in ICP pulse amplitude, depending on the degree of intracranial compliance.[21]

The RAP index (a correlation coefficient between AMP and mean ICP) is a useful indicator of this relationship. It is derived by calculating the linear correlation between consecutive time-averaged data points of AMP and ICP (40 samples, each over a 6–10 second time-averaging period are typically taken).[25] It directly reflects the relationship between mean ICP and corresponding intracranial compliance, such that a low RAP reflects the early relatively flat part of the pressure–volume curve, corresponding to the 'normal' physiological working range. A rising RAP (tending towards +1) reflects the exponentially rising part of the curve, corresponding to exponential transmission of changes in CBV to ICP, where

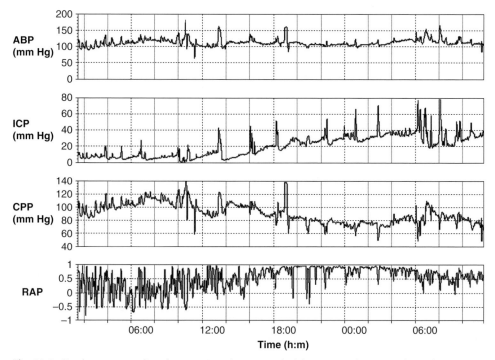

**Fig. 11.9.** Simultaneous recordings from a patient showing gradual deterioration from around 20:00 hours – note this is preceded by a tendency of RAP to increase towards 1. ABP, mean arterial blood pressure; CPP, cerebral perfusion pressure; RAP, indicator of compensatory reserve.

compensatory volume buffering is lost. Finally, the terminal portion of the curve (associated with collapse of the vascular bed where ICP critically overcomes MAP and further vasodilatation is impossible), is reflected by negative values of RAP (Fig. 11.9). Thus RAP tells us the position of a patient on the pressure-volume curve at any given time, allowing prediction of imminent decompensation.

Direct invasive methods of measuring intracranial compliance, which stemmed from earlier work looking into the volume pressure response have also shown promise.[29,30] An automated continuous assessment of intracranial compliance in the form of the Spiegelberg monitor is currently under evaluation for neuromonitoring in a number of scenarios, including head trauma.[27] These also aim to predict decompensation based on observed trends.

### PRx index

The Pressure Reactivity Index (PRx) looks at the slow waves of the ICP waveform, that is changes in cerebrovascular reactivity.[18] It is a correlation coefficient between ABP and ICP (again using around 40 time-averaged data points of each variable). PRx relates changes in arterial blood pressure to corresponding slow changes in ICP. In the normal state, fluctuations in arterial blood pressure (and hence cerebral perfusion pressure) are compensated by reactive changes in vasomotor tone, and therefore in vascular resistance. Thus, a reduction in perfusion pressure, for example, would induce relative vasodilatation, leading to an increase in CBV and hence in ICP (Fig. 11.10).

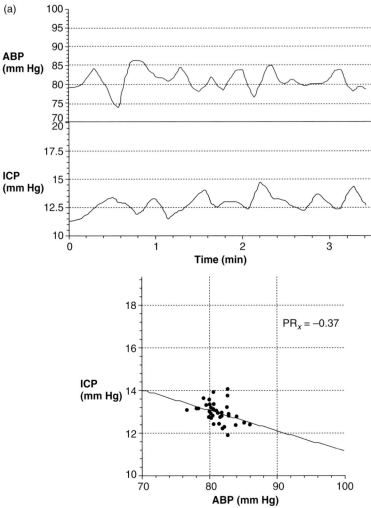

**Fig. 11.10.** ABP, ICP and PRx. Relationship between ABP and ICP in a normal individual (a): PRx = –0.37; and in a patient with deranged cerebrovascular reactivity (b): PRx = +0.42. ABP, mean arterial blood pressure; PRx, pressure reactivity index (gradient of ABP-ICP graph).

If cerebrovascular reactivity were functioning as normal in this way, one would expect a negative correlation between ABP and ICP (and therefore a negative PRx). Conversely, if the cerebrovascular bed were to be non-responsive, changes in arterial blood pressure would be passively transmitted to the ICP waveform (thus giving a positive correlation between ABP and ICP).

Cerebrovascular reactivity is a key component of cerebral autoregulation and, although the two are not the same, this index provides insight into the state of autoregulation and changes in it. Following decompressive craniectomy, there is a partial deterioration in PRx as a result of the influence of mechanical decompression, at which point its validity may be questionable.[28]

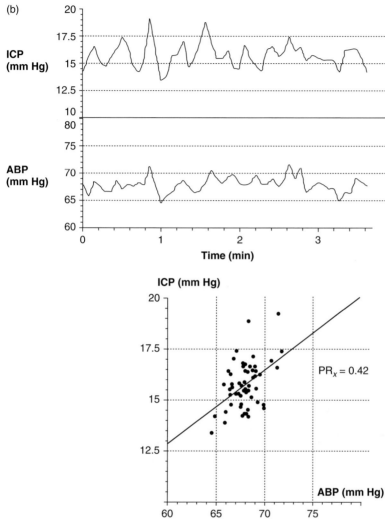

**Fig. 11.10.** (cont.)

## High-frequency centroid

Complementary to recent findings of high slow-wave content being predictive of favourable outcome, it has been found in the past that higher activity at the upper end of the frequency spectrum correlates with worse outcome and higher mortality.[19] This phenomenon, known as high frequency centroid (HFC), has been defined as the power-weighted average frequency within the 4- to 15-Hz band of the ICP spectrum.[15,24] HFC inversely correlates with ICP volume index (PVI). Indeed, there has been demonstration that a HFC value with an upper threshold of 9.0 Hz coincided with a reduction in the PVI to a critical level, indicating exhaustion of intracranial volume-buffering capacity. Mortality has also been shown to correlate with mean HFC, length of time HFC remained greater than the 'threshold' value of 9.0Hz and with more rapid rises in HFC.[24] These findings are consistent with current interpretations of the components of the ICP waveform.

ICP (mm Hg)

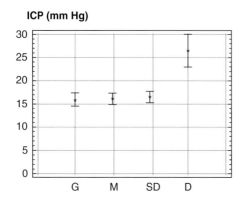

**Fig. 11.11.** ICP and outcome. Mean and 95% confidence intervals of ICP in different outcome groups. G, good outcome; M, moderate outcome; SD, severe disability; D, death. From ref. 17 with permission.

## Other avenues

In patients with hydrocephalus, the ratio of the gradient of the pulse wave during inspiration and expiration (I:E ratio) has been a useful differentiator between hydrocephalic and non-hydrocephalic patients, based on the effect of varying intracranial venous venting during the respiratory cycle on compliance and hence on the ICP waveform.[29] This measure, in effect, looks at the degree of venous volume buffering available and can conceivably be used as an indicator of a critical change in intracranial volume prior to the point at which ICP rises rather steeply with further increases in volume (Fig. 11.8). More specifically it has been predicted that values of I:E ratio approaching unity may be used as a herald of loss in intracranial volume buffering and hence imminent exhaustion of compliance.[29] This has yet to be formally tested in the context of head injury.

The concept of cerebrovascular pulse transmission (CVPT) has been studied by several groups as a means of assessing changes in the cerebrovascular bed.[26,30–32] This is done by direct comparison of the frequency spectrum of the ICP waveform with that of arterial blood pressure by means of a transfer function. More recent studies have aimed to classify these transfer functions as a means of predicting deterioration in intracranial compensatory mechanisms, although this is yet to be demonstrated clinically.[26,32]

# ICP-derived predictors of clinical outcome

One of the main objectives in brain monitoring and research is to develop a method of predicting imminent decompensation. Thus, all novel techniques developed for brain monitoring ought to be tested against this litmus of clinical application. So far, four of these measures have proved useful as predictors of clinical outcome: mean ICP, RAP, PRx and slow wave content.

Elevated mean ICP correlates with mortality rate following head injury. Remarkably, no difference in averaged ICP is seen between those with severe disability and favourable outcome (Fig. 11.11).[17] This has prompted the introduction of decompressive craniectomy as a life-saving procedure for patients with intracranial hypertension. Current evidence suggests that CPP on the other hand is not always predictive of outcome (except at very high values, where the incidence of favourable outcome decreases) and as a predictor of mortality carries less significance than ICP.[17] Thus it seems that CPP as an independent parameter, where CPP-orientated protocols are in place, would not be useful without also incorporating measures and trends in ICP.

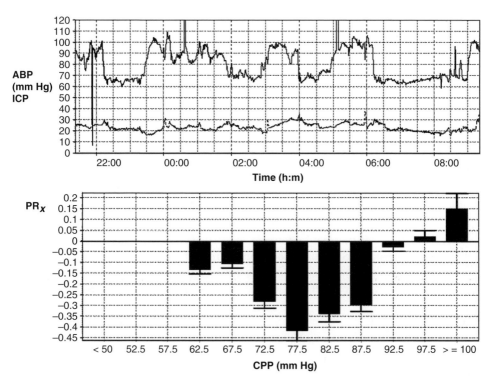

**Fig. 11.12.** Pressure reactivity, PRx and CPP. Studying CPP vs PRx, reveals a defined range of CPP over which PRx is optimal (lower panel).

RAP has been a useful tool in indicating the patient's position on the pressure–volume curve. Low average RAP has been shown to be associated with worse outcome when it is detected along with raised ICP.[25] More specific predictions have also been made using RAP; these include prediction of ICP response to hyperventilation (in a preliminary study[33]) and recovery of good compensatory reserve after decompressive craniectomy.[34] Furthermore, significant correlation between RAP and CBF (as assessed by positron emission tomography) and width of ventricles and contusion size in closed head injury have been observed.[15,35]

PRx as a measure of pressure-reactivity in the cerebrovascular bed has shown a number of useful clinical correlates. PRx has been shown to be predictive of outcome in head injury, independently of mean ICP, age or severity of injury.[36] It has been shown that PRx correlates with CBF (as predicted by PET and $CMRO_2$[37]); PRx has also been demonstrated as an indicator of loss of autoregulatory reserve in ICP-plateau waves and in refractory intracranial hypertension.[38]

Plotting PRx against CPP, reveals a U-shaped curve, suggesting a defined range of CPP over which PRx is optimal (Fig. 11.12). Based on early evidence that an optimum range of CPP does indeed exist (in terms of brain tissue oxygenation) it has been suggested that PRx might be used as an indicator of the optimum CPP, to guide CPP-orientated therapy.[15,19] Incidentally, PRx-based predictions have also found agreement with biochemical markers of deterioration as found by microdialysis-based studies.[15]

## Clinical usefulness of ICP monitoring

ICP monitoring has long become an established modality of brain monitoring, particularly in head injury. This is in view of its essential role in directing therapeutic interventions such as CPP-orientated protocols, osmotherapy and decompressive craniectomy.[34,39–41] Furthermore, it has been shown that ICP, along with CPP are useful as predictors of outcome in the brain injured.[17]

As well as trends in absolute values of ICP, it has been shown that parameters derived from the ICP waveform provide quite reliable insights into the state of intracranial homeostatic mechanisms, including autoregulatory reserve.[3,15] This allows prediction of developing events and would better inform clinical practice. These latter variables have also been shown to be predictive of outcome in head injury.

The natural conclusion is that the use of ICP-monitoring as a therapeutic guide is itself compatible with lower mortality and better outcomes in the head injured, and the bulk of recent evidence points to that fact.[42] However, the lack of class I evidence as proof and some studies refuting a benefit keeps this a moot point.[43] Indeed, monitoring ICP itself is unlikely to improve a patient's management; more crucial is what we do with this information and how we incorporate it into clinical practice in order to form effective management protocols.

## Acknowledgement

With thanks to Mick Cafferkey who helped produce the figures in this chapter.

## References

1. Lundberg N. Continuous recording and control of ventricular fluid pressure in neurosurgical practice. *Acta Psych Neurol Scand* 1960; **36**(Suppl 149): 1–193.

2. Steiner LA, Andrews PJD. Monitoring the injured brain: ICP and CBF. *Br J Anaesth* 2006; **97**(1): 26–38.

3. Czosnyka M, Pickard JD. Monitoring and interpretation of intracranial pressure. *J Neurol Neurosurg Psychiatry* 2004; **75**: 813–21.

4. Aucoin PJ, Kotilainen HR, Gantz NM, Davidson R, Kellogg P, Stone B. Intracranial pressure monitors. Epidemiologic study of risk factors and infections. *Am J Med* 1986; **80**: 369–76.

5. Mayhall CG, Archer NH, Lamb VA *et al.* Ventriculostomy related infections. A prospective epidemiologic study. *N Engl J Med* 1984; **310**: 553–9.

6. Citerio G, Andrews PJ. Intracranial pressure. Part two: clinical applications and technology. *Intens Care Med* 2004; **30**: 1882–5.

7. Citerio G, Piper I, Cormio M *et al.* Bench test assessment of the new Raumedic Neurovent-P ICP sensor: a technical report by the BrainIT group. *Acta Neurochir (Wien)* 2004; **146**: 1221–6.

8. Wolfla CE, Luerssen TG, Bowman RM *et al.* Brain tissue pressure gradients created by expanding frontal epidural mass lesion. *J Neurosurg* 1996; **84**: 642–7.

9. Chambers IR, Siddique MS, Banister K *et al.* Clinical comparison of the Spiegelberg parenchymal transducer and ventricular fluid pressure. *J Neurol Neurosurg Psychiatry* 2001; **71**: 383–5.

10. Schmidt B, Klingelhofer J, Schwarze JJ *et al.* Noninvasive prediction of intracranial pressure curves using transcranial Doppler ultrasonography and blood pressure curves. *Stroke* 1997; **28**: 2465–72.

11. Shimbles S, Dodd C, Banister K, Mendelow AD, Chambers IR. Clinical comparison of tympanic membrane displacement with invasive intracranial pressure measurements. *Physiol Meas* 2005; **26**: 1085–92.

12. Albeck MJ, Borgesen SE, Gjerris F *et al.* Intracranial pressure and cerebrospinal fluid outflow conductance in healthy subjects. *J Neurosurg* 1991; **74**: 597–600.

13. Chapman PH, Cosman ER, Arnold MA. The relationship between ventricular fluid pressure and body position in normal subjects and subjects with shunts: a telemetric study. *Neurosurgery* 1990; **26**: 181–9.

14. Mazzola CA, Adelson PD. Critical care management of head trauma in children. *Crit Care Med* 2002; **30**: S393–401.

15. Czosnyka M, Smielewski P, Timoveev I *et al.* Intracranial pressure: more than a number. *Neurosurg Focus* 2007; **22**(5): E10.

16. Avezaat CJ, van Eijndhoven JH, Wyper DJ. Cerebrospinal fluid pulse pressure and intracranial volume–pressure relationships. *J Neurol Neurosurg Psychiatry* 1979; **42**: 687–700.

17. Balestreri M, Czosnyka M, Hutchinson P *et al.* Impact of intracranial pressure and cerebral perfusion pressure on severe disability and mortality after head injury. *Neurocritical Care* 2006; **4**: 8–13.

18. Czosnyka M, Smielewski P, Kirkpatrick P, Laing RJ, Menon D, Pickard JD. Continuous assessment of the cerebral vasomotor reactivity in head injury. *Neurosurgery* 1997; **41**(1): 11–17.

19. Steiner LA, Czosnyka M, Piechnik SK *et al.* Continuous monitoring of cerebrovascular pressure reactivity allows determination of optimal cerebral perfusion pressure in patients with traumatic brain injury. *Crit Care Med* 2002; **30**: 733–8.

20. Lofgren J, von Essen C, Zwetnow NN. The pressure-volume curve of the cerebrospinal fluid space in dogs. *Acta Neurol Scand* 1973; **49**: 557–74.

21. Avezaat CJ, van Eijndhoven JH, Wyper DJ. Cerebrospinal fluid pulse pressure and intracranial volume–pressure relationships. *J Neurol Neurosurg Psychiatry* 1979; **42**: 687–700.

22. Shapiro K, Marmarou A, Shulman K. Characterization of clinical CSF dynamics and neural axis compliance using the pressure–volume index: I. The normal pressure-volume index. *Ann Neurol* 1980; **7**: 508–14.

23. Gray WJ, Rosner MJ. Pressure–volume index as a function of cerebral perfusion pressure. Part 2: the effects of low cerebral perfusion pressure and autoregulation. *J Neurosurg* 1987; **67**: 377–80.

24. Robertson CS, Narayan RK, Contant CF *et al.* Clinical experience with a continuous monitor of intracranial compliance. *J Neurosurg* 1989; **71**: 673–80.

25. Czosnyka M, Guazzo E, Whitehouse M *et al.* Significance of intracranial pressure waveform analysis after head injury. *Acta Neurochir (Wien)* 1996; **138**: 531–41.

26. Piper I, Miller JD, Dearden M, Leggate JRS, Robertson I. System analysis of cerebrovascular pressure transmission: an observational study in head injured patients. *J Neurosurg* 1990; **73**: 871–80.

27. Yau Y, Piper I, Contant C *et al.* Multi-centre assessment of the Spiegelberg compliance monitor: interim results. *Acta Neurochir* 2002; Suppl **81**: 167–70.

28. Wang EC, Ang BT, Wong J, Lim J, Ng I. Characterization of cerebrovascular reactivity after craniectomy for acute brain injury. *Br J Neurosurg* 2006; **20**: 24–30.

29. Foltz EL, Blanks JP, Yonemura K. CSF pulsatility in hydrocephalus: respiratory effect on pulse wave slope as an indicator of intracranial compliance. *Neurol Res* 1990; **12**(2): 67–74.

30. Portnoy HD, Chopp M, Branch C, Shannon MB. Cerebrospinal fluid pulse waveform as an indicator of cerebral autoregulation. *J Neurosurg* 1982; **56**(5): 666–78.

31. Takizawa H, Gabra-Sanders T, Miller JD. Changes in the cerebrospinal fluid pulse wave spectrum associated with raised intracranial pressure. *Neurosurgery* 1987; **20**(3): 355–61.

32. Lewis SB. Cerebrovascular pressure transmission analysis as a guide to the pathophysiology of raised intracranial pressure. *Clin Exp Pharmacol Physiol* 1998; **25**(11): 947–50.

33. Steiner LA, Balestreri M, Johnston AJ *et al.* Predicting the response of intracranial pressure to moderate hyperventilation. *Acta Neurochir (Wien)* 2005; **147**: 477–83.

34. Whitfield PC, Patel H, Hutchinson PJ *et al.* Bifrontal decompressive craniectomy in the management of posttraumatic intracranial hypertension. *Br J Neurosurg* 2001; **15**: 500–7.

35. Hiler M, Czosnyka M, Hutchinson P, *et al.* Predictive value of initial computerized tomography scan, intracranial pressure, and state of autoregulation in patients with traumatic brain injury. *J Neurosurg* 2006; **104**: 731–7.

36. Balestreri M, Czosnyka M, Steiner LA *et al.* Association between outcome, cerebral pressure reactivity and slow ICP waves following head injury. *Acta Neurochir* 2005; Suppl **95**: 25–8.

37. Steiner LA, Coles JP, Johnston AJ *et al.* Assessment of cerebrovascular autoregulation in head-injured patients. A validation study. *Stroke* 2003; **34**: 2404–9.

38. Balestreri M, Czosnyka M, Steiner LA *et al.* Intracranial hypertension: what additional information can be derived from ICP waveform after head injury? *Acta Neurochir (Wien)* 2004; **146**: 131–41.

39. Rosner MJ, Rosner SD, Johnson AH. Cerebral perfusion pressure: Management protocol and clinical results. *J Neurosurg* 1995; **83**: 949–62.

40. Patel HC, Menon DK, Tebbs S *et al.* Specialist neurocritical care and outcome from head injury. *Intens Care Med* 2002; **28**: 547–53.

41. Bullock R. Mannitol and other diuretics in severe neurotrauma. *New Horizons* 1995; **3**: 448–52.

42. Patel HC, Bouamra O, Woodford M, King AT, Yates DW, Lecky FE. Trauma Audit and Research Network. Trends in head injury outcome from 1989 to 2003 and the effect of neurosurgical care: an observational study. *Lancet* 2005; **366**: 1538–44.

43. Cremer OL, van Dijk GW, van Wensen E *et al.* Effect of intracranial pressure monitoring and targeted intensive care on functional outcome after severe head injury. *Crit Care Med* 2005; **33**(10): 2207–13.

# Chapter 12

# Multimodality monitoring in head injury

I. Timofeev, Adel Helmy, Egidio J. da Silva, Arun K. Gupta, Peter J. Kirkpatrick and Peter J. Hutchinson

## Introduction

The application of intracranial pressure (ICP) monitoring to patients with severe head injury in intensive care is recommended by both European and North American guidelines and is now well established. The ability to measure ICP as part of the escalating cycle of brain swelling, raised pressure, reduced cerebral blood flow, cerebral hypoxia, energy failure and further swelling forms the cornerstone of cerebral monitoring. In addition, there are several other techniques that can be applied to monitor the brains of patients following acute brain injury. These techniques include measurement of cerebral chemistry (microdialysis), cerebral oxygenation (jugular venous oxygenation, brain tissue oxygen, near infrared spectroscopy) and cerebral blood flow (extrapolated from cerebral blood velocity measurements from transcranial Doppler, laser Doppler and thermal diffusion). These techniques continue to undergo evaluation and have contributed to our understanding of the pathophysiology of acute brain injury. Current efforts are being made to determine their utility in terms of assisting in the management of patients on an individual basis (intention to treat). This chapter describes the principles of these techniques and their application following head injury.

## Cerebral metabolism

### Microdialysis

Microdialysis is a tool for sampling the brain extracellular fluid for a range of molecules including fundamental substrates and metabolites, cytokines and drugs. It enables monitoring of the chemical milieu within the brain providing information on the underlying physiological and pathological processes that follow neuronal injury. Initially envisaged as a research tool, it is gradually entering the clinical arena in a number of centres across the world. As well as head injury, microdialysis has also been used in other neurosurgical conditions such as monitoring of ischaemia during temporary clip placement in cerebral aneurysm surgery.

The intensive care management of traumatic brain injury focuses on the prevention of secondary injury. Traditionally, this has led to a focus on intracranial pressure monitoring and maintenance of cerebral perfusion pressure. The ideal cerebral perfusion pressure for an individual patient is still contentious, with the latest recommendations from the Brain Trauma Foundation recommending a range (50–70 mmHg) as opposed to an individual value. One potential application of microdialysis is to assist in establishing the optimal CPP for a given patient.

### Principles of microdialysis

The microdialysis catheter is a flexible plastic probe inserted into the brain parenchyma. It consists of two concentric tubes ending in a dialysis membrane at the tip. A physiological

*Head Injury: A Multidisciplinary Approach*, ed. Peter C. Whitfield, Elfyn O. Thomas, Fiona Summers, Maggie Whyte and Peter J. Hutchinson. Published by Cambridge University Press. © Cambridge University Press 2009.

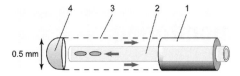

**Fig. 12.1.** Microdialysis catheter. The catheter consists of outer (1) and inner (2) concentric tubes with a semipermeable dialysis membrane at the distal end (3). A golden tip (4) facilitates visualization on CT. Perfusion fluid circulation via the catheter is indicated by arrows with extracellular molecules entering the perfusate by a process of diffusion across the dialysis membrane.

fluid (the 'perfusate') is pumped down one tube to the dialysis membrane which is exposed to the surrounding extracellular fluid. This fluid then travels back up the other tube where it is collected and termed the microdialysate (Fig. 12.1). Typical flow rates for this process are 0.3–2 μl/minute allowing time for molecules in the extracellular space to diffuse from the extracellular space into the fluid within the catheter. Thus, the constitution of the microdialysate reflects that of the extracellular space.

The molecules that are recovered by the microdialysis catheter are limited to those that can diffuse across the microdialysis membrane. The most important practical considerations are the molecular weight of the molecule of interest and its hydrophobicity. The efficiency of recovery of a molecule of interest by microdialysis is termed the 'relative recovery' for that molecule.[1] It is defined as the concentration of a molecule in the microdialysate divided by the concentration in the external solution multiplied by 100%. Relative recovery can be calculated *in vitro* or *in vivo* and can allow direct quantification of the concentration in the extracellular fluid from microdialysis data. As one would expect, small molecular weight hydrophilic molecules such as lactate and pyruvate have high relative recoveries of the order of 95%, while larger molecules such as cytokines have relative recoveries around only 40% with the same catheter.[2] Several other factors impact on relative recovery such as the size of the pores on the dialysis membrane and the flow rate of the perfusate. These variables can be manipulated to allow a range of molecules to be recovered at sufficient concentration for assay.

## Microdialysis markers of cerebral metabolism and injury

Cerebral metabolism is an intricate process involving numerous molecular intermediaries, many of which are shuttled between neurones and the surrounding glial matrix. The clinical application of microdialysis focuses on just a few key molecules in this complex process in order to determine the balance between aerobic and anaerobic metabolism (Fig. 12.2).

Cells metabolise glucose to pyruvate (a process termed glycolysis). During aerobic metabolism, pyruvate enters the tricarboxylic acid (TCA) cycle and is ultimately metabolized to carbon dioxide and water. Reducing equivalents produced by the TCA cycle generate ATP molecules from ADP via the electron transport chain on the mitochondrial membrane. However, if oxygen delivery becomes restricted and tissue hypoxia supervenes, the pyruvate molecules can no longer enter the TCA cycle. In this circumstance pyruvate is diverted down a separate anaerobic pathway to be metabolized to lactate. The absolute amount of lactate generated cannot be used as a marker of anaerobic metabolism as this also depends on how much glucose enters the metabolic pathway. In order to compensate for this dynamic variation, a ratio of recovered lactate to recovered pyruvate is used.[3]

Lactate and pyruvate are small molecules that can be readily taken up using microdialysis. The lactate : pyruvate ratio is commonly used as a marker of anaerobic metabolism in clinical studies.

(a)                                        (b)

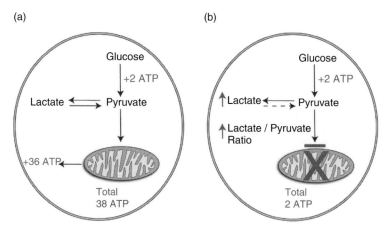

**Fig. 12.2.** Intracellular production of energy under aerobic and anaerobic conditions
(a)  Aerobic metabolism: glycolysis produces pyruvate which enters the TCA cycle. This requires adequate delivery of oxygen and normal mitochondrial function.
(b)  Anaerobic metabolism: ischaemia or hypoxia lead to reduced availability of tissue oxygen and/or impaired mitochondrial function. Pyruvate is therefore metabolised to lactate with an increase in the lactate/pyruvate ratio. Cellular damage will release glycerol from the cell membrane; this can also be measured using microdialysis.

Another commonly assayed molecule following TBI is glycerol. The cell membrane is largely made up of a bi-layer of phospholipids, which act as a hydrophobic barrier for the cell and suspend a range of membrane-bound signalling proteins. Following cellular death, the phospholipids within the membrane are enzymatically digested into their constituent components, fatty acid and glycerol. Thus glycerol levels are therefore thought to reflect cell death.[4]

Glucose, lactate, pyruvate and glycerol can all be monitored following head injury using portable real time analysers at the bedside.

## Microdialysis catheter placement

A key factor in basing clinical decisions on microdialysis-derived data is the exact positioning of the microdialysis catheter. The microdialysis catheter is a focal probe, which can only sample a small volume of brain tissue, limited by the diffusion distance of the molecules of interest.

The microdialysis catheter can be inserted through a bolt or through a burr hole. Alternatively, it can be placed into tissue at risk at the time of open surgery. The triple-lumen cranial access device (Fig. 12.3) enables the microdialysis catheter to be inserted in conjunction with a brain tissue oxygen sensor and ICP transducer.[5] In terms of catheter location, a consensus statement recommends that, for diffuse injury, the microdialysis catheter should be inserted into the non-dominant frontal cortex, and for focal injury, in peri-contusional/haematoma tissue with the option of a second catheter to monitor 'normal' brain as determined by CT scan.[6] It is essential to take account of the location of the catheter when interpreting the microdialysis data.

## Pathological thresholds and intensive care interventions

A number of observational studies in TBI have identified a pathological threshold for lactate/pyruvate ratio of >25. Lactate/pyruvate ratios above this threshold correlate with a worsening

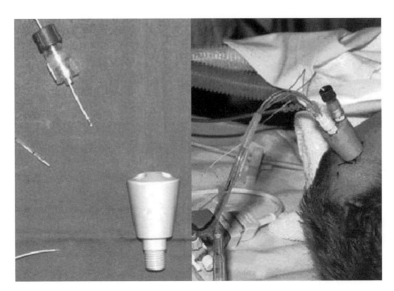

**Fig. 12.3.** Cranial access device. This screws into a twist drill hole and enables three different intraparenchymal probes to be placed in close proximity (e.g. ICP, $P_{bt}O_2$ and microdialysis).

outcome and increased mortality. Possible interventions under investigation to promote aerobic metabolism include hyperoxia and increasing cerebral perfusion pressure.

A glycerol level of >200 µmol/l has also been used as a pathological threshold, which reflects neuronal death. As this may reflect established damage, it may predict outcome but not add additional information to guide management.

## The future of microdialysis in TBI

As an increasing number of molecules are being recovered by microdialysis from the human brain after TBI, there are ever more innovative uses for this technique. For example, microdialysis can be used to determine pharmacokinetic data for centrally acting drugs including antibiotics. Endogenous molecules such as cytokines are also being increasingly investigated as potential biomarkers of injury severity.[6]

Microdialysis is a versatile technique that is being increasingly used in neuro-intensive care. It has the potential to become an important part of the monitoring armamentarium for the individualization of therapy following severe TBI.

## Cerebral oxygenation

A substantial body of experimental and clinical evidence supports the assumption that cerebral ischaemia and hypoxia can be responsible for a large proportion of primary and secondary brain injury following head trauma. These pathophysiological events are common, particularly early after an injury, and they are not easily detected by conventional imaging and physiological monitoring, including ICP measurement.[7]

While the routine assessment of general oxygenation and gas exchange using $PaO_2$ and oxygen saturation helps to detect global hypoxia, it does not provide accurate information about the state of cerebral oxygenation. This can be measured by three methods: jugular venous oximetry, brain tissue oxygen sensors and near infrared spectroscopy.

### Jugular venous oximetry

Jugular venous oximetry ($SjvO_2$) is performed by inserting a catheter into the internal jugular vein with its tip positioned in the jugular bulb. Placement in the right internal jugular vein is

**Table 12.1.** Causes of changes in global ($S_{jv}O_2$) and focal ($P_{bt}O_2$) brain tissue oxygenation.

| Change in monitoring parameter | | | |
|---|---|---|---|
| **Low $S_{jv}O_2$ or $P_{bt}O_2$** | | **High $S_{jv}O_2$ or $P_{bt}O_2$** | |
| Reduced delivery | Increased consumption | Increased delivery or by-pass | Decreased consumption |
| $\downarrow PaO_2$ | Seizures | High $FiO_2 \rightarrow \uparrow PaO_2$ | Deep sedation (e.g. barbiturates) |
| Anaemia | Fever | $\uparrow CBF$ | Hypothermia |
| Hypotension | Inadequate sedation or analgesia | Hypertension or impaired autoregulation with $\uparrow CPP$ | Hypometabolism, e.g. cerebral infarction, brain death |
| Vasospasm | Hypermetabolism | $\uparrow PaCO_2$ | |
| $\uparrow ICP / \downarrow CPP$ | | Arterio-venous shunt | |
| $\downarrow PaCO_2$ | | Impaired diffusion | |

In addition to the data in the table, probe misplacement or technical failure can cause artefactual measurements.

the most common site in clinical practice, as right cerebral venous outflow is believed to be dominant in most patients. However, such dominance is not universal and left-sided placement is also acceptable, although technically less easy to perform. Intermittent sampling of venous blood allows direct estimation of the partial pressure of oxygen in the blood leaving the brain ($P_{jv}O_2$). Modern fibreoptic jugular venous catheters allow continuous assessment of jugular venous saturation ($S_{jv}O_2$) following initial calibration without the need for frequent repeated sampling. Normal values for $S_{jv}O_2$ are in the range of 60%–75% and represent the balance between cerebral oxygen delivery and consumption. Substantial deviation from these levels may indicate technical issues, inadequacy of oxygen supply, an increased cerebral demand or a metabolically suppressed brain.

- Reduction in $SjvO_2$ values (desaturation) can be caused by reduced oxygen delivery or its increased cerebral consumption (Table 12.1). The common causes for the former are extracerebral hypoxaemia (decreased $PaO_2$, low haemoglobin and haematocrit), and inadequacy of cerebral blood flow (hypotension, vasospasm, elevated intracranial pressure, hypocapnia due to hyperventilation). Increased consumption can be due to an increase in cerebral metabolism (seizures, fever, inadequate analgesia and sedation, uncoupling between metabolism and cerebral blood flow).

- High values of $SjvO_2$ may represent excessive oxygen delivery or reduced consumption (Table 12.1). Excessive delivery is often linked to an increased fraction of inspired oxygen with high $PaO_2$ as part of treating a patient's cardio-respiratory insufficiency. However, it may also represent pathologically increased cerebral blood flow and impaired cerebral autoregulation, with more oxygen than required by cerebral metabolism passing via cerebral circulation. Impaired diffusion of oxygen into tissue due to oedema or other pathological barriers may also play a role. Decreased consumption is seen with deeper sedation (e.g. barbiturate coma), hypothermia, large cerebral infarcts and brain death.

Many of the above mentioned clinical situations can be established and corrected at the bedside, making jugular oximetry a useful monitoring modality to guide treatment of patients with head injury. The main current practical applications of jugular venous oximetry include assessing the adequacy of cerebral perfusion pressure target driven therapy and preventing excessive hypocapnia, during controlled therapeutic hyperventilation. In addition, combining jugular venous and arterial blood gas measurements allows calculation of the arterio-jugular difference for oxygen and lactate; parameters which have been linked to both severity of injury and neurological outcome after head injury.[8,9]

While complications related to the insertion and use of the $SjvO_2$ catheters are similar to central venous line placement and are relatively infrequent, the main limitations of this method are in its lack of sensitivity for focal or regional cerebral hypoxia. In addition, the commonly used threshold of SjvO2 <55%, below which significant global ischaemia was thought to occur, has been shown to underestimate the volume of brain which may be at risk.[10] Furthermore, fibreoptic catheters are subject to calibration drift and misplacement and may provide false values, unless due attention to their day-to-day running is paid.

## Brain tissue oxygenation

The direct, invasive measurement of the partial pressure of oxygen in the cerebral tissue $(P_{bt}O_2)$ requires direct placement of the sensor into cerebral tissue either via cranial access device or following craniotomy with tunnelling under skin. Most currently commercially available devices utilize a Clark electrode principle. The sensor consists of two electrodes and an outer polyethylene membrane, permeable to oxygen. Following insertion of the catheter, oxygen, driven by its partial pressure, diffuses from the tissue into the internal compartment of the sensor. Oxygen is reduced at the internal cathode generating a voltage difference with the second reference electrode. This difference is proportional to the $P_{bt}O_2$. Some probes allow concomitant measurement of cerebral temperature and/or ICP.

Following insertion, the sensor provides continuous measurement of $P_{bt}O_2$ with recordings on the bedside monitor. While $S_{jv}O_2$ is a 'global' monitoring technique, brain tissue oximetry provides information only about several $mm^3$ of cerebral tissue. However, when placed in non-contused areas of brain, changes in $PbtO_2$ have been shown to reflect global changes in brain oxygen when compared with $SjvO_2$.[11] Most sensors can be easily identified on conventional cerebral CT scans (Fig. 12.4) and location of the probe and its relation to cerebral parenchymal or extra-axial lesions need to be recorded. In most cases it can be assumed that a sensor located in radiologically 'normal' brain, with predominantly diffuse injury, provides values which correlate well with regional and global oxygenation values measured by other monitoring and imaging modalities and can therefore be used as an equivalent of 'global' monitoring technique.[12] Although at present it is virtually impossible to accurately define an area of 'penumbra' around traumatic parenchymal lesions, sensors placed in the immediate vicinity of such lesions are more likely to provide very 'focal' information on oxygen levels, albeit from the most vulnerable tissue. There are pros and cons for targeting 'normal' and 'perilesional' brain tissue during the placement of the sensors. In certain cases there may be a need for more than one catheter. Interpretation of the $P_{bt}O_2$ values and their integration with other monitoring modalities for optimization of the therapy need to be based on clear acknowledgement of probe position and sampled tissue.

The interpretation of reduced $P_{bt}O_2$ values follows a pattern very similar to $S_{jv}O_2$ with reduction representing reduced delivery or increased consumption. Currently recommended clinical thresholds are, by and large, based on observational evidence and assume 'safe' cerebral oxygenation levels above 20–25 mmHg, with levels below 10 mmHg considered pathological by most authors. Theoretically higher than 'normal' values of $PbtO_2$ can also occur due to reasons similar to high $SjvO_2$; however, much less is known about their practical

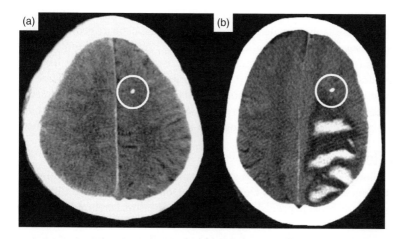

**Fig. 12.4.** Sensor locations on CT. (a) Diffusely injured brain. (b) Pericontusional tissue.

significance. Current clinical uses of $P_{bt}O_2$ include detection of cerebral ischaemia, optimization of CPP and protecting from deleterious effects of hyperventilation.

Invasiveness of brain tissue oxygen sensors limits their widespread use, although the level of haemorrhagic and infectious complications is very low. Focal artefacts (microhaematomas during insertion, proximity to a large vessel, local inflammatory response, etc.) and probe displacement during prolonged use may also affect accuracy of recordings.

Further prospective evidence that invasive monitoring of cerebral oxygenation and 'oxygen-driven' therapy can influence outcome after traumatic brain injury is required to support wider use of these monitoring modalities. At present, they provide a useful adjunct to the multimodality monitoring and provide unique information for better individualization of patients' therapy.

## Near infrared spectroscopy

Near infrared spectroscopy (NIRS) is a non-invasive method of estimating regional cerebral oxygenation, in the areas of the brain targeted by scalp optode placement. Each optode is known to illuminate a volume of about $10 \, cm^3$ of cerebral tissue. Light from the NIR portion of the spectrum (700–1000 nm) is both scattered and absorbed by its transition through tissue, bone and skin. The partial absorption of the NIR light results in a change in the intensity (concentration of the light beam). A modified version of the Beer–Lambert Law that is used to describe optical attenuation is used to quantify the change of concentration of near infrared light as it passes through various compounds. The readings are also dependent on the consistency of the tissues being monitored. In brain injury, the tissue geometry does not stay consistent and hence can render the continuous trace unreliable due to the changes in swelling of the underlying brain tissue.

The absorption of NIR light is proportional to the tissue concentration of certain chromophores, i.e. copper in cytochrome aa3 and iron in haemoglobin. Cytochrome aa3, deoxygenated and oxygenated haemoglobin have different absorption spectra. In the NIR range there is only one isobestic point at 805 nm. This is the point at which both deoxygenated and oxygenated haemoglobin have exactly the same light absorption ability. Above 805 nm, oxyhaemoglobin provides more effective absorption and below 805 nm, deoxygenated haemoglobin has a higher light absorption. It must be remembered that this part of the graph is only a small segment of the graph of molar extinction coefficient against wavelength (ranging from 200 nm–1000 nm). Transmission spectroscopy is a form of transiluminescence of the skull and is possible in neonates. Unfortunately, as the neonate grows and the skull thickness and soft tissue increase in size and amount, this method becomes increasingly less possible. NIRS measurements in older children and adults use the principle of reflectance spectroscopy. The optodes are placed 4–7 cm apart on the same side of the forehead. They are kept away from the midline and the temporalis muscles and are directed at a relatively acute angle to each other. The normal range for readings is 60%–80% where 47% is considered the ischaemic threshold, whereby deoxygenated haemoglobin has a major impact on reflectance.

# Cerebral blood flow

Cerebral blood flow following trauma is an important parameter that is frequently inferred by a variety of methods such as transcranial Doppler, laser Doppler and thermal diffusion. TCD is a non-invasive simple bedside procedure that does not measure cerebral blood flow directly but provides calculated data based on the velocity of blood in large arteries. It is operator dependent, and requires training and experience to perform and interpret results. Quantitative methods of measuring cerebral blood flow were described as early as 1945.[13] Several imaging or tracer-based methods have been developed, allowing accurate estimation of global or regional cerebral blood flow. These techniques are technically challenging and can only provide intermittent assessment.

## Transcranial Doppler (TCD)

TCD requires ultrasound to penetrate thin bone without being excessively damped. Measurements are based upon the Doppler shift of the ultrasound waveform by moving red blood cells. There are three main windows of access:

1. Transtemporal: found above the zygomatic arch. There are four different locations of the temporal window (frontal, anterior, middle and posterior).

2. Transorbital

3. Transforaminal (foramen magnum)

Accurate identification of the arteries is helped by: spatial orientation of the signal to other intracranial signals (including information on the depth and angle of the probe), direction of blood flow (away or towards the transducer) and the signal response to compression or vibration manoeuvres.

The main landmark for orientation is the branching of the supraclinoid internal carotid artery into the anterior cerebral artery and middle cerebral artery. TCD sonography measures the flow velocity in cerebral arteries, which changes with the phases of the cardiac cycle. The Doppler signals are used to derive systolic, average mean flow and end-diastolic flow velocities. The mean carries the highest physiological significance as it correlates with perfusion better than the peak and trough values. Once the flow velocity is known, the CBF can be calculated, provided the angle and area of insonation are measured:

*Cerebral blood flow = mean flow velocity × area of insonated vessel*
*× cosine angle of insonation*

TCD measurements are comparable to xenon computed tomography and PET cerebral blood flow measurements.[14,15] There are several clinical applications of TCD,[16,17] but it is mostly used to evaluate and manage patients with suspected vasospasm following subarachnoid haemorrhage using the Lindegaard index and mean flow velocity.[18] Although it can provide indirect information on cerebral blood flow and state of autoregulation after head injury, technical difficulties of continuous reliable TCD monitoring limit its practical applications in patients with TBI.

# Laser Doppler and thermal diffusion techniques

The search for continuous methods of CBF monitoring led to development of invasive parenchymal sensors, which currently utilize two different principles to measure focal blood flow.

## Laser Doppler flowmetry

Laser Doppler flowmetry, like TCD, is based on the Doppler principle, but uses monochromatic laser light instead of an ultrasound wave. Light that is scattered by the moving red blood cells undergoes a frequency shift. Conversely, static tissue does not change the light frequency, but leads to randomization of light directions, impinging on red blood cells. Hence, red blood cells receive light from numerous random directions. Since the frequency shift is dependent not only on the velocity of the red blood cells but also on the angle between the wave vectors of the incident and the scattered light, scattering of the light in tissue broadens the Doppler-shift power spectrum. From this spectrum the average velocity of red blood cells, the volume of red blood cells and the local cerebral blood flow can be determined based on a theory of light scattering in tissue in relative units.[19,20] Laser Doppler does not allow direct measurement of CBF in conventional units (ml/100 g per min) but provides a qualitative assessment of CBF expressed in arbitrary units. Current laser Doppler probes are small enough to be directly implanted into brain parenchyma during a craniotomy or bolt device (via burr hole) and can be used to continuously monitor focal cerebral blood flow. Recent studies conclude that laser Doppler perfusion monitoring has the potential to be used as an intracerebral guidance tool.[21]

The second category of continuous CBF measurement devices employs the principles of thermodilution or thermal diffusion.

## Thermodilution or thermal diffusion

The former requires placement of a specialized catheter into a blood vessel in the circulatory territory of interest. The cold indicator (cold normal saline) is then injected upstream and the sequential change in blood temperature downstream is evaluated by a thermistor in the distal catheter tip, allowing calculation of regional blood flow. Jugular vein thermodilution can be used to evaluate global cerebral CBF; however, this technique has not found widespread use in the monitoring of patients with head injury, possibly due to the prevalence of jugular bulb oximetry and TCD.

More recently, the similar principle of **thermal diffusion** has been employed to monitor focal cortical blood flow.[22] Brain tissue has the ability to dissipate heat, which is in turn directly related to local cerebral blood flow. Thermal diffusion intraparenchymal sensors contain two thermistors.[23] The proximal one is kept at physiological temperature and the distal one is heated. The heat dissipation in the tissue between thermistors reflects local blood flow and the latter can be estimated quantitatively in conventional units (ml/100 g per min). This method is advantageous by its ability to provide near continuous measurements (4/min) within the immediate vicinity of measurement.[24] The intraparenchymal probes provide continuous quantitative data that are comparable with results obtained by xenon-CT for a volume of approximately 5 cm$^3$ around the probe tip.[23]

Although numerous animal studies exist, the translation of laser Doppler flowmetry and thermal diffusion technology to human studies is still required to provide clinical validation and better evaluation of the utility of these devices. CBF probes are also subject to the same limitations as other intracerebral devices (microdialysis, brain tissue oximetry). These, in particular, provide very focal measures, which need to be interpreted carefully and in the context of the presenting clinical situation. The major drawback is the potential need for multiple probes to monitor multiple areas of perfusion simultaneously. Nevertheless, these devices may find a niche in multimodality monitoring by providing additional useful information for optimizing and individualizing therapy of a patient with traumatic brain injury.

## Conclusion

The application of multimodality monitoring to patients with head injury enables the continuous measurement of fundamental parameters such as intracranial pressure, cerebral oxygenation and cerebral metabolism. These techniques, from a research perspective, are increasing our understanding of the pathophysiology of acute brain injury. Current efforts are directed at refining the methodology and determining their clinical utility to assist in the management of individual patients on intensive care.

## References

1. Ungerstedt U. Microdialysis – principles and applications for studies in animals and man. *J Intern Med* 1991; **230**(4): 365–73.

2. Hutchinson PJ, O'Connell MT, Nortje J *et al.* Cerebral microdialysis methodology – evaluation of 20 kDa and 100 kDa catheters. *Physiol Meas* 2005; **26**(4): 423–8.

3. Persson L, Valtysson J, Enblad P *et al.* Neurochemical monitoring using intracerebral microdialysis in patients with subarachnoid hemorrhage. *J Neurosurg* 1996; **84**(4): 606–16.

4. Hillered L, Valtysson J, Enblad P, Persson L. Interstitial glycerol as a marker for membrane phospholipid degradation in the acutely injured human brain. *J Neurol Neurosurg Psychiatry* 1998; **64**(4): 486–91.

5. Hutchinson PJ, Hutchinson DB, Barr RH, Burgess F, Kirkpatrick PJ, Pickard JD. A new cranial access device for cerebral monitoring. *Br J Neurosurg* 2000; **14**(1): 46–8.

6. Winter CD, Ianotti F, Pringle A, Trikkas C, Clough GF, Church MK. A microdialysis method for the recovery of IL-1beta, IL-6 and nerve growth factor from human brain in vivo. *J Neurosci Methods* 2002; **119**(1): 45–50.

7. Coles JP, Fryer TD, Smielewski P *et al.* Incidence and mechanisms of cerebral ischemia in early clinical head injury. *J Cereb Blood Flow Metab* 2004; **24**(2): 202–11.

8. Stocchetti N, Canavesi K, Magnoni S *et al.* Arterio-jugular difference of oxygen content and outcome after head injury. *Anesth Analg* 2004; **99**(1): 230–4.

9. Artru F, Dailler F, Burel E *et al.* Assessment of jugular blood oxygen and lactate indices for detection of cerebral ischemia and prognosis. *J Neurosurg Anesthesiol* 2004; **16**(3): 226–31.

10. Coles, JP, Regional ischemia after head injury. *Curr Opin Crit Care* 2004; **10**(2): 120–5.

11. Gupta AK, Hutchinson PJ *et al.* Measurement of brain tissue oxygenation compared with jugular venous oxygen saturation for monitoring cerebral oxygenation after traumatic brain injury: *Anesth Analg* 1999; **88**(3): 549–53.

12. Gupta AK, Hutchinson PJ, Fryer T *et al.* Measurement of brain tissue oxygenation performed using positron emission tomography scanning to validate a novel monitoring method. *J Neurosurg* 2002; **96**(2): 263–8.

13. Kety SS, Schmidt CF. The determination of cerebral blood flow in man by the use of nitrous oxide in low concentrations. *Am J Physiol* 1945; **143**: 53–66.

14. Steiner LA, Coles JP, Johnston AJ *et al.* Predicting the response of intracranial

pressure to moderate hyperventilation. *Acta Neurochir (Wien)* 2005; **147**: 477–83

15. Brauer P, Kochs E, Werner C *et al.* Correlation of transcranial Doppler sonography mean flow velocity with cerebral blood flow in patients with intracranial pathology. *J Neurosurg Anesthesiol* 1998; **10**: 80–5.

16. Sloan MA, Alexandrov AV, Tegeler CH *et al.* Assessment: transcranial Doppler ultrasonography: report of the Therapeutics and Technology Assessment Subcommittee of the American Academy of Neurology. *Neurology* 2004; **62**(9): 1468–81.

17. Alexandrov AV, Joseph M. Transcranial Doppler: an overview of its clinical applications. *Internet J Emerg Intens Care Med* 2000; **4**(1).

18. Lindegaard KF, Nornes H, Bakke SJ, Sorteberg W, Nakstad P. Cerebral vasospasm after subarachnoid haemorrhage investigated by means of transcranial Doppler ultrasound. *Acta Neurochir Suppl (Wien)* 1988; **42**: 81–4.

19. Bonner RF, Nossal R. *Principles of laser-Doppler flowmetry.* In: Shepherd AP, Oberg P, eds. *Laser-Doppler Blood Flowmetry.* Boston, Kluwer Academic Publishers; 1990: 17–46.

20. Riva CE, Cranstoun SD, Grunwald JE, Petrig BL. Choroidal blood flow in the foveal region of the human ocular fundus. *Invest Ophthalmol Vis Sci* 1994; **35**: 4273–81.

21. Wårdell K, Blomstedt P, Richter J *et al.* Intracerebral microvascular measurements during deep brain stimulation implantation using laser Doppler perfusion monitoring. *Stereotact Funct Neurosurg* 2007; **85**(6): 279–86.

22. Steiner LA, Andrews PJ. Monitoring the injured brain: ICP and CBF. *Br J Anaesth* 2006; **97**(1): 26–38.

23. Vajkoczy P, Roth H, Horn P *et al.* Continuous monitoring of regional cerebral blood flow: experimental and clinical validation of a novel thermal diffusion microprobe. *J Neurosurg* 2000; **93**: 265–74.

24. Delhomme G, Newman WH, Roussel B *et al.* Thermal diffusion probe and instrument system for tissue blood flow measurements: validation in phantoms and in vivo organs. *IEEE Trans Biomed Eng* 1994; **41**(7): 656–62.

# Chapter 13

# Therapeutic options in neurocritical care: optimizing brain physiology

Rowan Burnstein and Joseph Carter

Although the major determinant of outcome from traumatic brain injury (TBI) is the severity of the primary injury, a plethora of factors that can occur in the post-injury phase have also been independently demonstrated to contribute to 'secondary brain injury', thereby worsening morbidity and mortality. These include intracranial hypertension, systemic hypotension, hypoxaemia, hyperpyrexia, hypocapnoea, hyper- and hypoglycaemia. Many of these factors are amenable to clinical manipulation. The exact mechanisms leading to 'secondary brain injury' are not yet fully elucidated, but exacerbation of cerebral ischaemia is thought to be central. The integrated management of these factors forms the basis for specialist neurocritical care.

## Protocol-driven therapy

The development of clinical protocols based on both laboratory and clinical data has underpinned the success of neurocritical care in the management of severe TBI. There is now good evidence that such protocol-based treatments lead to improved outcomes after TBI. The evidence for the superiority of any one protocol over other regimes remains controversial.[1–3] Further improvement in outcomes may also be associated with treatment within a specialist neurocritical care unit.[4]

Most protocols developed for the critical care management of TBI incorporate both surgical and non-surgical components. All rely on the provision of good basic intensive care. They are essentially divided into two 'schools'. Those, such as the Rosner and Addenbrooke's protocol, hold maintenance of cerebral perfusion pressure (CPP) as central to the management of TBI.[2,5] Such CPP-driven protocols also recognize that intracranial pressure (ICP) is an independent predictor of outcome after TBI, and incorporate pathological thresholds for ICP.[6–9] Alternately, the 'Lund protocol' focuses on brain volume regulation, differing from CPP-orientated protocols in the details of ICP and arterial pressure management.[10,11] In recent years the distinction between such approaches has become increasingly blurred. Improvements in monitoring and imaging of brain tissue and their interpretation are likely to lead to further refinement of protocols and the development of a more individualized approach to TBI management.

## CPP-based therapy

Cerebral ischaemia is the single most important secondary factor to influence outcome after severe TBI and this is the basis from which CPP-driven protocols, such as the Addenbrooke's protocol (Fig. 13.1) have developed.[12,13] Cerebral perfusion pressure is defined as the difference between mean arterial pressure (MAP) and ICP. Low CPP (<60 mmHg) has been

*Head Injury: A Multidisciplinary Approach*, ed. Peter C. Whitfield, Elfyn O. Thomas, Fiona Summers, Maggie Whyte and Peter J. Hutchinson. Published by Cambridge University Press. © Cambridge University Press 2009.

## Addenbrooke's NCCU: ICP/CPP management algorithm

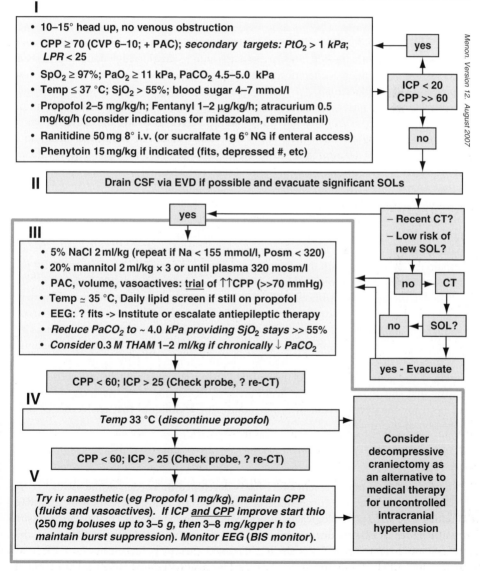

**Fig. 13.1.** Management algorithm for the management of raised intracranial pressure in patients with severe traumatic brain injury used in the Neurocritical Care Unit at Addenbrooke's Hospital, Cambridge. (Reproduced with permission of Professor DK Menon.)

associated with a poor outcome after TBI.[14–16] Rosner et al. first demonstrated, in a retrospective study, an improvement in outcome after TBI with maintenance of CPP > 70mmHg.[4] The first and second Brain Trauma Foundation (BTF) guidelines, published in 1996 and 2000 respectively, adopted a CPP of 70 mmHg as a target for management after severe TBI. This was subsequently revised to 60 mmHg in 2003 and the third edition suggests a general threshold in the realm of 60 mmHg but qualifies this with a statement that the CPP target requires individualization and lies within the range of 50–70 mmHg.[17–19]

CPP maintenance is initially focused on ensuring an appropriate MAP. Hypotension is avoided at all costs, and haemodynamic stability is desirable. In the first instance intravascular volume should be maintained by targeting a central venous pressure of 5–10 mmHg with isotonic crystalloids and colloids.[20] If an adequate MAP cannot be achieved, vasopressors should be instituted. There is some evidence that the response to noradrenaline may be less variable than to dopamine in terms of tissue oxygenation.[21] Adrenal insufficiency is not uncommon after severe TBI and in patients with escalating/high ionotrope and/or vasopressor requirements consideration should be given, following a short synacthen test, to empirical steroid replacement.[22]

The ideal target for post-traumatic CPP has long been a source of contention. Definition of the lower limit in terms of ischaemic threshold has been elusive and the degree to which CPP augmentation might be beneficial is not well established. The ischaemic threshold is likely to be between 50–60 mmHg.[19] However, the situation is not simple. The significant metabolic heterogeneity within the injured brain may render some areas ischaemic at a CPP value that appears to be globally sufficient.[23–26] In addition, if vascular autoregulation is impaired, increasing CPP will result in increased cerebral blood volume and hence ICP. Furthermore, the increased hydrostatic pressure across the capillary bed may exacerbate vasogenic oedema particularly in regions with poor autoregulation. Howells et al. reported that patients appeared to have worse outcomes using a CPP-based protocol if autoregulation was impaired.[27] In keeping with this, Steiner et al. reported favourable outcomes if CPP was tailored to the level at which cerebral autoregulation was intact in individual patients.[28]

CPP-based therapy is not without its hazards; in particular it has been associated with an increased risk of cardiorespiratory complications as discussed in Chapter 14.[29,30] The current BTF guidelines make a level II recommendation that aggressive attempts to maintain a CPP > 70 mmHg with fluid and vasopressors should be avoided because of the risk of developing acute respiratory distress syndrome (ARDS). The recommended CPP target range of 50–70 mmHg, with a general threshold in the realm of 60 mmHg, does not take into account data suggesting that this may lead to significant areas of ischaemia.[19,25,26] As such, there is an urgent need for the development of brain monitoring techniques that enable better individualization of therapy for TBI.

## Lund therapy

The 'Lund concept' of management of TBI was developed in Sweden in the 1990s.[10,31] As with CPP-based therapy, the cornerstone of Lund therapy is the prevention of secondary brain injury. The pathophysiological basis is a reduction in the capillary hydrostatic pressure and maintenance of plasma oncotic pressure to support brain volume regulatory mechanisms, primarily targeting ICP (hence 'ICP-targeted therapy'). In contrast to CPP-based therapy, proponents of Lund therapy accept lower levels of CPP (down to 50–60 mmHg).[11,24] Lund therapy is a treatment package which targets an ICP <20 mmHg utilizing a variety of surgical and non-surgical treatments.[32] Surgical options include early evacuation of mass lesions but, in contrast to CPP-based therapy, drainage of cerebrospinal fluid (CSF) is generally avoided. A decompressive craniectomy may be performed after failed medical therapy to attempt reduction of ICP. The non-surgical element of Lund therapy includes maintenance of normocapnoea, normal $PaO_2$ and normothermia. Euvolaemia is mandatory and red cell and albumin transfusions are used to normalize haemoglobin (12–14 g/dl) and plasma oncotic pressure. The overall aim is for a negative fluid balance. Effective sedation and stress reduction is achieved by a combination of sedatives, α-2 agonists and β-1 blockade. Sedation is achieved with propofol, midazolam and thiopentone either alone or in combination; the latter is used in 'low doses' of 2–3 mg/kg to avoid barbiturate side effects. ICP is controlled by optimizing plasma oncotic pressure and by blood pressure control using antihypertensive and catecholamine controlling agents (α-2 agonists, e.g. clonidine, dexmedetomidine; β-1 blockade, e.g. metoprolol and angiotensin II antagonists). Prostacyclin may also be used to improve the microcirculation in pericontusional areas.[33] Sustained ICP rises may also be treated with dihydroergotamine which is a last option before craniectomy.[11]

Outcome studies for Lund therapy have indicated favourable results.[10,34–36] The incidence of cardiorespiratory complications appears to be lower than that seen with CPP-targeted therapy.

## Which therapy?
In recent years the distinction between the different approaches to the management of severe TBI has become increasingly blurred. Data suggest that, if pressure autoregulation is intact, CPP-driven therapy may be associated with a better outcome but that ICP-based therapy is associated with better outcomes where autoregulation is lost.[27] However, a significant 'cost' of CPP driven therapy appears to be a higher incidence of cardiorespiratory complications. It is likely in the years to come that improvements in monitoring and imaging will lead to further protocol refinement and the development of a more individualized approach to TBI management.

## Sedation, analgesia and muscle relaxants
Adequate sedation and analgesia are one of the cornerstones of post-traumatic ICP control. Inadequate analgesia and sedation are associated with waves of elevated ICP, partly related to an increased cerebral metabolic rate for oxygen ($CMRO_2$). Furthermore, a number of the sedative drugs have additional benefits in terms of seizure reduction/control. Muscle relaxants are important to optimize ventilation in patients with severe TBI, as well as to minimize coughing and straining, which may be associated with increased ICP.

No single agent has all the desirable characteristics needed for sedation and analgesia in patients with severe TBI. The ideal agent would have a rapid onset and recovery, allowing assessment of neurological status, be easily titrated to achieve the desired level of sedation, reduce ICP, cerebral blood flow (CBF) and $CMRO_2$ whilst maintaining flow-metabolism coupling, cerebral autoregulation and normal cerebral vascular reactivity to $PaCO_2$. Minimal adverse cardiovascular effects and predictable clearance independent of end organ function are favoured qualities.[37]

The most common agents used for sedation in severe TBI are propofol or the short-acting benzodiazepine, midazolam. Both drugs cause dose-dependent reductions in $CMRO_2$ and CBF, whilst flow-metabolism coupling remains intact.[38] Midazolam is usually administered as an infusion and is effective as a sedative and an anticonvulsant. Accumulation of the drug can be a problem after infusions of greater than 24 hours' duration.[39,40] Midazolam has little effect on haemodynamics in euvolaemic patients. Propofol has a relatively rapid onset and short duration of action, which allows rapid assessment of neurological status. It is administered by continuous infusion and can be given for long periods with little change in its pharmacokinetic profile.[37] It has no active metabolites. The duration of action is dependent on the redistribution of propofol into the peripheral tissues – emergence is slightly prolonged after infusions of more than 12 hours. There is less certainty relating to seizure control with propofol, mainly because changes in cerebral concentrations at induction or emergence from sedation may induce seizure-like phenomena.[41] However, propofol infusions are regularly and successfully used in the management of status epilepticus. A number of problems have been associated with propofol, including precipitous cardiovascular collapse and propofol infusion syndrome.[42,43] Propofol is not recommended in hypothermic patients due to the risk of hyperlipidaemia.[44]

Adequate analgesia is provided with regular doses of acetaminophen and infusion of an opioid (e.g. morphine, fentanyl or remifentanil).[45] Opioids have minimal effects on cerebral haemodynamics in adequately resuscitated patients but a number of studies have suggested that some opioids can cause a mild increase in ICP.[46] Whilst morphine does not have any direct cerebrovascular effect, it is probably not the ideal agent for use in this setting due to its prolonged duration of action and its pro-convulsant metabolite normeperidine.[37] Fentanyl is a shorter-acting alternative, although with prolonged infusions it too can have a protracted effect due to accumulation in peripheral tissues. Remifentanil has appeal as an analgesic drug after TBI. It has an ultra-short duration of action with a context sensitive half life of less than 5 minutes due to rapid metabolism by plasma esterases. This avoids accumulation of the drug. Large feasibility studies for this drug are required in the neurocritical care setting.

Assessment of depth of sedation can be problematical in patients with severe TBI. Patients who have appropriate sedation and analgesia should not have waves of elevated ICP in response to stimulation such as endotracheal suctioning. More recently there has been interest in the use of bi-spectral index (BIS) monitoring for depth of sedation. Although there is some evidence that this processed EEG derived parameter can be useful, further study is required before it can be recommended as a standard of care.[47,48]

## Barbiturate coma

Many laboratory and clinical studies demonstrate a beneficial effect of barbiturates in lowering ICP in severe TBI. Despite this, the use of barbiturates in TBI remains controversial because of the lack of outcome data, concerns that barbiturates may reduce mortality but not morbidity and the incidence of serious side effects.[44,49] The BTF guidelines make a level II recommendation that high-dose barbiturates can be used to control ICP in patients who have refractory intracranial hypertension despite otherwise maximal therapy.[49]

High-dose barbiturates such as thiopentone can be administered as bolus doses of 250 mg up to 3–5 g until burst suppression is achieved, followed by an infusion of 3–8 mg/kg per h to maintain burst suppression with a goal of 3–5 bursts per minute (Addenbrooke's protocol). In the absence of EEG monitoring, CFAM or BIS monitoring can be used.[50] In some units serum levels are used to monitor infusion rates but the correlation between serum level, therapeutic benefit and systemic complications is poor.[49] Barbiturates have a long half-life due to their slow hepatic metabolism combined with high lipid solubility. Therefore, prolonged sedation is often seen after the cessation of barbiturate infusions and is particularly disadvantageous following TBI, since clinical assessment becomes difficult. Barbiturates have been used prophylactically, i.e. as first-line sedative agents.[51,52] However, no clinical benefit has been demonstrated and the BTF make a level II recommendation against this practice.[49]

Barbiturates lower ICP by a number of mechanisms, including reduced cerebral metabolism, altered cerebral vascular haemodynamics, reduced intracellular acidosis, inhibition of excitotoxicity and inhibition of free radical-mediated lipid peroxidation.[53–55]

Serious complications have been described with high dose barbiturate infusions. Hypotension is due to a combination of impaired venous return, inhibition of baroreflexes and myocardial depression.[56] A pronounced fall in serum potassium is common during barbiturate infusions, but significantly, this is not accompanied by increased urinary losses, and is likely to represent increased intracellular uptake of potassium. Sudden cardiovascular collapse and severe hyperkalaemia have been reported following cessation of barbiturate infusions.[57] Other complications of barbiturate therapy include immunosuppression and hepatic dysfunction. Renal dysfunction has been described but is difficult to explain and may be a function of other elements of patient care at the time.[58]

In summary, although barbiturates are effective at reducing ICP, their use is associated with a number of potentially serious side effects. Administration should be confined to the management of refractory intracranial hypertension, unresponsive to other therapies. The prophylactic administration of thiopentone is not recommended.

# Ventilatory support

To avoid hypoxaemia and intracranial hypertension secondary to hypercarbia, hyperventilation (using mechanical ventilation) was traditionally part of the acute management of patients with TBI.[20] However, the BTF guidelines make a level II recommendation that prophylactic hyperventilation should be avoided and a level III recommendation that hyperventilation be specifically avoided during the first 24 hours when CBF is often critically reduced.[59] Although a level III recommendation supports temporary hyperventilation to reduce ICP, this is now being challenged.[60]

Mechanical ventilation should be instituted early in the management of TBI. Normal values of arterial oxygen and carbon dioxide partial pressures ($PaO_2$ >11 kPa, $PaCO_2$ 4.5–5 kPa) should be aggressively maintained. Following adequate sedation, muscle relaxants should be used to achieve this, particularly in the early stages of TBI, to eliminate the work of breathing and ensure consistency of $PaCO_2$. However, the use of muscle relaxants reduces the ability to detect seizures, and their long-term use is associated with significant problems, including critical illness polyneuromyopathy. There is no evidence that positive end expiratory pressure (PEEP) is deleterious in TBI and this should be instituted as necessary.[61] $CO_2$ is a potent cerebral vasodilator; Figure 13.2 illustrates the relationship between CBF and $PaCO_2$ at normal MAP. Hypocapnoea results in cerebral vasoconstriction and a reduction in cerebral blood volume.[60,62] At normal arterial pressures, CBF decreases in a linear fashion between a $PaCO_2$ of 10 kPa and 2.5 kPa. The reduction in CBF and the concomitant reduction in cerebral blood volume is the most likely explanation for the potent reduction in ICP seen with hyperventilation, and the original basis for its use as part of TBI management. Provided $CMRO_2$ is preserved and the metabolic demand remains fixed, oxygen requirements can be met by increasing oxygen extraction as CBF is reduced. However, in the first 24 hours following TBI, CBF is often critically reduced and the institution of hyperventilation can compound cerebral ischaemia;[63] hence the BTF recommendation.[59]

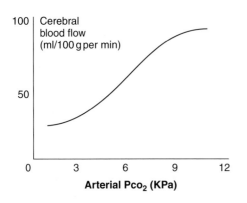

**Fig. 13.2.** The relationship between cerebral blood flow and arterial $PaCO_2$.

More contentious is the subsequent use of hyperventilation to control ICP. There are no trials evaluating the direct effect of hyperventilation on TBI patients' outcome. If hyperventilation is used, the BTF currently make a level III recommendation that jugular venous oximetry ($SjO_2$) or brain tissue oxygen tension ($PbtO_2$) measurements are used to monitor cerebral oxygen delivery.[59] Difficulties in defining clear evidence of critically ischaemic brain and the limitations of current modes of intracerebral monitoring remain a barrier. Thus, defining the ischaemic threshold in any individual is difficult. It is likely that the ischaemic threshold varies across the brain following TBI. A series of PET studies found no evidence of post-hyperventilation cerebral ischaemia or reduced $CMRO_2$, even in regions with low CBF.[64,65] However, more recent PET studies have demonstrated that the response to hyperventilation is heterogeneous and that levels of hypocapnoea deemed permissible within current guidelines may result in significant regional ischaemia, which is not detected by common bedside monitors for cerebral ischaemia, e.g. $SjvO_2$.[60,66,67]

The use of hyperbaric oxygen (HBO) in the management of severe TBI has also been proposed. Rockswold *et al.* demonstrated an improvement in survival, but no difference in functional recovery in patients receiving hyperbaric oxygen.[68] A subsequent study demonstrated a reduction in CSF lactate following HBO, suggesting that it may have an effect on cerebral flow–metabolism coupling in these patients.[69] However, HBO is not widely available and difficulties in the practical management of this therapy limit its mainstream use.

## THAM

CSF acidosis can cause irreversible damage to potentially viable brain cells in TBI patients. One suggested benefit of hyperventilation is considered to be the minimization of CSF acidosis. However, due to the loss of bicarbonate buffer the effect on CSF pH may not be sustained. Tromethamine (THAM) is a buffer which is more effective than bicarbonate at improving CSF pH. The only randomized controlled trial of the use of THAM in head injured patients failed to show a positive outcome benefit for its use but suggested that THAM is useful in preventing elevations in ICP.[70] Its effect in reducing ICP has been shown to be more prolonged than that following an infusion of mannitol.

## Hyperosmolar therapy

Osmotic diuretics have long been used to manage acute rises in ICP.

## Mannitol

Mannitol is currently the only osmotic diuretic used clinically in the management of severe TBI, although a number of others have been described, e.g. urea, glycerol.[71,72] The effectiveness of mannitol in the treatment of acutely raised ICP is considered to be well established without the need for randomized controlled trials.[73] In recent years, with the introduction of hypertonic saline for the management of raised ICP, the place of mannitol is being challenged. Controversy still exists over the mechanism of action of mannitol in reducing ICP. Its immediate effect is likely to arise from improved blood rheology due to a reduction in viscosity, and a plasma-expanding effect which increases cerebral blood flow and oxygen delivery.[74] Mannitol also creates an osmotic gradient across the intact blood–brain barrier, reducing cerebral oedema by drawing water into the vascular compartment.[75] An effect of mannitol on ICP is usually seen within 10–20 minutes of a bolus administration and lasts variably from 90 minutes to 6 hours. The effectiveness of repeated administration of mannitol is not established. It is contraindicated in patients whose serum osmolality is >320 mOsm/l in whom it is associated with an increased incidence of neurological and renal side effects.[76] Other side effects of mannitol include hypotension, intravascular volume depletion, profound diuresis, hyperkalaemia and rebound increase in ICP.[77,78]

Mannitol is most frequently prescribed as a single bolus dose of 0.25–1 g/kg body weight, administered often as a 20% solution. This is effective in reducing ICP provided that arterial hypotension is avoided.[79] Mannitol has been compared with thiopentone in a randomized controlled trial to control high ICP after TBI.[51] It was found to be superior in terms of improving ICP, CPP and mortality. High dose mannitol (1.4 g/kg body weight) in severe TBI has been demonstrated to be beneficial when given within 80–90 minutes of initial evaluation.[80] However, major concerns regarding the validity of this study exist such that further studies are required.[73] The BTF guidelines make a level III recommendation that the use of mannitol prior to the institution of ICP monitoring should be restricted to patients with signs of transtentorial herniation or deteriorating neurology not attributable to extracranial causes.[79] There is little evidence to support regular administration of mannitol over several days.

## Hypertonic saline

Interest in the use of hypertonic saline for the acute management of raised ICP after TBI, arose from studies for trauma resuscitation.[81–83] In recent years hypertonic saline has increasingly been used as an alternative to mannitol, although current evidence is not strong enough to make recommendations on the use, concentration or method of administration.[79] Hypertonic saline has been demonstrated to reduce ICP as effectively as mannitol in both the experimental and clinical settings.[84,85] Hypertonic saline has an osmotic effect with water extracted down an osmotic gradient from the brain parenchyma to the intravascular space, so reducing tissue pressure and cell size, and hence brain volume.[86] This is effectively demonstrated on serial CT imaging by a reduction in lateral displacement of the brain following hypertonic saline administration.[87] Mobilization of fluid into the vascular compartment helps maintain blood pressure and CPP. Effects of the vascular endothelium and erythrocytes are also of relevance. Vasodilatation and reduction in endothelial oedema may improve cerebral perfusion and reduce leukocyte adherence.[88,89] Reduction in erythrocyte volume also contributes to improved rheology.[88,90] Hypertonic saline may also induce reuptake of the glutamate which accumulates after neuronal damage.[91]

Hypertonic saline has been administered in a wide range of concentrations (1.7%–29.2%) and numerous regimes are described, making it difficult to draw conclusions about optimal doses, concentrations or treatment. It has a rapid onset of action. Battison *et al*. reported a greater reduction of ICP as compared to mannitol and a more prolonged duration of action.[84] Vialet *et al*. reported a reduction in the ICP spikes following an infusion of hypertonic saline as compared to mannitol.[92] Unlike mannitol, rebound intracranial hypertension is not a problem after repeated administration.[93,94] Hypertonic saline has also proven to be effective in the management of intracranial hypertension refractory to mannitol.[95]

Treatment with hypertonic saline is generally well tolerated. In contrast to mannitol, it is effective as a volume expander without the problems of hyperkalaemia and impaired renal function. There is a risk of central pontine myelinolysis when hypertonic saline is administered to patients with pre-existing hyponatraemia, and this must be excluded prior to administration.[96] Hypertonic saline administration also carries a risk of inducing or aggravating pulmonary oedema in patients with underlying cardiac or pulmonary dysfunction.[87]

# Control of temperature

Homeostasis normally maintains the human body at a temperature of 36.5–37.5 °C. Hypothermia is defined as a core temperature of less than 35 °C. It has long been hypothesized that cooling patients might have a neuro-protective effect and this has been demonstrated in numerous animal experiments.

The BTF guidelines state that current evidence is insufficient to make recommendations regarding the use of prophylactic hypothermia in TBI.[97] As such, the use of induced hypothermia in the treatment of TBI remains controversial but is widely practised in neurocritical care units. It has an unequivocal effect in reducing the ICP.[98]

In the 1990s, several single centre trials investigating the neuroprotective effect of hypothermia after severe head injury were carried out. These mostly demonstrated a benefit in those patients who were cooled – especially in those who had a GCS of 4–7 on admission.[99–101] In 2001 the results of a large multi-centre randomized controlled trial was published, which demonstrated a reduction in the ICP for those patients who were cooled but no benefit to those patients in terms of neurological outcome or survival.[102] There was actually an increase in 'days with complications' amongst patients who were cooled. Proponents of induced hypothermia have criticised this study because some of the units involved had little prior experience in the use of therapeutic hypothermia, the speed at which hypothermia was induced was slow and there were significant differences in results between centres. Other studies have, however, shown favourable outcomes in TBI and it is possible that the benefit is only seen when it is performed by experienced units with expertise in the management of the hypothermic period. Post-hoc analysis of the data seems to suggest that the period of hypothermia should be maintained for more than 48 hours in order to improve outcome.

There are many proposed mechanisms by which hypothermia may exert a potentially beneficial effect. These include but are not limited to a reduction in $CMRO_2$ (decreases by 5%–7% for each °C), prevention of apoptosis, improved cellular homeostasis particularly with respect to a reduction of intracellular calcium, suppression of ischaemia-induced inflammatory reactions, decreased free radical production and an alteration in the pattern of cerebral thermo-pooling. In the reverse circumstance of pyrexia, these are all increased.

The induction of therapeutic hypothermia (31–35 °C) is not without complications, although these become more pronounced as core temperature decreases below 29 °C.[98,103,104] Shivering may be seen with temperatures as high as 35 °C. This causes an increase in oxygen consumption, $CO_2$ production and cardiac output and potentially arterial oxygen desaturation and haemodynamic instability. The use of muscle relaxants limits these effects in cooled patients. Blood pressure and cardiac output drop at temperatures below 32 °C. This is partly a function of the reduced metabolic rate and oxygen consumption, but is also due to a direct effect on the myocardium and is the basis of 31–32 °C being the lower limit for therapeutic hypothermia in this group of patients. The reduction of cardiac output is also reflected in a reduction in renal perfusion and glomerular filtration rate. Tubular reabsorption of water also declines, both as a result of reduced cellular activity, and possibly also as a result of resistance to antidiuretic hormone. In mild to moderate hypothermia, tubular dysfunction tends to predominate and large volumes of hyposmolar urine are secreted (so-called 'cold diuresis'), which may render the patient both hypovolaemic and hypokalaemic. The former particularly becomes evident on rewarming to normothermia. Prolonged bleeding times and platelet dysfunction tend only to be seen in patients who are profoundly hypothermic.

Hypothermia may be achieved in various ways and numerous devices are available to facilitate cooling. These include ice packs, sponge water baths, air-cooled circulating blankets, ice water-circulating blankets, infusion of cooled fluids (30 ml/kg of 4 °C lactated Ringer's solution), helmets and caps with cooling properties, iced nasal or peritoneal lavage, extracorporeal circuits and intravascular catheter-based heat exchange systems.

Pyrexia is a frequent complication in the brain-injured patient. There is good evidence that pyrexia worsens outcome in patients with traumatic brain injury.[105] Following head injury, brain temperature exceeds core temperature and this gap is further increased as core temperature rises. Active cooling of patients to normothermia using acetaminophen and mechanical cooling aids should be pursued.

# References

1. Elf K, Nilsson P, Enblad P. Outcome after traumatic brain injury improved by an organized secondary insult program and standardized neurointensive care. *Crit Care Med* 2002; **30**: 2129–34.

2. Patel HC, Menon DK, Tebbs S, Hawker R, Hutchinson PJ, Kirkpatrick PJ. Specialist neurocritical care and outcome from head injury. *Intens Care Med* 2002; **28**: 547–53.

3. Clayton TJ, Nelson RJ, Manara AR. Reduction in mortality from severe head injury following introduction of a protocol for intensive care management. *Br J Anaesth* 2004; **93**: 761–7.

4. Patel HC, Bouamra O, Woodford M, King AT, Yates DW, Lecky FE. Trends in head injury outcome from 1989 to 2003 and the effect of neurosurgical care: an observational study. *Lancet* 2005; **366**: 1538–44.

5. Rosner MJ, Rosner SD, Johnson AH. Cerebral perfusion pressure: management protocol and clinical results. *J Neurosurg* 1995; **83**: 949–62.

6. Marshall LF, Smith RW, Shapiro HM. The outcome with aggressive treatment in severe head injuries. Part I: the significance of intracranial pressure monitoring. *J Neurosurg* 1979; **50**: 20–5.

7. Robertson CS, Valadka AB, Hannay HJ *et al.* Prevention of secondary ischemic insults after severe head injury. *Crit Care Med* 1999; **27**: 2086–95.

8. Czosnyka M, Balestreri M, Steiner L *et al.* Age, intracranial pressure, autoregulation, and outcome after brain trauma. *J Neurosurg* 2005; **102**: 450–4.

9. Hiler M, Czosnyka M, Hutchinson P *et al.* Predictive value of initial computerized tomography scan, intracranial pressure, and state of autoregulation in patients with traumatic brain injury. *J Neurosurg* 2006; **104**: 731–7.

10. Eker C, Asgeirsson B, Grände PO, Schalén W, Nordström CH. Improved outcome after severe head injury with a new therapy based on principles for brain volume regulation and preserved microcirculation. *Crit Care Med* 1998; **26**: 1881–86.

11. Grände PO. The 'Lund Concept' for the treatment of severe head trauma: physiological principles and clinical application. *Intens Care Med* 2006; **32**: 1475–84.

12. Chesnut RM, Marshall LF, Klauber MR *et al.* The role of secondary brain injury in determining outcome from severe head injury. *J Trauma* 1993; **34**: 216–22.

13. Chesnut RM, Marshall SB, Piek J, Blunt BA, Klauber MR, Marshall LF. Early and late systemic hypotension as a frequent and fundamental source of cerebral ischemia following severe brain injury in the Traumatic Coma Data Bank. *Acta Neurochir Suppl (Wien)* 1993; **59**: 121–5.

14. Clifton GL, Miller ER, Choi SC *et al.* Fluid thresholds and outcome from severe brain injury. *Crit Care Med* 2002; **30**: 739–45.

15. Juul N, Morris GF, Marshall SB *et al.* Intracranial hypertension and cerebral perfusion pressure: influence on neurological deterioration and outcome in severe head injury. The Executive Committee of the International Selfotel Trial. *J Neurosurg* 2000; **92**: 1–6.

16. Andrews PJ, Sleeman DH, Statham PF *et al.* Predicting recovery in patients suffering from traumatic brain injury by using admission variables and physiological data: a comparison between decision tree analysis and logistic regression. *J Neurosurg* 2002; **97**: 326–36.

17. Brain Trauma Foundation, American Association of Neurological Surgeons, Joint Section on Neurotrauma and Critical Care. Guidelines for the management of severe head injury. *J Neurotrauma* 1996; **13**: 641–734.

18. Brain Trauma Foundation, American Association of Neurological Surgeons, Joint Section on Neurotrauma and Critical Care. Guidelines for the management of severe traumatic brain injury. *J Neurotrauma* 2000; **17**: 449–554.

19. Brain Trauma Foundation, American Association of Neurological Surgeons, Joint Section on Neurotrauma and Critical Care. 3rd edition. IX Cerebral Perfusion Thresholds. *J Neurotrauma* 2007; **24**: S59–64.

20. Ghajar J. Traumatic brain injury. *Lancet* 2000; **356**: 923–9.

21. Johnston AJ, Steiner LA, Chatfield DA *et al.* Effect of cerebral perfusion pressure augmentation with dopamine and norepinephrine on global and focal brain oxygenation after traumatic brain injury. *Intens Care Med* 2004; **30**: 791–7.

22. Bernard F, Outtrim J, Menon DK, Matta BF. Incidence of adrenal insufficiency after severe traumatic brain injury varies according to definition used: clinical implications. *Br J Anaesth* 2006; **96**: 72–6.

23. Gupta AK, Hutchinson PJ, Al-Rawi P *et al.* Measuring brain tissue oxygenation compared with jugular venous oxygen saturation for monitoring cerebral oxygenation after traumatic brain injury. *Anesth Analg* 1999; **88**: 549–53.

24. Nordström CH, Reinstrup P, Xu W, Gärdenfors A, Ungerstedt U. Assessment of the lower limit for cerebral perfusion in severe head injuries by bedside monitoring of regional energy metabolism. *Anesthesiology* 2003; **98**: 809–14.

25. Coles JP, Fryer TD, Smielewski P et al. Defining ischemic burden after traumatic brain injury using 15O PET imaging of cerebral physiology. *J Cereb Blood Flow Metab* 2004; **24**: 191–201.

26. Coles JP, Fryer TD, Smielewski P *et al.* Incidence and mechanisms of cerebral ischemia in early clinical head injury. *J Cereb Blood Flow Metab* 2004; **24**: 202–11.

27. Howells T, Elf K, Jones PA *et al.* Pressure reactivity as a guide in the treatment of cerebral perfusion pressure in patients with brain trauma. *J Neurosurg* 2005; **102**: 311–17.

28. Steiner LA, Czosnyka M, Piechnik SK *et al.* Continuous monitoring of cerebrovascular pressure reactivity allows determination of optimal cerebral perfusion pressure in patients with traumatic brain injury. *Crit Care Med* 2002; **30**: 733–8.

29. Robertson CS, Valadka AB, Hannay HJ *et al.* Prevention of secondary ischemic insults after severe head injury. *Crit Care Med* 1999; **27**: 2086–95.

30. Contant CF, Valadka AB, Gopinath SP *et al.* Adult respiratory distress syndrome: a complication of induced hypertension after severe head injury. *J Neurosurg* 2001; **95**: 560–8.

31. Asgeirsson B, Grände PO, Nordström CH. A new therapy of post-trauma brain oedema based on haemodynamic principles for brain volume regulation. *Intens Care Med* 1994; **20**: 260–7.

32. Grände PO, Asgeirsson B, Nordström CH. Volume-targeted therapy of increased

intracranial pressure: the Lund concept unifies surgical and non-surgical treatments. *Acta Anaesthesiol Scand* 2002; **46**: 929–41.

33. Grände PO, Möller AD, Nordström CH, Ungerstedt U. Low-dose prostacyclin in treatment of severe brain trauma evaluated with microdialysis and jugular bulb oxygen measurements. *Acta Anaesthesiol Scand* 2000; **44**: 886–94.

34. Naredi S, Eden E, Zall S, Stephensen H, Rydehag B. A standardized neurosurgical neurointensive therapy directed towards vasogenic oedema after severe traumatic brain injury: clinical results. *Intens Care Med* 1998; **24**: 446–51.

35. Naredi S, Olivecrona M, Lindgren C, Ostlund AL, Grände PO, Koskinen LO. An outcome study of severe traumatic head injury using the 'Lund therapy' with low dose prostacyclin. *Acta Anaesthesiol Scand* 2001; **45**: 402–6.

36. Elf K, Nilsson P, Ronne-Engstrom E, Howells T, Enblad P. Cerebral perfusion pressure between 50 and 60 mm Hg may be beneficial in head-injured patients: a computerized secondary insult monitoring study. *Neurosurgery* 2005; **56**: 962–71.

37. Citerio G, Cormio M. Sedation in neurointensivecare: advances in understanding and practice. *Curr Opin Crit Care* 2003; **9**: 120–26.

38. Johnston AJ, Steiner LA, Chatfield DA *et al.* Effects of propofol on cerebral oxygenation and metabolism after head injury. *Br J Anaesth* 2003; **91**: 781–6.

39. Hanley DF Jr, Pozo M. Treatment of status epilepticus with midazolam in the critical care setting. *Int J Clin Pract* 2000; **54**: 30–5.

40. Shafer A. Complications of sedation with midazolam in the intensive care unit and a comparison with other sedative regimes. *Crit Care Med* 1998; **26**: 947–56.

41. Walder B, Tramer MR, Seeck, M. Seizure-like phenomena and propofol: a systematic review. *Neurology* 2002; **58**: 1327–32.

42. Warden JC, Pickford DR. Fatal cardiovascular collapse following propofol induction in high-risk patients and dilemmas in the selection of a short-acting induction agent. *Anaesth Intensive Care* 1995; **23**: 485–7.

43. Kumar MA, Urrutia VC, Thomas CE, Abou-Khaled KJ, Schwartzman RJ. The syndrome of irreversible acidosis after prolonged propofol infusion. *Neurocrit Care* 2005; **3**: 257–9.

44. Helmy A, Vizcaychipi M, Gupta AK. Traumatic brain injury: intensive care management. *Br J Anaesth* 2007; **99**: 32–42.

45. Karabinis A, Mandragos K, Stergiopoulos S *et al.* Safety and efficacy of analgesia-based sedation with remifentanil versus standard hypnotic-based regimens in intensive care unit patients with brain injuries: a randomised, controlled trial. *Crit Care* 2004; **8**: R268–80.

46. Sperry RT, Bailey PL, Reichman MV. Fentanyl and sufentanyl increase intracranial pressure in head trauma patients. *Anesthesiology* 1992; **77**: 416–20.

47. Consales G, Chelazzi C, Rinaldi S, de Gaudio AR. Bispectral Index compared to Ramsay score for sedation monitoring in intensive care units. *Minerva Anestesiol* 2006; **72**: 329–36.

48. Le Blanc JM, Dasta JF, Kane-Gill SL. Role of the bispectral index in sedation monitoring in the ICU. *Ann Pharmacother* 2006; **40**: 490–500.

49. Brain Trauma Foundation, American Association of Neurological Surgeons, Joint Section on Neurotrauma and Critical Care. 3rd edition. XI Anesthetics, Analgesics and Sedatives. *J Neurotrauma* 2007; **24**: S71–6.

50. Riker RR, Fraser GL, Wilkins ML. Comparing the bispectral index and suppression ratio with burst suppression of the electroencephalogram during pentobarbital infusions in adult intensive care patients. *Pharmacotherapy* 2003; **23**: 1087–93.

51. Schwartz ML, Tator CH, Rowed DW, Reid SR, Meguro K, Andrews DF. The University of Toronto head injury treatment study: a prospective, randomized comparison of pentobarbital and mannitol. *Can J Neurol Sci* 1984; **11**: 434–40.

52. Ward JD, Becker DP, Miller JD *et al.* Failure of prophylactic barbiturate coma in the treatment of severe head injury. *J Neurosurg* 1985; **62**: 383–8.

53. Demopoulos HB, Flamm ES, Pietronigro DD, Seligman ML. The free radical pathology and the microcirculation in the major central nervous system trauma. *Acta Physiol Scand Suppl* 1980; **492**: 91–119.

54. Kassell NF, Hitchon PW, Gerk MK, Sokoll MD, Hill TR. Alterations in cerebral blood flow, oxygen metabolism, and electrical activity produced by high-dose thiopental. *Neurosurgery* 1980; **7**: 598–603.

55. Goodman JC, Valadka AB, Gopinath SP, Cormio M, Robertson CS. Lactate and excitatory amino acids measured by microdialysis are decreased by pentobarbital coma in head-injured patients. *J Neurotrauma* 1996; **13**: 549–56.

56. Schalén W, Messeter K, Nordström CH. Complications and side effects during thiopentone therapy in patients with severe head injuries. *Acta Anaesthesiol Scand* 1992; **36**: 369–77.

57. Cairns CJ, Thomas B, Fletcher S, Parr MJ, Finfer SR. Life-threatening hyperkalaemia following therapeutic barbiturate coma. *Intens Care Med* 2002; **28**: 1357–60.

58. Cruz J. Adverse effects of pentobarbital on cerebral venous oxygenation of comatose patients with acute traumatic brain swelling: relationship to outcome. *J Neurosurg* 1996; **85**: 758–61.

59. Brain Trauma Foundation, American Association of Neurological Surgeons, Joint Section on Neurotrauma and Critical Care. 3rd edition. XIV Hyperventilation. *J Neurotrauma* 2007; **24**: S87–90.

60. Coles JP, Fryer TD, Coleman MR *et al.* Hyperventilation following head injury: Effect on ischemic burden and cerebral oxidative metabolism. *Crit Care Med* 2007; **35**: 568–78.

61. Huynh T, Messer M, Sing RF, Miles W, Jacobs DG, Thomason MH. Positive end-expiratory pressure alters intracranial and cerebral perfusion pressure in severe traumatic brain injury. *J Trauma* 2002; **53**: 488–92.

62. Madden JA. The effect of carbon dioxide on cerebral arteries. *Pharmacol Ther* 1993; **59**: 229–250.

63. Muizelaar JP, Marmarou A, Ward JD *et al.* Adverse effects of prolonged hyperventilation in patients with severe head injury: a randomized clinical trial. *J Neurosurg* 1991; **75**: 731–9.

64. Diringer MN, Yundt K, Videen TO *et al.* No reduction in cerebral metabolism as a result of early moderate hyperventilation following severe traumatic brain injury. *J Neurosurg* 2000; **92**: 7–13.

65. Diringer MN, Videen TO, Yundt K *et al.* Regional cerebrovascular and metabolic effects of hyperventilation after severe traumatic brain injury. *J Neurosurg* 2002; **96**: 103–8.

66. Coles JP, Minhas PS, Fryer TD *et al.* Effect of hyperventilation on cerebral blood flow in traumatic head injury: clinical relevance and monitoring correlates. *Crit Care Med* 2002; **30**: 1950–9.

67. Imberti R, Bellinzona G, Langer M. Cerebral tissue $PO_2$ and $SjvO_2$ changes during moderate hyperventilation in patients with severe traumatic brain injury. *J Neurosurg* 2002; **96**: 97–102.

68. Rockswold GL, Ford SE, Anderson DC, Bergman TA, Sherman RE. Results of a prospective randomized trial for treatment of severely brain-injured patients with hyperbaric oxygen. *J Neurosurg* 1992; **76**: 929–34.

69. Rockswold, SB, Rockswold GL, Vargo JM *et al.* Effects of hyperbaric oxygenation therapy on cerebral metabolism and intracranial pressure in severely brain injured patients. *J Neurosurg* 2001; **94**: 403–11.

70. Wolf AL, Levi L, Marmarou A, Ward JD *et al.* Effect of THAM upon outcome in severe head injury: a randomized prospective clinical trial. *J Neurosurg* 1993; **78**: 54–9.

71. Ghajar J, Hariri RJ, Narayan RK, Iacono LA, Firlik K, Patterson RH. Survey of critical care management of comatose, head-injured patients in the United States. *Crit Care Med* 1995; **23**: 560–7.

72. Matta B, Menon DK. Severe head injury in the United Kingdom and Ireland: a survey of practice and implications for management. *Crit Care Med* 1996; **24**: 1743–8.

73. Wakai A, Roberts I, Schierhout G. Mannitol for acute traumatic brain injury. *Cochrane Database of Systematic Reviews* 2007; **1**: CD001049.

74. Mendelow AD, Teasdale GM, Russell T, Flood J, Patterson J, Murray GD. Effect of mannitol on cerebral blood flow and cerebral perfusion pressure in human head injury. *J Neurosurg* 1985; **63**: 43–8.

75. Nath F, Galbraith S. The effect of mannitol on cerebral white matter water content. *J Neurosurg* 1986; **65**: 41–3.

76. Bullock R. Mannitol and other diuretics in severe neurotrauma. *New Horizons* 1995; **3**: 448–52.

77. Manninen PH, Lam AM, Gelb AW, Brown SC. The effect of high dose mannitol on serum and urine electrolytes and osmolality in neurosurgical patients. *Can J Anaesth* 1987; **34**: 442–6.

78. Marshall LF, Smith RW, Rauscher LA, Shapiro HM. Mannitol dose requirements in brain-injured patients. *J Neurosurg* 1978; **48**: 169–72.

79. Brain Trauma Foundation, American Association of Neurological Surgeons, Joint Section on Neurotrauma and Critical Care. 3rd edition. II Hyperosmolar Therapy. *J Neurotrauma* 2007; **24**: S14–20.

80. Cruz J, Minoja G, Okuchi K, Facco E. Successful use of the new high-dose mannitol treatment in patients with Glasgow Coma Scale scores of 3 and bilateral abnormal pupillary widening: a randomized trial. *J Neurosurg* 2004; **100**: 376–83.

81. Mattox KL, Maningas PA, Moore EE *et al.* Prehospital hypertonic saline/dextran infusion for post-traumatic hypotension. The USA Multicenter Trial. *Ann Surg* 1991; **213**: 482–91.

82. Shackford SR. Effect of small-volume resuscitation on intracranial pressure and related cerebral variables. *J Trauma* 1997; **42**: S48–53.

83. Shackford SR, Bourguignon PR, Wald SL, Rogers FB, Osler TM, Clark DE. Hypertonic saline resuscitation of patients with head injury: a prospective, randomized clinical trial. *J Trauma* 1998; **44**: 50–8.

84. Battison C, Andrews PJ, Graham C, Petty T. Randomized, controlled trial on the effect of a 20% mannitol solution and a 7.5% saline/6% dextran solution on increased intracranial pressure after brain injury. *Crit Care Med* 2005; **33**: 196–202.

85. Harutjunyan L, Holz C, Rieger A, Menzel M, Grond S, Soukup J. Efficiency of 7.2% hypertonic saline hydroxyethyl starch 220/0.5 versus mannitol 15% in the treatment of increased intracranial pressure in neurosurgical patients – a randomised controlled trial. *Crit Care* 2005; **9**: 530–40.

86. Schmoker JD, Shackford SR, Wald SL, Pietropaoli JA. An analysis of the relationship between fluid and sodium administration and intracranial pressure after head injury. *J Trauma* 1992; **33**: 476–81.

87. Qureshi AI, Suarez JI, Bhardwaj A *et al.* Use of hypertonic (3%) saline/acetate infusion in the treatment of cerebral edema: effect on intracranial pressure and lateral displacement of the brain. *Crit Care Med* 1998; **26**: 440–6.

88. Shackford SR, Zhuang J, Schmoker J. Intravenous fluid tonicity: effect on intracranial pressure, cerebral blood flow, and cerebral oxygen delivery in focal brain injury. *J Neurosurg* 1992; **76**: 91–8.

89. Doyle JA, Davis DP, Hoyt DB. The use of hypertonic saline in the treatment of traumatic brain injury. *J Trauma* 2001; **50**: 367–83.

90. Kreimeier U, Brückner UB, Messmer K. Improvement of nutritional blood flow using hypertonic-hyperoncotic solutions for primary treatment of hemorrhagic hypotension. *Eur Surg Res* 1988; **20**: 277–9.

91. Qureshi AI, Suarez JI. Use of hypertonic saline solutions in the treatment of cerebral edema and intracranial hypertension. *Crit Care Med* 2000; **28**: 3301–13.

92. Vialet R, Albanese J, Thomachot L *et al.* Isovolume hypertonic solutes (sodium chloride or mannitol) in the treatment of refractory posttraumatic intracranial hypertension: 2 mL/kg 7.5% saline is more effective than 2 mL/kg 20% mannitol. *Crit Care Med* 2003; **31**: 1683–7.

93. Härtl R, Medary M, Ruge M *et al.* Hypertonic / hyperoncotic saline attenuates microcirculatory disturbances after traumatic brain injury. *J Trauma* 1977; **42**: S41–7.

94. Horn P, Munch E, Vajkoczy P *et al.* Hypertonic saline solution for control of elevated intracranial pressure in patients with exhausted response to mannitol and barbiturates. *Neurol Res* 1999; **21**: 758–64.

95. Suarez JI, Qureshi AI, Bhardwaj A *et al.* Treatment of refractory intracranial hypertension with 23.4% saline. *Crit Care Med* 1998; **26**: 1118–22.

96. Kleinschmidt-DeMasters BK, Norenberg MD. Rapid correction of hyponatremia causes demyelination: relation to central pontine myelinolysis. *Science* 1981; **211**: 1068–70.

97. Brain Trauma Foundation, American Association of Neurological Surgeons, Joint Section on Neurotrauma and Critical Care. 3rd edition. III Prophylactic Hypothermia. *J Neurotrauma* 2007; **24**: S21–5.

98. Polderman KH, Tjong Tjin Joe R, Peerdeman SM, Vandertop WP, Girbes AR. Effects of therapeutic hypothermia on intracranial pressure and outcome in patients with severe head injury. *Intens Care Med* 2002; **28**: 1563–67.

99. Clifton GL, Allen S, Barrodale P *et al.* A phase II study of moderate hypothermia in severe brain injury. *J Neurotrauma* 1993; **10**: 263–71.

100. Marion DW, Penrod LE, Kelsey SF *et al.* Treatment of traumatic brain injury with moderate hypothermia. *N Engl J Med* 1997; **336**: 540–6.

101. Bernard S. Induced hypothermia in intensive care medicine. *Anaesth Intens Care* 1996; **24**: 382–8.

102. Clifton GL, Miller ER, Choi SC *et al.* Lack of effect of induction of hypothermia after acute brain injury. *N Engl J Med* 2001; **344**: 556–63.

103. Polderman KH. Application of therapeutic hypothermia in the ICU: opportunities and pitfalls of a promising treatment modality. Part 1: Indications and evidence. *Intens Care Med* 2004; **30**: 556–75.

104. Polderman KH. Application of therapeutic hypothermia in the ICU: opportunities and pitfalls of a promising treatment modality. Part 2: Practical aspects and side effects. *Intens Care Med* 2004; **30**: 757–69.

105. Stocchetti N, Rossi S, Zanier ER, Colombo A, Beretta L, Citerio G. Pyrexia in head-injured patients admitted to intensive care. *Intens Care Med* 2002; **28**: 1555–62.

# Therapeutic options in neurocritical care: beyond the brain

Matthew J. C. Thomas, Alexander R. Manara, Richard Protheroe and Ayan Sen

## Cardio-respiratory issues in head-injured patients

### Systemic complications of head injury

Systemic complications of head injury are common. A review of 209 patients admitted to intensive care with traumatic brain injury (TBI) showed that 89% developed non-neurological dysfunction in at least one other organ system, worsening the outcome.[1] This is a high incidence in a group of patients who are typically younger – the median age in this trial was 36 – and with less co-morbidity than other intensive care patients. The reasons for the increased incidence of complications after TBI may be due to the systemic effects of the brain injury itself, the presence of other associated injuries and the complications of treatment. The implications of systemic complications following head injury are increasingly recognized and attracting more attention.[2,3] The presence of one organ failure is reportedly associated with a mortality rate of 40% increasing to 47% with two organ failures and to 100% with three or more organs failing.[1] The commonest organ failures were cardiovascular and respiratory.

### Cardiovascular complications

Cardiac dysfunction is well documented following subarachnoid haemorrhage and can result in global dysfunction, regional wall abnormalities and subendocardial changes, presumably secondary to the accompanying catecholamine surge.[4] Cardiac dysfunction occurs less frequently following traumatic brain injury, despite it also being associated with a well-documented catecholamine surge. Studies of patients who died following TBI show that 16%–41% of patients had echocardiographic evidence of myocardial dysfunction thought to be due to release of catecholamines.[5,6] Post-mortem studies show a characteristic pattern of myocardial damage with contraction band necrosis and myocytolysis, a pattern that is distinct to that seen in myocardial ischaemia.[7] These changes may explain the common occurrence of haemodynamic instability and a relative hypotension requiring the use of vasoactive agents in patients with TBI.

Neurogenic hypotension as a result of disruption to brainstem pathways complicates head injury in 13% of cases.[3] However, this diagnosis should only be made after excluding other sources of hypotension, particularly other sources of bleeding.

Neurogenic pulmonary oedema (NPO) is another consequence of head injury that usually develops rapidly in the early stages following brain injury, but it has also been reported as late as 14 days after injury.[8] Certain patterns of TBI have been shown to cause more NPO in animal models, and Graf and Rossi showed that NPO was associated with medullary damage in human TBI.[9] The raised circulating levels of epinephrine and norepinephrine seen following TBI are thought to cause a sudden increase in both preload and afterload resulting initially in left ventricular failure and hydrostatic oedema. This is followed

*Head Injury: A Multidisciplinary Approach*, ed. Peter C. Whitfield, Elfyn O. Thomas, Fiona Summers, Maggie Whyte and Peter J. Hutchinson. Published by Cambridge University Press. © Cambridge University Press 2009.

by pulmonary capillary damage causing a permeability oedema exacerbated by the release of secondary mediators. In experimental animal work beta blockers have been shown to prevent NPO. In brain injured patients the problems are often magnified by the use of catecholamines as part of cerebral perfusion pressure (CPP) guided therapy and the possibility of myocardial injury as a result of trauma. The treatment of NPO is mainly supportive using oxygen and mechanical ventilation with positive end expiratory pressure (PEEP). It differs from the treatment of cardiogenic pulmonary oedema in that although dobutamine may be beneficial in improving ventricular function, indiscriminate use of diuretics or nitrates often causes an unwelcome reduction in blood pressure and potentially in CPP.[10]

## Vasoactive drugs following TBI

Vasoactive drugs are used frequently in head-injured patients most commonly to increase mean arterial pressure (MAP) and CPP, but occasionally they are required in patients who develop neurogenic pulmonary oedema, myocardial dysfunction or multiple organ dysfunction.

Before using vasoactive drugs to augment MAP and CPP in head-injured patients, it is important to ensure that hypovolaemia is excluded and adequate circulating volume achieved. The 2007 guidelines from the Brain Trauma Foundation (BTF) recommend that CPP should be maintained between 50 and 70 mm Hg in adults even if this means using vasoactive agents.[11] However, they also recommend that aggressive attempts to maintain CPP above 70 mm Hg with fluids and vasoactive drugs should be avoided as this may increase the incidence of acute respiratory distress syndrome (ARDS).[11]

The commonly used agents in neurosurgical intensive care practice are norepinephrine, epinephrine, dobutamine and dopamine. All are sympathomimetic agents acting by stimulating naturally occurring adrenoreceptors to exert an effect.

### Epinephrine

Epinephrine is a naturally occurring hormone that acts on α1, β1 and β2 adrenergic receptors. It increases the heart rate and force of cardiac contraction by its β1 effect and increases peripheral vasoconstriction by its α1 effect. This has the effect of increasing cardiac output (CO), systemic vascular resistance (SVR) and MAP. However, its use is associated with ventricular arrhythmias and with the development of lactic acidosis. For this reason, although it reliably increases MAP, it is not usually a first-line drug in intensive care. In addition, using epinephrine to increase CPP has been shown to be an independent risk factor for developing ARDS, although the authors make the point that raising the blood pressure by any means increases the risk of ARDS.[12]

### Norepinephrine

Norepinephrine is primarily an α1 adrenergic agonist, increasing SVR and MAP with little effect on cardiac contractility. Indeed, by increasing SVR, norepinephrine can worsen cardiac failure. Since most patients with head injuries are young and unlikely to have significant cardiac co-morbidities, cardiac failure is not usually an issue and norepinephrine can be used to reliably increase MAP. Whilst norepinephrine is the most reliable vasoactive drug for increasing CPP, and is used commonly in TBI, a recent review suggests that it may play a part in worsening multi-organ failure, possibly due to its adverse effects on thrombocytes and leukocytes.[13] Occasionally, other α1 agonists are used, particularly the synthetic drug metaraminol since it can be administered peripherally in the short term and has similar effects to norepinephrine. All adrenergic agents show some tachyphylaxis requiring increasing doses to achieve the same effect.

## Dobutamine

Dobutamine is a synthetic catecholamine that exerts its effect primarily via $\beta1$ adrenergic receptors, increasing cardiac contractility and heart rate. Peripheral $\beta_2$ stimulation can also cause vasodilatation with the resulting effect that, whilst dobutamine improves blood flow, it may cause hypotension and tachycardia. Dobutamine is a useful drug in the management of cardiac failure, sepsis and in NPO where it improves myocardial function, but it is less reliable than other drugs at increasing CPP in head injured patients and therefore is used infrequently for this purpose.[10]

## Dopamine

Dopamine is a naturally occurring substance that exerts its effects via $\alpha1$, $\beta1$ and $\beta2$ adrenergic receptors as well as via specific dopaminergic receptors. It therefore has a similar effect to epinephrine in increasing both CO and SVR with a rise in CPP. Dopamine also has effects on the neuro-endocrine system, suppressing the release of most anterior pituitary hormones. It is used widely in general intensive care practice in Europe but the results of the recent SOAP study, showing an increased mortality in patients with sepsis receiving dopamine, may limit its use in the future.[14] Furthermore, a recent study comparing the cerebrovascular effects of dopamine and norepinephrine in head-injured patients showed that norepinephrine was more predictable and efficient at augmenting CPP suggesting that it should be considered the drug of choice for this purpose.[15]

## Other vasoactive agents

Vasopressin has also been used to increase MAP when first line vasopressors have failed to do so, particularly in the setting of septic shock where its addition to norepinephrine may reduce mortality.[16,17] There is also increasing interest in its use as an alternative to norepinephrine in head-injured patients in whom it has been used successfully,[18] although concerns regarding its potential to induce unwanted cerebral ischaemia may limit its more widespread use.[19] The use of vasopressin in combination with tri-iodothyronine (T3) is recommended by several transplant centres to manage the neuro-endocrine failure following brainstem death in potential organ donors.

# Deleterious effects of vasoactive agents in TBI

No vasoactive drugs can be given without risk of side effects. Both dopamine and epinephrine have been shown to increase the risk of ARDS probably as a result of increasing MAP.[12] Epinephrine also causes lactic acidosis.[20] All the drugs that increase blood pressure by vasoconstriction will increase CPP but at the possible expense of cerebral blood flow. Norepinephrine has been shown to have benefits over dopamine, but recent evidence suggests a deleterious effect on the immune system possibly increasing the risk of multiple organ dysfunction syndrome.[13]

# Respiratory complications

The respiratory system is the organ system most likely to develop complications following TBI. The commonest complications are pneumonia, pulmonary aspiration and ARDS.

## Pneumonia

Pneumonia following TBI occurs earlier and tends to be associated with different pathogens than ventilator associated pneumonia developing during the course of other critically ill patients. The incidence of early onset pneumonia (<5 days) is 41%–44% in comatose patients requiring ventilation.[21,22] The commonest organisms isolated are *Staphylococcus aureus* and *Haemophilus influenzae*, both of which are common nasopharyngeal commensals, suggesting a primary endogenous source of infection. All patients who are comatose following TBI are likely to aspirate substantial quantities of oropharyngeal secretions and these may contain potentially pathogenic commensal organisms. Clinical aspiration before intubation has been shown to be an independent predictor of early onset pneumonia.[22] Other risk factors include older age, nasal carriage of *S. aureus*, barbiturate infusion, other sedation, and no antibiotic use in the first 24 hours. It is also interesting to note that interventions commonly used in TBI as part of CPP/ICP management increase the risk of pneumonia. Sedative infusions and barbiturates are immunosuppressive and have been shown to increase the incidence of pneumonia as has the use of induced hypothermia.[22,23] Since most aspiration occurs before the airway is protected with a cuffed endotracheal tube it can be difficult to prevent early onset pneumonia in head-injured patients. Manoeuvres to reduce further aspiration in patients being mechanically ventilated, including semi-recumbent positioning, subglottic suctioning and the use of low-volume low-pressure tracheal tube cuffs that stop microaspiration around the cuff but do not cause tracheal necrosis, have all been recommended in this patient population.[24–26]

The pneumonia should be treated with appropriate antibiotics. Empirical treatment whilst awaiting the results of sputum culture and sensitivities should include antibiotics active against local strains of *S. aureus* and *H. influenzae*. Early onset pneumonia can result in pyrexia, hypotension and hypoxaemia, all of which require aggressive management in their own right since they have been shown to worsen outcome in head injury. Pneumonia *per se*, however, has not been shown to be an independent risk factor for mortality after TBI.

The use of antibiotic prophylaxis to prevent early onset pneumonia remains controversial. Patients who receive antibiotics for other reasons such as open fractures develop less pneumonia. Two trials have shown that prophylactic administration of cefuroxime or ampicillin and sulbactam reduces the incidence of early onset pneumonia in head-injured patients.[21,27] Despite this, prophylactic antibiotics are not routinely used after head injury as they have not been shown to reduce mortality and they increase the risk of subsequent colonization with resistant organisms.[21] In their 2007 guidelines the BTF, however, based only on the study of Sirvent *et al.*, make a level II recommendation for periprocedural antibiotics for intubation to reduce the incidence of pneumonia.[28] The use of prophylactic antibiotics in the form of selective decontamination of the digestive tract has been reviewed in multiple trials with a lot of evidence of a mortality benefit, but it is not widely used due to fears of multi-resistant organisms.[29,30] Oral decontamination with both antibiotics and antiseptics without parenteral drugs has been shown to reduce the risk of pneumonia but without a mortality benefit.[31]

### Acute lung injury

Acute lung injury (ALI) is described as the presence of diffuse parenchymal infiltrates on chest X-ray (three or four quadrants) and hypoxaemia as manifested by a $PaO_2/FiO_2$ ratio of <300 mmHg (<40 kPa) in the absence of left heart failure. Acute respiratory distress syndrome (ARDS) is a severe form of ALI with a $PaO_2/FiO_2$ ratio of <200 mmHg (<27 kPa). ALI is one of the more common systemic complications after TBI with an incidence of 20%–50%.[2,32,33] Patients with TBI who develop ARDS are three times more likely to die or have a poor neurological outcome on discharge than those who do not.[11] The development of ALI is multifactorial with NPO, aspiration pneumonitis, associated chest injuries and early pneumonia all contributing. Multivariate analysis also identified the severity of injury and administration of dopamine and norepinephrine as risk factors for developing ALI after TBI.[12] This latter study suggests that aggressive CPP targeted therapy with inotropes and fluids, as opposed to ICP-directed therapy, is associated with a higher rate of ARDS in patients with TBI.

The outcome of patients with ARDS is improved if a lung protective ventilation strategy is used.[34] This includes the use of low tidal volumes and low inspiratory pressures combined with the use of high levels of PEEP to maintain oxygenation, and permissive hypercarbia. The latter and other aspects of current ARDS management such as fluid restriction are at odds with CPP/ICP management goals in head-injured patients. Some techniques to improve oxygenation in ARDS, such as prone position ventilation, have been shown to be associated with an increased ICP, whereas others such as PEEP below $12\,cmH_2O$ do not affect ICP and may in fact decrease it by improving cerebral oxygenation.[35,36] Other promising techniques that may be useful in the management of ARDS in TBI include using high frequency ventilation to maintain oxygenation whilst controlling $CO_2$,[37] and extracorporeal $CO_2$ removal devices, including the recently reported Novalung,[38] allowing the use of a low tidal volume lung protective ventilatory strategy without the fear of causing hypercapnoea. The conflicting therapeutic requirements of maintaining CPP or lowering ICP versus those required to manage concomitant systemic organ dysfunction or failure remain a challenging aspect of the intensive care management of patients with TBI.

## Venous thromboembolism

Thromboprophylaxis is effective and has been repeatedly shown to reduce the risks of deep vein thrombosis (DVT), pulmonary embolism (PE) and fatal PE, the most common cause of preventable hospital death. There is grade I evidence that DVT prophylaxis with low molecular weight heparin improves outcome in the general intensive care population.[39] The absolute risk of venous thromboembolism (VTE) in patients with major trauma not receiving prophylaxis is 40%–80%, with pulmonary embolism occurring in approximately 2%, but it is difficult to predict who will develop symptomatic thromboembolic disease, meaning that prophylaxis should be used in all. It is important to recognize that the recommendations for patients with trauma and head injury are different to those for patients undergoing elective neurosurgery. The latter can be effectively managed using intermittent pneumatic compression devices with or without graduated compression stockings (grade IA recommendation), whereas for trauma patients routine use of thromboprophylaxis has become a standard of care, with low molecular weight heparin (LMWH) being recommended for all patients when it is considered safe to do so (grade IA recommendation).[40] If the risk of haemorrhage is considered high, then graduated compression stockings or intermittent pneumatic compression should be used until LMWH can be started (grade IB). The question in the context of head injuries is at what stage is the risk of haemorrhage low enough to contemplate using LMWH? VTE is a real risk to patients with head injuries, DVT being reported in up to 17% despite the use of conventional methods of prophylaxis.[41] Unfortunately, most major trials of LMWH have excluded patients with head injury due to fear of bleeding and a study by Dickinson using preoperative LMWH that showed an increased risk of intracranial bleeding in patients undergoing craniotomy for brain tumours appeared to justify these concerns.[42] More recently, however, Norwood and colleagues showed that it is safe to administer LMWH to these patients as long as it is prescribed a minimum of 24 hours after a head injury associated with intracranial haemorrhage and that it is withheld for 24 hours after any subsequent craniotomy or cranioplasty.[43] The overall evidence would point to minimal risk in brain trauma and a significant benefit in reducing the incidence of VTE.

# Tracheostomy in head injury

Tracheostomy is a procedure undertaken commonly in the ICU, 12.6% of over 10 000 patients in European ICUs having a tracheostomy in the EPIC study in the early 1990s.[44] This is not surprising considering that many intensivists believe that tracheostomy facilitates nursing care, improves comfort and mobility, allows speech and oral nutrition, and speeds weaning from mechanical ventilation. Since then, a report from a neuroscience ICU in the UK suggests that, since the introduction of percutaneous techniques, tracheostomy is being undertaken more frequently and performed earlier.[45] This may reflect a relaxation of the indications for tracheostomy, a previous under-utilization of tracheostomy, or alternatively done to allow safe discharge of patients to a lower dependency environment. Many patients with head injury will undergo tracheostomy, occasionally because they require prolonged mechanical ventilation, but more commonly as a means of securing the airway, allowing pulmonary toilet and preventing aspiration in patients who breathe spontaneously and adequately but who continue to have a reduced level of consciousness, poor bulbar function or associated facial trauma.

Until recently the timing of tracheostomy was mainly influenced by the 1989 Consensus Conference on Artificial Airways that recommended that tracheostomy should be performed if the need for mechanical ventilation is likely to exceed 21 days.[46] However, a recent meta-analysis suggests that early tracheostomy may shorten the duration of mechanical ventilation by a mean of 8 days and reduce the length of ICU stay by a mean of 15 days, but not reduce mortality or the incidence of nosocomial pneumonia.[47] A reduction in the duration of mechanical ventilation from 12 days to 6 days and a reduction in ICU length of stay were also shown in a study specifically of patients with TBI undergoing early (day 5 or 6) tracheostomy compared with prolonged endotracheal intubation,[48] but was not demonstrated in another study that excluded patients with TBI.[49] The latest BTF guidelines make a level II recommendation that early tracheostomy should be performed to reduce mechanical ventilation days.[28] The question on the optimal timing of tracheostomy, however, remains unanswered and is currently being addressed by the TracMan study, a multicentre UK trial, aiming to resolve whether early tracheostomy is beneficial or not.[50]

Percutaneous dilatational tracheostomy (PDT) has become the technique of choice in the UK being undertaken by 86% of all ICUs.[51] The procedure can be performed rapidly on the ICU, as safely as open surgical tracheostomy, without the need for surgical staff or a transfer to the operating theatre. A large meta-analysis showed no apparent difference in complications between the two techniques.[52] It should also be remembered that PDT is a semi-elective procedure and not an emergency one and should only be undertaken when the patient is stable. PDT is often associated with periods of hypoventilation, hypercarbia and occasionally hypoxaemia and it has been shown that the ICP may increase and CPP may fall when PDT is undertaken in patients with TBI.[53] When PDT is undertaken using bronchoscopic guidance, the hypercarbia is even more pronounced and the potential for cerebral ischaemia potentially more significant.[54] Bronchoscopy should therefore only be used for as short a time as possible to confirm correct position of the needle, guidewire and tube, and meticulous care should be taken to maintain MAP and CPP during the procedure. On current evidence there is little to suggest that one technique of PDT is superior to another in terms of early complications, although it should be remembered that published experience is greatest with the Ciaglia technique, accounting for approximately 70% of all patients in the literature.[55]

Some concern has been raised about the incidence of tracheal stenosis following PDT and that stenosis may occur at a higher level and be more difficult to treat.[56] Most follow-up studies have so far shown very low rates of symptomatic stenosis and it has been estimated that a study with 80% power to show a difference in the rate of stenosis between PDT and open tracheostomy would need to recruit a minimum of 500 patients.[57] Patients with brain injuries who have undergone tracheostomy because of prolonged coma are often considered to have a worse prognosis, but a study of 277 brain-injured patients showed that, whilst prolonged coma was associated with a poor outcome, tracheostomy *per se* was not.[58] Furthermore, less than 10% of patients continue to require the tracheostomy after 3 months and 66% of patients who had undergone tracheostomy were discharged from hospital and able to return to their previous vocation.[58] The requirement to keep patients intubated when they meet standard criteria for extubation but remain unconscious is also being challenged. A study of 136 brain-injured patients with a continuing reduced level of consciousness found that the 99 patients who were extubated within 48 hours of meeting the defined criteria had less pneumonia and a shorter ICU stay than those in whom extubation was delayed.[59] Only 17 of the 99 patients required re-intubation, suggesting that a trial of extubation when patients meet standard weaning criteria is justified, and that perhaps tracheostomy should be reserved for those who fail extubation. In fact, the latest BTF guidelines make a level III recommendation that early extubation can be safely performed in suitable patients.[28]

Many aspects of tracheostomy remain unresolved in intensive care practice and decisions regarding the indications and timing of tracheostomy will continue to be made on an individual patient basis.

## Nutritional issues in head-injured patients

### Introduction

Patients with severe head injury have altered metabolic homeostasis, resulting in increased energy expenditure and protein catabolism. In the early 1980s, several studies were conducted to assess the metabolic effect of severe head injury.[60–62] These showed that hypermetabolism and nitrogen wasting were common. The consequent depletion of muscle mass and depressed immunofunction was reported to increase complication rates and worsen long-term outcome. Although one suggested preventive approach is to provide nutrition in accordance with the accelerated metabolism, evidence-based guidelines in this respect are lacking.[63–70] There is, however, some evidence supporting early institution of feeding in patients with severe brain injury. Indeed, one prospective randomized controlled trial demonstrated that early enteral nutrition accelerated neurological recovery and reduced major complications.[71] Of note, most studies in this area only report nutritional and not clinical outcomes.

### Options for delivery of nutritional support: enteral versus parenteral

Enteral feeding is preferred not only during rehabilitation but also in intensive care settings. The advantages of enteral nutrition over total parenteral nutrition (TPN) are lower risks of hyperglycaemia and infection at a lower cost. Increased intracranial pressure and the severity of the brain injury may affect the ability to initiate enteral feeding.[72] This delay in feeding has been attributed to larger gastric residuals, delay in gastric emptying, prolonged paralytic ileus, abdominal distension, aspiration pneumonitis and diarrhoea.[60,73–77] The use of sedating agents exacerbates these motility problems. Indeed, barbiturates have been associated with a failure in enteral feeding in virtually 100% of patients.[78] Pro-kinetic agents such as metoclopramide or erythromycin may help establish early enteral nutrition in patients with large gastric residuals, but a few will require post-pyloric feeding and occasionally TPN.[74,79]

The initiation and absorption of enteral feeds in the clinical setting are determined by measurements of gastric residual volume along with other clinical signs of impairment. The reported criteria of gastrointestinal intolerance varies between studies, with most recommending a residual volume below 200 ml and checking every 2–8 hours or a total amount of residual volumes per day of 500–700 ml.[66,69,71,76] There are several options available to administer enteral support. Apart from the oro/naso-gastric route, percutaneous endoscopic gastrostomy or jejunostomy tubes are currently the standard, although percutaneous gastro-jejunostomy tubes are gaining favour.[80–82] Radiological guidance with insufflation of the upper gastrointestinal tract via a nasogastric tube (RIG) can be used as an alternative to the endoscopic approach (PEG) for placement of percutaneous feeding tubes.

## Stress ulceration prophylaxis

The increased incidence of ileus in patients with traumatic brain injury also increases the risk of stress ulceration. Meta analysis has suggested that, until critically ill patients are absorbing enteral nutrition, ulcer prophylaxis should be prescribed.[83] The anti-histamine ranitidine has been shown to be more effective than sucralfate.[84] Proton pump inhibitors like omeprazole have not been compared to ranitidine in this group of patients but their superiority in other areas of clinical practice makes them a popular choice.

## Total parenteral nutrition

Some investigators report that early parenteral nutritional support improves the outcome after head injury.[85] Others have shown that, with nearly equivalent quantities of feeding, the mode of administration has no effect on neurologic outcome and either parenteral or enteral support is equally effective.[66,86,87] Animal data has suggested that administration of hyper-osmolar total parenteral nutrition and resultant hyperglycaemia may potentiate cerebral vasogenic oedema and increase neuronal damage after head injury.[88] However, clinical studies have shown that total parenteral nutrition can be given safely without causing serum hyperosmolality or affecting intracranial-pressure levels.[89] Since hyperglycaemia is associated with worse neurological outcome following brain injury, tight glycaemic control is essential regardless of nutritional route employed.[90–93]

## Early feeding and relation of caloric intake to patient outcome

Current data suggest that nutritional replacement should usually begin no later than 48 hours after injury, and full caloric replacement should be achieved by day 7.[63] In one study, the consequence of not meeting the metabolic needs for a 2-week period after injury was increased mortality when compared with patients who received full nutritional replacement of measured caloric expenditures by day 7.[85] In a subsequent study of brain-injured patients, full replacement at day 3 after injury versus late feeding by day 9 showed no changes in morbidity, but the outcomes after 3 months were better.[86]

A recent Cochrane review of nutritional support in head-injured patients, based on 11 RCTs, concluded that early feeding may be associated with a trend towards better outcomes in terms of survival and disability.[64] Early nutrition was associated with relative risk of death of 0.67 (0.41–1.07) and a relative risk of death or disability at the end of follow-up of 0.75 (0.50–1.11). The latest BTF guidelines make a level II recommendation that severely brain-injured patients should be fed to attain full calorific replacement by day 7 post injury.[65]

## Nitrogen losses

Nitrogen balance is usually defined as the difference between nitrogen intake and nitrogen excretion. For each gram of nitrogen measured in urine, 6.25 g of protein is catabolized. Optimal protein use has been found to be heavily dependent on the adequacy of caloric intake. After severe brain injury, energy requirements rise and nitrogen excretion increases.[87] In severely brain-injured patients, nitrogen catabolism is 14 to 25 g N/d.[80,92] The average nitrogen loss of a fasting, head-injured patient is double or triple that of a normal patient. This loss will produce a 10% decrease in lean mass in 7 days, and under-feeding for 2 to 3 weeks could result in a 30% weight loss.[94,95]

At a high range of nitrogen intake (>17 g/d), less than 50% of administered nitrogen is retained after head injury. Therefore, the level of nitrogen intake that generally results in less than 10 g of nitrogen loss per day is 15 to 17 g N/d. This is about 20% of the caloric composition of a 50 kcal/kg per day feeding protocol. Nitrogen equilibrium is seldom achieved; however, increasing the nitrogen content of feed from 14% to 20% does result in improved nitrogen retention.[96] The survival rate is better when an increased protein diet is begun within 1 to 10 days of injury versus the same diet administered more gradually or after a longer period.[66,86] Current recommendations for nutritional support in severe head injury include a high-protein diet (2 g/kg per d or about 15% of the total calorie value), which helps with nitrogen retention.

## Immune-enhancing nutrition

No studies to date have been published on the effects of immune-enhancing feeds in brain-injured patients.[97] The theoretical concepts involved are sound and animal data in head injury models are supportive of immune-enhancing diets. Further clinical investigations are needed in the area of isolated head injury using immune enhancing diets with an iso-nitrogenous control before any definitive conclusion can be made.

## Conclusion

Initiation of early feeding within the first 24 hours of head injury seems to reduce the relative risk of morbidity and mortality. Enteral feeding is the preferred mode of nutritional support, but data suggest that both parenteral and enteral modes are equally effective. A high protein diet is recommended.

## Fluid balance in head-injured patients

Fluid, electrolyte and metabolic consequences of severe head injury are profound. The goal of fluid management is homeostasis, i.e. to provide appropriate parenteral and/or enteral fluid to maintain intravascular volume, left ventricular filling pressure, cardiac output, blood pressure and ultimately oxygen delivery to the tissues, when normal physiological functions are often altered by surgical and traumatic stress as well as drugs. A specific aim is to prevent secondary neuronal damage due to inadequate oxygen delivery to the brain; this not only requires ventilation and oxygenation but an adequate cardiac output.

## Effects of intravenous fluids on the brain

Historically, fluid restriction was part of the management of head injury due to inherent fears about the possibilities of development of cerebral oedema due to damage of the blood–brain barrier and alteration of cerebral autoregulation. The reduction of oedema formation has been the mainstay of the 'Lund protocol' of head injury management with its emphasis on reduction of capillary hydrostatic pressure by reducing mean arterial pressure, cerebral blood volumes and negative fluid balance by the use of diuretics.[98,99] Clifton's work looked at critical factors associated with poor outcomes in a post-hoc analysis of the NABISH study.[100] It found that fluid balance less than – 594 ml in a 24 h period exerted significantly poorer outcome (P<0.001). Stepwise logistic regression showed effects of negative fluid balance were similar to GCS at admission when looking at outcome measures. However, the reasons ascribed were the purported increased mannitol use in patients who had higher intracranial pressures and lack of fluid replacement and thereby indicating more severe brain injuries. There are little data, apart from the Lund protocol, to support dehydration in brain injuries. Little rationale exists for dehydrating patients. There is no good evidence supporting fluid restriction as a means of limiting cerebral oedema after brain injury.[101] Dehydration increases sympathetic stimulation, metabolism and oxygen demand.[102] Some data exist as to the maintenance of euvolaemia avoiding predisposition to problems with elevated intracranial pressures. Indeed, adequate fluid replacement after head injury would maintain euvolemia and electrolyte levels. The therapeutic aim is now to maintain euvolemia and normal physiological indices, especially cerebral perfusion pressure. Animal studies support this approach.[103,104]

## Hypernatraemia in head-injured patients

Head injuries lead to altered homeostasis with the impairment of sodium regulation as one of the most common and significant abnormalities. Hypernatraemia is defined as plasma sodium concentration greater than 145 mmol/l. It is always associated with hyperosmolality and is caused by water depletion, excessive administration of sodium salts or a combination of the two.

Thirst mechanisms are absent in head-injured patients, which can lead to water-depleted states (renal, enteral and insensible). Head-injured patients may develop diabetes insipidus (DI) due to pituitary or hypothalamic dysfunction, and increased insensible water loss from central fever may also result in hypernatraemia. Other causes include the use of iodinated contrast media and severe hyperglycaemia.

Excessive administration of sodium salts may cause hypernatraemia through therapeutic misadventure or over-zealous administration of sodium in isotonic intravenous fluids.[105–113] In patients with raised ICP, hypernatraemia can result from the therapeutic use of osmotic diuretics by relative water loss (mannitol) as well as sodium ion administration (hypertonic saline).

Hypernatraemia due to osmotic therapy has been associated with an increased incidence of renal dysfunction, and is an independent predictor of morbidity and mortality, particularly when the peak serum sodium exceeds 160 mmol/l.[114–116]

Cranial DI following head injury leads to complete or partial failure of antidiuretic hormone (ADH) secretion. A very early onset is characteristic of major hypothalamic damage and is associated with a high mortality.[117] Head-injured patients with fractures involving the base of the skull and sella turcica appear to be at increased risk of DI.[118,119] The time of onset is variable, sometimes as early as 12–24 hours, but usually around 5–10 days after the injury.[120] In most cases onset is characterized by polyuria, hypernatraemia and plasma hyperosmolality. If the damage is limited to the pituitary or lower pituitary stalk, DI may only be transient. High stalk lesions or injury to the hypothalamus may cause permanent DI and the incidence of pituitary dysfunction in patients with mild, moderate and severe TBI has been reported to be 37.5%, 57.1% and 59.3%, respectively.[121]

Hypernatraemia leads to increased plasma osmolarity that leads to shrinkage of brain cells due to loss of water. With prolonged high plasma osmolarity, brain cells accumulate organic osmolytes such as polyols (e.g. sorbitol and myo-inositol), amino acids (e.g. alanine, glutamine, glutamate, taurine), and methylamines (e.g. glycerylphosphorylcholine and betaine). Rapid correction of chronic hypernatraemia can lead to the shift of water into the hyperosmolar brain cells and thus exacerbate cerebral edema.[122–124] A correction rate of hypernatraemia of about 12 mmol/l per day is recommended to avoid rebound cerebral oedema.[125]

## Diagnosis

Measuring serum and urine osmolalities facilitates diagnosing the cause of a hypernatraemic state.

### Normal concentration of urine (urine osmolality > 700 mosmol/l)

This suggests insufficient water intake, with or without excessive extrarenal water loss.

### Urine osmolality between 700 mosmol/l and plasma osmolality

This suggests partial cranial DI, osmotic diuresis, diuretic therapy, nephrogenic DI or renal failure.

### Urine osmolality below that of plasma

This suggests either complete cranial DI or nephrogenic DI. In milder cases urine osmolality may not be below that of plasma, and may be 300–600 mosmol/l.

Patients with cranial DI remain sensitive to exogenous ADH. Patients with partial DI have urinary volumes much less than those with complete DI.

In contrast to DI, a solute diuresis is usually accompanied by a higher urinary osmolality (between 250 and 320 mosmol/l).[126]

## Treatment

Pure water depletion is treated by water administration (NG route or intravenous fluids 5% dextrose). The rate of decrease in serum osmolality should be no greater than 2 mosmol/kg per h.[127,128] Hypernatraemia due to excess sodium is treated similarly with water/dextrose and a thiazide diuretic to encourage renal sodium loss.[129]

1. Calculate free water deficit:

    Free $H_2O$ deficit (litres) $= 0.6 \times$ (body weight [kg]) $\times$ ([[$Na^+$]/140] $-$ 1)

    e.g. if serum [$Na^+$] $= 154$ mmol/l in 75 kg male then deficit $= 4.5$ l of water.

2. Parenteral replacement of half of deficit immediately; remainder over 24–36 hours. Use 5% dextrose, **not** saline solutions.

3. Calculate maintenance fluid requirements and hourly urine output. Replace with 5% dextrose.

4. Aqueous vasopressin (AVP): If urine output remains excessive (>200–250 ml/h) in the absence of diuretics, or if maintenance of fluid balance is difficult or hyperosmolality is present give AVP 5–10 U s.c. or i.m.

5. Desmopressin (DDAVP) Synthetic analogue of AVP with longer half-life and fewer vasoconstrictive effects: 1–2 μg s.c. or i.v. every 12–24 h or by nasal insufflation of 5–20 μg every 12 h.

# Hyponatraemia in head-injured patients

Hyponatraemia (plasma [Na$^+$] <135 mmol/L) is seen in 5–12% of patients with severe head injury.[130] Severe hyponatraemia (<120 mmol/l) can cause significant and permanent neurological injury and death. Hyponatraemia may be isotonic, hypertonic or hypotonic, based on the measured plasma osmolality. The risk of hyponatraemia seems greater in those with severe head injuries, chronic subdural haematoma and basal skull fractures.[130,131] Deterioration in the level of consciousness, new focal deficits, myoclonus, seizures or increasing ICP could indicate the possibility of hyponatraemia in the brain-injured patient.

## Hypertonic hyponatraemia

Hyperglycaemia is common after head injuries and mannitol is used to control increased ICP. In patients with an increased amount of an impermeant solute, such as glucose or mannitol in extracellular fluid (ECF), osmotic equilibration occurs. Water moves down the osmotic gradient from the intracellular fluid (ICF) to the ECF, thus diluting the ECF (i.e. serum) sodium. In such circumstances, hyponatraemia is often associated with an elevated measured serum osmolality and treatment will depend on the value of the corrected [Na$^+$]. In the presence of hyperglycaemia this is derived from the formula:[132–135]

$$\text{Corrected } [Na^+] = \text{measured serum } [Na^+] + ([\text{serum glucose mmol/L} - 5.6] \times 0.288)$$

## Hypotonic hyponatraemia

Hypotonic hyponatraemia is a consequence of relative or absolute water excess, which can be iatrogenic in origin, or a relative excessive loss of sodium compared to water. Head injured patients are particularly susceptible to the detrimental effects of intravenous fluids such as 5% dextrose and 0.45% saline as they have an increase in the stimulation of ADH from hypovolemia, hypotension, pain, nausea or postoperative stress.[136–138] Low plasma osmolality causes osmotic pressure gradients across the brain cell membranes and leads to cellular swelling that may exacerbate contusions and diffuse axonal injuries. Hyponatraemic encephalopathy and cerebral oedema may eventually occur and result in centrally mediated non-cardiogenic pulmonary oedema, respiratory failure or cerebral herniation. Many changes in brain architecture are irreversible and therefore, prevention is the key. Normally the brain partially adapts to the hypo-osmolality within 24 hours, reducing the cerebral water excess by losing or inactivating intracellular osmotically active solutes but, in head-injured patients, re-adaptation may take some time (5–7 days).[127,139]

### Syndrome of inappropriate antidiuretic hormone secretion (SIADH)

This syndrome is defined as hypotonic hyponatraemia due to an elevated level of ADH non-commensurate with the prevailing osmotic or volume stimuli.[140,141] ADH secretion from the neurohypophysis is no longer under normal regulatory influences. SIADH is a form of dilutional hyponatraemia; ECF volume is usually increased by 3–4 litres but interstitial shifts do not occur and peripheral oedema is not seen due to unknown reasons. It is hypothesized that, due to the expanded ECF volume, glomerular filtration rate is increased and the renin – angiotensin – aldosterone mechanism is suppressed resulting in a decrease in the renal reabsorption of sodium.

### Cerebral salt wasting syndrome (CSW)

Peters et al. introduced the term cerebral salt wasting in 1950.[142] Some authors have doubted the existence of CSW as an independent entity.[143] However, it seems to be increasingly described in medical literature in the form of case series and anecdotal reports. Welt and Cort hypothesized in the 1950s that CSW was caused by a defect in direct neural regulation of renal tubular activity in the presence of intact hypothalamic–pituitary–adrenal axis.[144,145] It was also noted that patients were hypovolaemic as compared to euvolaemic or hypervolaemic. Cerebral infarction has also been reported in patients who have been fluid restricted due to hyponatraemia.[146]

The mechanism by which intracranial disease leads to CSW is not well understood. Many physicians have postulated that the most probable process involves the disruption of neural input into the kidney and/or the central elaboration of a circulating natriuretic factor.[147–152] Natriuretic peptides, direct neural effects and an ouabain-like compound have been implicated in the pathogenesis of CSW. Decreased sympathetic input to the kidney directly and indirectly alters salt and water management and may explain the natriuresis and diuresis seen within CSW.[147,150] A decrease in sympathetic tone leads to a decreased glomerular filtration rate, decreased renin release and a decrease in renal tubular sodium resorption.[153–156] In addition to a decreased neural input to the kidney, an ouabain-like compound in the brain may play a role in renal salt wasting though studies have shown that it may not be the sole intermediary of CSW. Circulating natriuretic peptides could contribute to the picture. Other mediators producing natriuresis are being investigated for their role in CSW.

## Diagnosis of hyponatraemia

The evaluation of hypotonic hyponatraemia requires clinical assessment of volume status and measurement of urinary indices. However, volume status can be difficult to assess clinically in a critically ill patient. Fall in body weight, large negative fluid balance, decrease in skin turgor and increase of blood urea nitrogen/creatinine ratio >20:1 may reflect fluid depletion. However, ECF volume may be affected by blood loss, the amount and type of fluid administered and the use of diuretics. Urinary [$Na^+$] measurements are affected by the use of osmotic and non-osmotic diuretics. When making the diagnosis of SIADH, it is essential to exclude other causes of hyponatraemia that commonly occur in neurological diseases such as oedematous states, recent diuretic therapy and hypovolaemic states. Moreover, the diagnosis of SIADH cannot be made in the presence of severe pain, nausea, stress or hypotension as these conditions can stimulate ADH secretion even in the presence of serum hypotonicity. All the changes in electrolyte imbalances observed in SIADH have also been described in CSW; however, the presence of signs of volume depletion (for example, decreased skin turgor or low central venous pressure) with salt wasting distinguishes CSW from SIADH.[157] In essence, the primary distinction between SIADH and CSW lies in the assessment of extracellular volume (ECV) status. SIADH is an expanded state of ECV due to ADH-mediated renal water retention; whereas CSW is characterized by a contracted state of ECV due to renal salt wasting. Additional laboratory evidence that relates to the ECV may also help distinguish SIADH from CSW. These include haemoconcentration, albumin concentration, blood urea nitrogen/creatinine ratio, potassium concentration, plasma rennin and aldosterone levels, atrial natriuretic factor, plasma urea concentration and central venous pressure.

# Treatment of hyponatraemia

Management of hyponatraemia depends on the presence and assessment of severity of symptoms (acute, chronic) and determination of the most appropriate treatment strategy based on volume status. It can include:

- Fluid restrict to 500 ml/day or less (in SIADH if possible, **not** CSW)
- Hypertonic saline (50–70 mmol/h)
- Diuresis of 160 ml/h or greater
- Rate of correction: no greater than 20 mmol/l per day (1–2 mmol/l per h)
- Seizures: 100–250 mmol hypertonic saline over 10 min

The rate of correction of acute hyponatraemia should be no greater than 1–2 mmol/l per h of sodium until the plasma level has increased to 120 mmol/l or by a maximum of 20 mmol/l during the first 24 hours.[127] This is achieved initially by intravenous administration of hypertonic saline given at 50–70 mmol/h. It is important to note that the purpose of using hypertonic saline is not to correct a saline deficit, as there is no deficit in total body sodium, but rather the hypertonicity draws water into the intravascular compartment and reduces brain oedema. A spontaneous or loop diuretic-induced diuresis is then required to excrete the water load.

If the hyponatraemia presents with convulsions, then urgent correction of the cerebral oedema using 250 mmol of hypertonic saline over 10 minutes can be used. This will immediately elevate the plasma sodium in adults by about 7 mmol/l.[148]

If fluid deprivation is difficult to sustain in patients with SIADH, then patients with hyponatraemia and chronic congestive cardiac failure may benefit from an angiotensin converting enzyme inhibitor added to the loop diuretic. This will inhibit the stimulation of thirst and ADH release by angiotensin II.[158,159] However, in these patients a direct ADH inhibitor such as phenytoin may be of greater value.[160] This has been used to reduce ADH release from the hypophysis in patients with SIADH due to CNS disorders including head injury.[161] Pharmacological treatment has been tried with demeclocycline, which inhibits ADH action on renal tubules and increases excretion of solute-free urine but is slow and associated with nephrotoxicity. Lithium has been considered but is associated with numerous side effects.

The objectives of treatment of CSW are volume replacement and maintenance of a positive salt balance. Intravenous hydration with normal saline, hypertonic saline or oral salt may be used alone or in combination.[162–166] Rapid correction of hyponatraemia is associated with pontine myelinolysis but the optimum rate is unclear. A cautious approach is to raise the serum sodium by 0.5–1 mmol/l per h for a maximum total daily change not exceeding 20 mmol/l. Management aims primarily at repletion of plasma volume. It should be kept in mind that signs of volume depletion may be masked by the high catecholamine state of the patient. Volume restriction (as for SIADH) is definitely contraindicated. The hypotonic state should be treated with additional sodium, often requiring the administration of hypertonic saline. The concomitant administration of a loop diuretic and saline is rarely adequate. The administration of 5% albumin may be beneficial.

Increasing salt intake during CSW may further enhance salt excretion and some authors advise the use of fludrocortisone to enhance renal tubular sodium reabsorption and hence reduce the incidence of a negative sodium balance.[146] Careful observation and monitoring is required as fludrocortisone use is associated with pulmonary oedema, hypokalaemia and hypertension.

# Complications of treatment of hyponatraemia

The complications reported with the use of hypertonic saline include congestive cardiac failure, intracerebral and subdural haemorrhages and cerebral pontine myelinolysis. To reduce the incidence of congestive cardiac failure, invasive haemodynamic monitoring should occur throughout its administration.

Rapid correction of hyponatraemia may lead to central pontine and extrapontine myelinolysis. The lesions of central pontine myelinolysis are caused by the destruction of myelin sheaths in the centre of the basilar portion of the pons and may extend from the midbrain to the lower pons. The clinical features range from coma, flaccid quadriplegia, facial weakness and pseudobulbar palsy to minor behavioural changes without focal findings. The onset may be from one to several days after the hyponatraemia has been corrected and may require MRI to confirm the diagnosis.[167]

# New therapies

New AVP receptor antagonists are undergoing trials in the treatment of hyponatraemia. Conivaptan which blocks V1 and V2 receptors has received FDA approval for treatment of euvolemic hyponatraemia in hospitalized patients, especially those with SIADH.[168] It acts by stimulating free water excretion and has been shown to improve plasma sodium concentration. Randomized controlled trials have shown significant improvement after its use at intravenous doses of 40 or 80 mg/day via infusion in one i.v. and two oral studies.[168] Lixivaptan and tolvaptan, which inhibit V2 receptors only, are undergoing phase III trials.

# Conclusion

Deranged fluid homeostasis is a common occurrence after severe head injury. Careful examination supplemented with plasma and urinary analysis enables the pathophysiology to be understood, permitting a logical management pathway to be implemented.

# References

1. Zygun DA, Kortbeek JB, Fick GH, Laupland KB, Doig CJ. Non-neurologic organ dysfunction in severe traumatic brain injury. *Crit Care Med* 2005; **33**: 654–60.
2. Zygun D. Non-neurological organ dysfunction in neurocritical care: impact on outcome and etiological considerations. *Curr Opin Crit Care* 2005; **11**: 139–43.
3. Lim HB, Smith M. Systemic complications after head injury: a clinical review. *Anaesthesia* 2007; **62**: 474–82.
4. Macmillan CS, Grant IS, Andrews PJ. Pulmonary and cardiac sequelae of subarachnoid haemorrhage: time for active management? *Intens Care Med* 2002; **28**: 1012–23.
5. Dujardin KS, McCully RB, Wijdicks EF *et al.* Myocardial dysfunction associated with brain death: clinical, echocardiographic, and pathologic features. *J Heart Lung Transpl* 2001; **20**: 350–7.
6. Huttemann E, Schelenz C, Chatzinikolaou K, Reinhart K. Left ventricular dysfunction in lethal severe brain injury: impact of transesophageal echocardiography on patient management. *Intens Care Med* 2002; **28**: 1084–8.
7. Connor RC. Myocardial damage secondary to brain lesions. *Am Heart J* 1969; **78**: 145–8.
8. Cohen HB, Gambill AF, Eggers GW Jr. Acute pulmonary edema following head injury: two case reports. *Anesth Analg* 1977; **56**: 136–9.
9. Graf CJ, Rossi NP. Catecholamine response to intracranial hypertension. *J Neurosurg* 1978; **49**: 862–8.
10. Deehan SC, Grant IS. Haemodynamic changes in neurogenic pulmonary oedema: effect of dobutamine. *Intens Care Med* 1996; **22**: 672–6.

11. The Brain Trauma Foundation and the Joint Section of the American Association of Neurological Surgeons and Congress of Neurological Surgeons on Neurotrauma and Critical Care. Guidelines for the Management of Severe Traumatic Brain Injury. 3rd edition. IX Cerebral Perfusion Thresholds. *J Neurotrauma* 2007; **24** (suppl 1): S59–64.

12. Contant CF, Valadka AB, Gopinath SP, Hannay HJ, Robertson CS. Adult respiratory distress syndrome: a complication of induced hypertension after severe head injury. *J Neurosurg* 2001; **95**: 560–8.

13. Stover JF, Steiger P, Stocker R. Controversial issues concerning norepinephrine and intensive care following severe traumatic brain injury. *Eur J Trauma* 2006; **32**: 10–27.

14. Sakr Y, Reinhart K, Vincent JL et al. Does dopamine administration in shock influence outcome? Results of the Sepsis Occurrence in Acutely Ill Patients (SOAP) Study. *Crit Care Med* 2006; **34**: 589–97.

15. Steiner LA, Johnston AJ, Czosnyka M et al. Direct comparison of cerebrovascular effects of norepinephrine and dopamine in head-injured patients. *Crit Care Med* 2004; **32**: 1049–54.

16. Patel BM, Chittock DR, Russell JA, Walley KR. Beneficial effects of short-term vasopressin infusion during severe septic shock. *Anesthesiology* 2002; **96**: 576–82.

17. Russell J. Hemodynamic support of sepsis. Vasopressin versus norepinephrine for septic shock. *Program and abstracts of the Society of Critical Care Medicine 36th Critical Care Congress*; 2007; Orlando, Florida.

18. Yeh CC, Wu CT, Lu CH, Yang CP, Wong CS. Early use of small-dose vasopressin for unstable hemodynamics in an acute brain injury patient refractory to catecholamine treatment: a case report. *Anesth Analg* 2003; **97**: 577–579.

19. Bradley P, Hiler M, Menon D, Yeh CC, Wu CT, Wong CS. Vasopressin in acute brain injury: a note of caution. *Anesth Analg* 2004; **98**: 872–3.

20. Totaro RJ, Raper RF. Epinephrine-induced lactic acidosis following cardiopulmonary bypass. *Crit Care Med* 1997; **25**: 1693–9.

21. Acquarolo A, Urli T, Perone G, Giannotti C, Candiani A, Latronico N. Antibiotic prophylaxis of early onset pneumonia in critically ill comatose patients: a randomized study. *Intens Care Med* 2005; **31**: 510–16.

22. Bronchard R, Albaladejo P, Brezac G et al. Early onset pneumonia: risk factors and consequences in head trauma patients. *Anesthesiology* 2004; **100**: 234–9.

23. Henderson WR, Dhingra VK, Chittock DR, Fenwick JC, Ronco JJ. Hypothermia in the management of traumatic brain injury. A systematic review and meta-analysis. *Intens Care Med* 2003; **29**: 1637–44.

24. Drakulovic MB, Torres A, Bauer TT, Nicolas JM, Nogue S, Ferrer M. Supine body position as a risk factor for nosocomial pneumonia in mechanically ventilated patients: a randomised trial. *Lancet* 1999; **354**: 1851–8.

25. Ewig S, Torres A. Prevention and management of ventilator-associated pneumonia. *Curr Opin Crit Care* 2002; **8**: 58–69.

26. Young PJ, Pakeerathan S, Blunt MC, Subramanya S. A low-volume, low-pressure tracheal tube cuff reduces pulmonary aspiration. *Crit Care Med* 2006; **34**: 632–9.

27. Sirvent JM, Torres A, El-Ebiary M, Castro P, de Batlle J, Bonet A. Protective effect of intravenously administered cefuroxime against nosocomial pneumonia in patients with structural coma. *Am J Respir Crit Care Med* 1997; **155**: 1729–34.

28. The Brain Trauma Foundation and the Joint Section of the American Association of Neurological Surgeons and Congress of Neurological Surgeons on Neurotrauma and Critical Care. Guidelines for the Management of Severe Traumatic Brain Injury. 3rd Edition. IV Infection Prophylaxis. *J Neurotrauma* 2007; **24** (suppl 1): S26–31.

29. de Jonge E, Schultz MJ, Spanjaard L et al. Effects of selective decontamination of digestive tract on mortality and acquisition of resistant bacteria in intensive care: a randomised controlled trial. *Lancet* 2003; **362**: 1011–16.

30. Liberati A, D'Amico R, Pifferi, Torri V, Brazzi L. Antibiotic prophylaxis to reduce respiratory tract infections and mortality in adults receiving intensive care. *Cochrane Database Syst Rev* 2004(**1**): CD000022.

31. Chan EY, Ruest A, Meade MO, Cook DJ. Oral decontamination for prevention of pneumonia in mechanically ventilated adults: systematic review and meta-analysis. *Br Med J* 2007; **334**: 889–900.

32. Bratton SL, Davis RL. Acute lung injury in isolated traumatic brain injury. *Neurosurgery* 1997; **40**: 707–12.

33. Holland MC, Mackersie RC, Morabito D, *et al.* The development of acute lung injury is associated with worse neurologic outcome in patients with severe traumatic brain injury. *J Trauma* 2003; **55**: 106–11.

34. The Acute Respiratory Distress Syndrome Network. Ventilation with lower tidal volumes as compared with traditional tidal volumes for acute lung injury and the acute respiratory distress syndrome. *N Engl J Med* 2000; **342**: 1301–8.

35. Caricato A, Conti G, Della Corte F *et al.* Effects of PEEP on the intracranial system of patients with head injury and subarachnoid hemorrhage: the role of respiratory system compliance. *J Trauma* 2005; **58**: 571–6.

36. Huynh T, Messer M, Sing RF, Miles W, Jacobs DG, Thomason MH. Positive end-expiratory pressure alters intracranial and cerebral perfusion pressure in severe traumatic brain injury. *J Trauma* 2002; **53**: 488–92.

37. Salim A, Miller K, Dangleben D, Cipolle M, Pasquale M. High-frequency percussive ventilation: an alternative mode of ventilation for head-injured patients with adult respiratory distress syndrome. *J Trauma* 2004; **57**: 542–6.

38. Mallick A, Elliot S, McKinlay J, Bodenham A. Extracorporeal carbon dioxide removal using the Novalung in a patient with intracranial bleeding. *Anaesthesia* 2007; **62**: 72–4.

39. Dellinger RP, Carlet JM, Masur H, *et al.* Surviving Sepsis Campaign guidelines for management of severe sepsis and septic shock. *Crit Care Med* 2004; **32**: 858–73.

40. Geerts WH, Pineo GF, Heit JA, *et al.* Prevention of venous thromboembolism: the Seventh ACCP Conference on Antithrombotic and Thrombolytic Therapy. *Chest* 2004; **126**: 338S–400S.

41. Kim J, Gearhart MM, Zurick A, Zuccarello M, James L, Luchette FA. Preliminary report on the safety of heparin for deep venous thrombosis prophylaxis after severe head injury. *J Trauma* 2002; **53**: 38–42.

42. Dickinson LD, Miller LD, Patel CP, Gupta SK. Enoxaparin increases the incidence of postoperative intracranial hemorrhage when initiated preoperatively for deep venous thrombosis prophylaxis in patients with brain tumors. *Neurosurgery* 1998; **43**: 1074–81.

43. Norwood SH, McAuley CE, Berne JD *et al.* Prospective evaluation of the safety of enoxaparin prophylaxis for venous thromboembolism in patients with intracranial hemorrhagic injuries. *Arch Surg* 2002; **137**: 696–701.

44. Vincent JL, Bihari DJ, Suter PM *et al.* The prevalence of nosocomial infection in intensive care units in Europe: results of the European Prevalence of Infection in Intensive Care (EPIC) Study. EPIC International Advisory Committee. *J Am Med Assoc* 1995; **274**: 639–44.

45. Simpson TP, Day CJ, Jewkes CF, Manara AR. The impact of percutaneous tracheostomy on intensive care unit practice and training. *Anaesthesia* 1999; **54**: 186–9.

46. Plummer AL, Gracey DR. Consensus conference on artificial airways in patients receiving mechanical ventilation. *Chest* 1989; **96**: 178–80.

47. Griffiths J, Barber VS, Morgan L, Young JD. Systematic review and meta-analysis of studies of the timing of tracheostomy in adult patients undergoing artificial ventilation. *Br Med J* 2005; **330**: 1243–8.

48. Bouderka MA, Fakhir B, Bouaggad A, Hmamouchi B, Hamoudi D, Harti A. Early tracheostomy versus prolonged endotracheal intubation in severe head injury. *J Trauma* 2004; **57**: 251–4.

49. Barquist ES, Amortegui J, Hallal A *et al.* Tracheostomy in ventilator dependent trauma patients: a prospective, randomized intention-to-treat study. *J Trauma* 2006; **60**: 91–7.

50. The Tracman Study http://www.tracman. org.uk/pdf/summary-protocol.pdf.

51. Patel C. The anaesthetic aspects of performing percutaneous tracheostomies in intensive care: report of a postal survey. *Brit J Anaesth* 2000; **84**: 684P–5P.

52. Freeman BD, Isabella K, Lin N, Buchman TG. A meta-analysis of prospective trials

comparing percutaneous and surgical tracheostomy in critically ill patients. *Chest* 2000; **118**: 1412–18.

53. Stocchetti N, Parma A, Lamperti M, Songa V, Tognini L. Neurophysiological consequences of three tracheostomy techniques: a randomized study in neurosurgical patients. *J Neurosurg Anesthesiol* 2000; **12**: 307–13.

54. Reilly PM, Sing RF, Giberson FA *et al.* Hypercarbia during tracheostomy: a comparison of percutaneous endoscopic, percutaneous Doppler, and standard surgical tracheostomy. *Intens Care Med* 1997; **23**: 859–64.

55. Byhahn C. A useful and safe intervention: current techniques of percutaneous tracheostomy. *Int J Intens Care* 2003; **10**: 155–65.

56. Koitschev A, Simon C, Blumenstock G, Mach H, Graumuller S. Suprastomal tracheal stenosis after dilational and surgical tracheostomy in critically ill patients. *Anaesthesia* 2006; **61**: 832–7.

57. Law RC, Carney AS, Manara AR. Long-term outcome after percutaneous dilational tracheostomy. Endoscopic and spirometry findings. *Anaesthesia* 1997; **52**: 51–6.

58. Keren O, Cohen M, Lazar-Zweker I, Groswasser Z. Tracheotomy in severe TBI patients: sequelae and relation to vocational outcome. *Brain Inj* 2001; **15**: 531–6.

59. Coplin WM, Pierson DJ, Cooley KD, Newell DW, Rubenfeld GD. Implications of extubation delay in brain-injured patients meeting standard weaning criteria. *Am J Respir Crit Care Med* 2000; **161**: 1530–6.

60. Ott L, Young B, McClain CJ. The metabolic response to brain injury. *J Parenter Enteral Nutr* 1987; **11**: 488–93.

61. Clifton GL, Robertson CS, Grossman RG, Hodge S, Foltz R, Garza C. The metabolic response to severe head injury. *J Neurosurg* 1984; **60**: 687–96.

62. Deutschman CS, Konstantinides FN, Raup S, Thienprasit P, Cerra FB. Physiological and metabolic response to isolated closed-head injury. Part 1: Basal metabolic state: correlations of metabolic and physiological parameters with fasting and stressed controls. *J Neurosurg* 1986; **64**: 89–98.

63. Twyman D. Nutritional management of the critically ill neurologic patient. *Crit Care Clin* 1997; **13**: 39–49.

64. Perel P, Yanagawa T, Bunn F, Roberts I, Wentz R, Pierro A. Nutritional support for head-injured patients. *Cochrane Database of Systematic Reviews* 2006; **4**: CD001530.

65. The Brain Trauma Foundation and the Joint Section of the American Association of Neurological Surgeons and Congress of Neurological Surgeons on Neurotrauma and Critical Care. Guidelines for the Management of Severe Traumatic Brain Injury. 3rd edition. XII Nutrition. *J Neurotrauma* 2007; **24**: S77–82.

66. Borzotta AP, Pennings J, Papasadero B, *et al.* Enteral versus parenteral nutrition after severe closed head injury. *J Trauma* 1994; **37**: 459–68.

67. Hatton J, Rapp RP, Kudsk KA *et al.* Intravenous insulin-like growth factor-I (IGF-I) in moderate-to-severe head injury: a phase II safety and efficacy trial. *J Neurosurg* 1997; **86**: 779–86.

68. Kudsk KA, Mowatt-Larssen C, Bukar J *et al.* Effect of recombinant human insulin-like growth factor I and early total parenteral nutrition on immune depression following severe head injury. *Arch Surg* 1994; **129**: 66–70.

69. Minard G, Kudsk KA, Melton S, Patton JH, Tolley EA. Early versus delayed feeding with an immune-enhancing diet in patients with severe head injuries. *J Parenter Enteral Nutr* 2000; **24**: 145–9.

70. Sacks GS, Brown RO, Teague D, Dickerson RN, Tolley EA, Kudsk KA. Early nutrition support modifies immune function in patients sustaining severe head injury. *J Parenter Enteral Nutr* 1995; **19**: 387–92.

71. Taylor SJ, Fettes SB, Jewkes C, Nelson RJ. Prospective, randomized, controlled trial to determine the effect of early enhanced enteral nutrition on clinical outcome in mechanically ventilated patients suffering head injury. *Crit Care Med* 1999; **27**: 2525–31.

72. Norton JA, Ott LG, McClain C *et al.* Intolerance to enteral feeding in the brain-injured patient. *J Neurosurg* 1988; **68**: 62–6.

73. Ott L, Young B, Phillips R *et al.* Altered gastric emptying in the head injured

patients: relationship to feeding intolerance. *J Neurosurg* 1991; **74**: 738–42.

74. Marino LV, Kiratu EM, French S, Nathoo N. To determine the effect of metoclopramide on gastric emptying in severe head injuries: a prospective, randomized, controlled clinical trial. *Br J Neurosurg* 2003; **17**: 24–8.

75. Kao CH, ChangLai SP, Chieng PU, Yen TC. Gastric emptying in head-injured patients. *Am J Gastroenterol* 1998; **93**: 1108–12.

76. Klodell CT, Carroll M, Carrillo EH, Spain DA. Routine intragastric feeding following traumatic brain injury is safe and well tolerated. *Am J Surg* 2000; **179**: 168–71.

77. Saxe JM, Ledgerwood AM, Lucas CE, Lucas WF. Lower esophageal sphincter dysfunction precludes safe gastric feeding after head injury. *J Trauma* 1994; **37**: 581–4.

78. Bochicchio GV, Bochicchio K, Nehman S, Casey C, Andrews P, Scalea TM. Tolerance and efficacy of enteral nutrition in traumatic brain-injured patients induced into barbiturate coma. *J Parenter Enteral Nutr* 2006; **30**: 503–6.

79. Reignier J, Bensaid S, Perrin-Gachadoat D, Burdin M, Boiteau R, Tenaillon A. Erythromycin and early enteral nutrition in mechanically ventilated patients. *Crit Care Med* 2002; **30**: 1237–41.

80. Akkersdijk WL, Roukema JA, van der Werken C. Percutaneous endoscopic gastrostomy for patients with severe cerebral injury. *Injury* 1998; **29**: 11–14.

81. McGonigal MD, Lucas CE, Ledgerwood AM. Feeding jejunostomy in patients who are critically ill. *Surg Gynecol Obstet* 1989; **168**: 275–7.

82. Kirby DF, Clifton GL, Turner H, Marion DW, Barrett J, Gruemer HD. Early enteral nutrition after brain injury by percutaneous endoscopic gastrojejunostomy. *J Parenter Enteral Nutr* 1991; **15**: 298–302.

83. Cook DJ, Reeve BK, Guyatt GH *et al.* Stress ulcer prophylaxis in critically ill patients. Resolving discordant meta-analyses. *J Am Med Assoc* 1996; **275**: 308–14.

84. Cook D, Guyatt G, Marshall J *et al.* A comparison of sucralfate and ranitidine for the prevention of upper gastrointestinal bleeding in patients requiring mechanical ventilation. *N Engl J Med* 1998; **338**: 791–7.

85. Rapp RP, Young B, Twyman D *et al.* The favorable effect of early parenteral feeding on survival in head-injured patients. *J Neurosurg* 1983; **58**: 906–12.

86. Young B, Ott L, Twyman D *et al.* The effect of nutritional support on outcome from severe head injury. *J Neurosurg* 1987; **67**: 668–76.

87. Hadley MN, Grahm TW, Harrington T, Schiller WR, McDermott MK, Posillico DB. Nutritional support and neurotrauma: a critical review of early nutrition in forty-five acute head injury patients. *Neurosurgery* 1986; **19**: 367–73.

88. Waters DC, Hoff JT, Black KL. Effect of parenteral nutrition on cold-induced vasogenic edema in cats. *J Neurosurg* 1986; **64**: 460–5.

89. Young B, Ott L, Haack D *et al.* Effect of total parenteral nutrition upon intracranial pressure in severe head injury. *J Neurosurg* 1987; **67**: 76–80.

90. Cherian L, Goodman JC, Robertson CS. Hyperglycaemia increases brain injury caused by secondary ischemia after cortical impact injury in rats. *Crit Care Med* 1997; **25**: 1378–83.

91. Lam AM, Winn HR, Cullen BF *et al.* Hyperglycaemia and neurological outcome in patients with head injury. *J Neurosurg* 1991; **75**: 545–51.

92. Young B, Ott L, Dempsey R *et al.* Relationship between admission hyperglycaemia and neurologic outcome of severely brain-injured patients. *Ann Surg* 1989; **210**: 466–73.

93. Van den Berhe G, Wouters P, Weekers F *et al.* Intensive insulin therapy in critically ill patients. *N Engl J Med* 2001; **345**: 1359–67.

94. Gadisseux P, Ward JD, Young HF, Becker DR. Nutrition and the neurosurgical patient. *J Neurosurg* 1984; **60**: 219–32.

95. Duke JH Jr, Jorgensen SB, Broell JR, Long CL, Kinney JM. Contribution of protein to caloric expenditure following injury. *Surgery* 1970; **68**: 168–74.

96. Clifton GL, Robertson CS, Contant CF. Enteral hyperalimentation in head injury. *J Neurosurg.* 1985; **62**: 186–93.

97. Montejo JC, Zarazaga A, Lopez-Martinez J *et al.* Immunonutrition in the intensive care unit. A systematic review and consensus statement. *Clin Nutr* 2003; **22**: 221–33.

**147**

98. Wahlstrom MR, Olivecrona M, Koskinen LO, Rydenhag B, Naredi S. Severe traumatic brain injury in pediatric patients: treatment and outcome using an intracranial pressure targeted therapy – the Lund concept. *Intens Care Med* 2005; **31**(6): 832–9.

99. Grande PO. Pathophysiology of brain insult. Therapeutic implications with the Lund Concept. *Schweiz Med Wochenschr* 2000; **130**(42): 1538–43.

100. Clifton GL, Miller ER, Choi SC, Levin HS. Fluid thresholds and outcome from severe brain injury. *Crit Care Med* 2002; **30**(4): 739–45.

101. Morse ML, Milstein JM, Haas JE *et al.* Effect of hydration on experimentally induced cerebral edema. *Crit Care Med* 1985; **13**(7): 563.

102. Beckstead JE, Tweed WA, Lee J *et al.* Cerebral blood flow and metabolism in man following cardiac arrest. *Stroke* 1978; **9**(6): 569.

103. Smith SD, Cone JB, Bowser BH *et al.* Cerebral edema following acute haemorrhage in a murine model: the role of crystalloid resuscitation. *J Trauma* 1982; **22**(7): 588.

104. Ito U, Ohno K, Nakamura R *et al.* Brain edema during ischaemia and after restoration of blood flow. *Stroke* 1979; **10**(5): 542.

105. Adrogue H, Madias N. Hypernatremia. *N Engl J Med* 2000; **342**; 1493–99.

106. Borra S, Beredo R, Kleinfeld M. Hypernatremia in the aging: causes, manifestations, and outcome, *J Natl Med Assoc* 1995; **87**: 220–4.

107. Kumar S, Berl T. Sodium. *Lancet* 1998; **352**: 220–8.

108. Long CA, Marin P, Bayer AJ *et al.* Hypernatraemia in an adult in-patient population. *Postgrad Med J* 1991; **67**: 643–5.

109. Palevsky P, Bhagrath R, Greenberg A. Hypernatremia in hospitalised patients. *Ann Intern Med* 1996; **124**: 197–203.

110. Palevsky P. Hypernatremia. *Semin Nephrol* 1998; **18**: 20–30.

111. Ross EJ, Christie SB. Hypernatremia. *Medicine (Baltimore)* 1969; **48**: 441–73.

112. Snyder N, Feigal DW, Arieff AI. Hypernatremia in elderly patients. A heterogeneous, morbid, and iatrogenic entity. *Ann Intern Med* 1987; **107**: 309–19.

113. Milionis HJ, Liamis G, Elisaf MS. Hypernatremia in hospitalised patients: a sequel of inadvertent fluid administration. *Arch Intern Med* 2000; **160**: 1541–2.

114. Valadka A, Robertson CS. Should we be using hypertonic saline to treat intracranial hypertension? *Crit Care Med* 2000; **28**: 1245–6.

115. Polderman KH, Schreuder WO, Strack van Schijndel RJ, Thijs LG. Hypernatremia in the intensive care unit: an indicator of quality of care? *Crit Care Med* 1999; **27**: 1105–8.

116. Aiyagari V, Deibert E, Diringer MN. Hypernatremia in the neurologic intensive care unit: how high is too high? *J Crit Care* 2006; **21**: 163–72.

117. Seckl JR, Dunger DB, Lightman SL. Neurohypophyseal function during early post-operative diabetes insipidus. *Brain* 1987; **110**: 737–46.

118. Crompton MR. Hypothalamic lesions following closed head injury. *Brain* 1971; **94**: 165–72.

119. Edwards OM, Clark JD. Post-traumatic hypopituitarism. Six cases and a review of the literature. *Medicine (Baltimore)* 1986; **65**: 281–90.

120. Kern K, Meislin H. Diabetes insipidus: occurrence after minor head trauma. *J Trauma* 1984; **24**: 69–72.

121. Bondanelli M, De Marinis L, Ambrosio MR *et al.* Occurrence of pituitary dysfunction following traumatic brain injury. *J Neurotrauma* 2004; **21**: 685–96.

122. De Petris L, Luchetti A, Emma F. Cell volume regulation and transport mechanisms across the blood-brain barrier: implications for the management of hypernatraemic states. *Eur J Pediatr* 2001; **160**: 71–7.

123. Gullans SR, Verbalis JG. Control of brain volume during hyperosmolar and hypoosmolar conditions. *Annu Rev Med* 1993; **44**: 289–301.

124. McManus ML, Churchwell KB, Strange K. Regulation of cell volume in health and disease. *N Engl J Med* 1995; **333**: 1260–6.

125. Oterno MH. Hypernatremia in the intensive care unit: instant quality – just add water. *Crit Care Med* 1999; **27**: 1041–2.

126. Shucart WA, Jackson I. Management of diabetes insipidus in neurosurgical patients. *J Neurosurg* 1976; **44**: 65–71.

127. Arieff AI. Central nervous system manifestations of disordered sodium metabolism. *Clin Endocrinol Metab* 1984; **13**: 269–94.

128. Arieff AI, Guisado R. Effects on the central nervous system of hypernatremic and hyponatremic states. *Kidney Int* 1976; **10**: 104–16.

129. Addleman M, Pollard A, Grossman RF. Survival after severe hypernatremia due to salt ingestion by an adult. *Am J Med* 1985; **78**: 176–8.

130. Steinbok P, Thompson GB. Metabolic disturbances after head injury: Abnormalities of sodium and water balance with special reference to the effects of alcohol intoxication. *Neurosurgery* 1978; **3**: 9–15.

131. Doczi T, Tarjanyi J, Huszka E, Kiss J. Syndrome of inappropriate secretion of antidiuretic hormone (SIADH) after head injury. *Neurosurgery* 1982; **10**: 685–8.

132. Katz MA. Hyperglycemia-induced hyponatraemia – calculation of expected serum sodium depression. *N Engl J Med* 1973; **289**: 843–4.

133. Crandall ED. Serum sodium response to hyperglycemia. *N Engl J Med* 1974; **290**: 465.

134. Jenkins PG, Larmore C. Hyperglycemia-induced hyponatremia. *N Engl J Med* 1974; **290**: 573.

135. Robin AP, Ing TS, Lancaster GA *et al.* Hyperglycemia-induced hyponatremia: a fresh look. *Clin Chem* 1979; **25**: 496–7.

136. Hayes MA. Water and electrolyte therapy after operation. *N Engl J Med* 1968; **278**: 1054–6.

137. Chung HM, Kluge R, Schrier RW, Anderson RJ. Postoperative hyponatraemia. A prospective study. *Arch Intl Med* 1986; **146**: 333–6.

138. Sinnatamby C, Edwards CRW, Kitau M, Irving MH. Antidiuretic hormone response to high and conservative fluid regimens in patients undergoing operation. *Surg Gynecol Obstet* 1974; **139**: 715–19.

139. Arieff AI, Llach F, Massry SG. Neurological manifestations and morbidity of hyponatraemia: correlation with brain water and electrolytes. *Medicine* 1976; **55**: 121–9.

140. Robinson, AG. Disorders of antidiuretic hormone secretion. *Clin Endocrinol Metabolism* 1985; **14**: 55–88.

141. Robertson GL. Syndrome of inappropriate antidiuresis. *N Engl J Med* 1989; **321**: 538–9.

142. Peters JP, Welt LG, Sims EA, Orloff J, Needham J. A salt-wasting syndrome associated with cerebral disease. *Trans Assoc Am Physicians* 1950; **63**: 57–64.

143. Oh MS, Carroll HJ. Disorders of sodium metabolism:hypernatraemia and hyponatraemia. *Crit Care Med* 1992; **20**: 94–103.

144. Welt LG, Seldin DW, Nelson WP, German WJ, Peters JP. Role of the central nervous system in metabolism of electrolytes and water. *AMA Arch Intern Med* 1952; **90**: 355–378.

145. Cort JH. Cerebral Salt Wasting. *Lancet* 1954; **266**: 752–4.

146. Wijdicks EF, Vermeulen M, Hijdra A, van Gijn J. Hyponatremia and cerebral infarction in patients with ruptured intracranial aneurysms: is fluid restriction harmful? *Ann Neurol* 1985; **17**: 137–40.

147. Harrigan MR. Cerebral salt wasting syndrome. *Crit Care Clin* 2001; **17**: 125–38.

148. Harrigan MR. Cerebral salt wasting syndrome: a review. *Neurosurgery* 1996; **38**: 152–60.

149. Lolin Y, Jackowski A. Hyponatraemia in neurosurgical patients: diagnosis using derived parameters of sodium and water homeostasis. *Br J Neurosurg* 1992; **6**: 457–66.

150. Palmer BF. Hyponatremia in patients with central nervous system disease: SIADH versus CSW. *Trends Endocrinol Metab* 2003; **14**: 182–7.

151. Weinand ME, O'Boynick PL, Goetz KL. A study of serum antidiuretic hormone and atrial natriuretic peptide levels in a series of patients with intracranial disease of hyponatremia. *Neurosurgery* 1989; **25**: 781–5.

152. Yamaki T, Tano-oka A, Takahashi A, Imaizumi T, Suetake K, Hashi K. Cerebral salt wasting syndrome distinct from the syndrome of inappropriate secretion of antidiuretic hormone (SIADH). *Acta Neurochir (Wien)* 1992; **115**: 156–62.

153. Berendes E, Walter M, Cullen P *et al.* Secretion of brain natriuretic peptide in

patients with aneurysmal subarachnoid haemorrhage. *Lancet* 1997; **349**: 245–9.

154. DiBona GF. Neural control of renal function in health and disease. *Clin Auton Res* 1994; **4**: 69–74.

155. Diringer M, Ladenson PW, Borel C, Hart GK, Kirsch JR, Hanley DF. Sodium and water regulation in a patient with cerebral salt wasting. *Arch Neurol* 1989; **46**: 928–30.

156. Ganong CA, Kappy MS. Cerebral salt wasting in children. The need for recognition and treatment. *Am J Dis Child* 1993; **147**: 167–9.

157. Cole CD, Gottfried ON, Liu JK, Couldwell WT. Hyponatremia in the neurosurgical patient: diagnosis and management. *Neurosurg Focus* 2004; **16**(4): E9.

158. Worthley, LI, Thomas PD. Treatment of hyponatraemic seizures with intravenous, 29.2% saline. *Br Med J(Clin Res Ed)* 1986; **292**: 168–70.

159. Packer M, Medina N, Yushak M. Correction of dilutional hyponatremia in severe chronic heart failure by converting-enzyme inhibition. *Ann Intern Med* 1984; **100**: 782–9.

160. Martinez-Maldonado M. Inappropriate antidiuretic hormone secretion of unknown origin. *Kidney Int* 1980; **17**: 554–67.

161. Mulinari RA, Gavras I, Wang YX, Franco R, Gavras H. Effects of a vasopressin antagonist with combined antipressor and antidiuretic activities in rats with left ventricular dysfunction. *Circulation* 1990; **81**: 308–11.

162. Adrogue HJ, Madias NE. Hyponatremia. *N Engl J Med* 2000; **342**: 1581–9.

163. Burke CW. Adrenocortical insufficiency. *Clin Endocrinol Metab* 1985; **14**: 947–76.

164. Diederich S, Franzen NF, Bahr V, Oelkers W. Severe hyponatremia due to hypopituitarism with adrenal insufficiency: report on 28 cases. *Eur J Endocrinol* 2003; **148**: 609–17.

165. Moro N, Katayama Y, Kojima J, Mori T, Kawamata T. Prophylactic management of excessive natriuresis with hydrocortisone for efficient hypervolemic therapy after subarachnoid hemorrhage. *Stroke* 2003; **34**: 2807–11.

166. Qureshi AI, Suri MF, Sung GY *et al.* Prognostic significance of hypernatremia and hyponatremia among patients with aneurysmal subarachnoid hemorrhage. *Neurosurgery* 2002; **50**: 749–56.

167. Brunner JE, Redmond JM, Haggar AM, Kruger DF, Elias SB. Central pontine myelinolysis and pontine lesions after rapid correction of hyponatraemia: a prospective magnetic resonance imaging study. *Ann Neurol* 1990; **27**: 61–6.

168. Munger MA. New agents for managing hyponatremia in hospitalised patients *Am J Health Syst Pharm* 2007; **64**: 253–65.

# Brainstem death and organ donation

Martin B. Walker

## Introduction

Death is a focus for many cultures and religions, but has no universal definition. It is not an event, but a process associated with irreversible and progressive loss of organ function. Progress of this process is very variable depending on complex patient and disease factors. Death requires the certain and irreversible cessation of the characteristics and processes that define life. In the United Kingdom (UK) there is no statutory definition of death. Criteria in the 1998 code of practice for the diagnosis of brain stem death are accepted as a viable definition.[1] The irreversible loss of consciousness with the irreversible loss of the capacity to breathe produced by brainstem death (BSD) is accepted in the UK as the death of the individual and can be diagnosed using clinical tests of brainstem function. Diagnosis of BSD facilitates the discontinuation of futile treatment, which is in the patient's best interests and thereby reduces distress to relatives and carers. It also minimizes futile use of healthcare resources. Diagnosing BSD on these ethical, humanitarian and utilitarian grounds facilitates organ donation when patients and families choose to donate.

## Brainstem death

### History

Mollaret and Goulon described brain death in 1959.[2] *Coma dépassé* ('beyond coma') was described as irreversible coma with loss of reflexes and electrical brain activity and was differentiated from *coma prolongé* (persistent vegetative state). In 1968, the Harvard Committee defined brain death using the criteria of unreceptivity and unresponsiveness with no movements or respirations and no reflexes during disconnection from the ventilator occurring in the presence of an isoelectric electroencephalogram (EEG).[3] In 1976, the Conference of Medical Royal Colleges stated that permanent functional death of the brainstem constituted brain death. This memorandum provided the foundations for the current UK code of practice for BSD testing, delineating the inclusion and exclusion criteria and describing the clinical tests of BSD function.[4]

### Anatomy and physiology

The brainstem is located between the cerebral hemispheres and the spinal cord; it comprises the mid-brain, pons and medulla. It contains the cranial nerve nuclei and transmits ascending and descending motor and sensory nerve impulses. Pontine reticular nuclei are vital for cortical arousal and conscious awareness. The medulla and pons (under influence of the hypothalamus) control and maintain cardiorespiratory function. Loss of brainstem controls and cranial nerve function form the basis of BSD testing.

*Head Injury: A Multidisciplinary Approach*, ed. Peter C. Whitfield, Elfyn O. Thomas, Fiona Summers, Maggie Whyte and Peter J. Hutchinson. Published by Cambridge University Press. © Cambridge University Press 2009.

**Table 15.1.** Common causes of brainstem death

| Aetiological condition | Features |
|---|---|
| Traumatic brain injury | Most common cause |
| Intracranial haemorrhage | |
| Tumours | |
| Infection | |
| Metabolic encephalopathy | e.g. hepatic |
| Hypoxaemia | More likely to result in persistent vegetative state |
| Ischaemia | |

## Pathophysiology

Brain tissue tolerates hypoxaemia and ischaemia poorly. The overlying brain tissue and skull provide some physical protection to the centrally located brainstem. However, the rigid cranium causes intracranial hypertension as brain swelling develops, regardless of the traumatic or non-traumatic aetiology of the primary brain injury. Secondary brain injury readily occurs with a vicious cycle of brain swelling causing tissue hypoxaemia from impaired oxygen delivery leading to worsening intracranial hypertension and ischaemia. Ultimately, this can cause downward pressure on the brainstem resulting in coning through the foramen magnum and BSD. The common causes of BSD are summarized in Table 15.1.

Profound brainstem injury results in unconsciousness, impaired homeostasis and variable cranial nerve lesions. Cushing's reflex (systemic hypertension and bradycardia) is not invariably observed. Indeed, almost any combination of cardiac rhythm and systemic pressure may occur. After BSD, systemic hypotension and tachycardia usually ensue with loss of all cranial nerve function. Loss of thermostatic homeostasis results in hypothermia. Cranial diabetes insipidus is common and results in profound polyuria, hypovolaemia and hypernatraemia unless treated vigorously.

## Brainstem death testing

### The UK code of practice for BSD testing

The 1998 code of practice for the diagnosis of BSD was prepared by a working party established on behalf of the Health Departments by the Royal College of Physicians for the Academy of Royal Colleges.[1] At the time of writing it is being updated. The code of practice emphasizes updating from 'brain death' to 'brain*stem* death' for clarity. Using 'BSD' demonstrates one brain structure is dead (not the entire brain) and the code of practice emphasizes that BSD is associated with certainty that recovery is impossible. Prior to BSD testing, mandatory inclusions and exclusions have to be considered (Table 15.2).

The timing of BSD testing is not mandated and, whilst it may be appropriate to test a few hours after an intracranial catastrophe (e.g. traumatic brain injury or spontaneous intracranial haemorrhage), it is preferable to wait for over 24 hours when the period of insult is more uncertain (e.g. cardiac arrest, circulatory insufficiency, hypoxaemia or air and fat embolism). The tests are performed by two medical practitioners who have been registered for over 5 years, are competent in the practice of the tests and are not members of the transplant team. At least one practitioner should be a consultant. Two sets of tests are

**Table 15.2.** Mandatory inclusions and exclusions to be considered prior to BSD testing

| *Prerequisite inclusions* |
| --- |
| 1. Patient is deeply unconscious |
| 2. Presence of severe irremediable brain damage of certain aetiology |
| 3. Patient is on a ventilator due to inadequate or absent spontaneous respiratory efforts |
| *Mandatory exclusions* |
| 1. Presence of sedative agents that might result in the comatose state of the patient<br>*Therapeutic or recreational drug effects can persist in critically ill patients* |
| 2. Primary hypothermia causing unconsciousness<br>*Core temperature <35 °C* |
| 3. Reversible circulatory, metabolic and endocrine abnormalities causing unconsciousness<br>*It is recognized that changes may occur as a result of BSD, but these effects rather than causes of the condition do not prevent BSD testing* |
| 4. Muscle relaxants or other drugs causing profound muscular weakness<br>*Determined by using a nerve stimulator or eliciting deep tendon reflexes* |

performed. These may be carried out by the two practitioners separately or together. Repetition of the tests avoids observer error. The time interval between tests is discretionary, dependent on the patient's pathology and clinical course. Although death is not pronounced until the second set of tests has been completed, the legal time of death is when the first set of tests was performed. The clinical BSD tests comprise a detailed assessment of cranial nerve function and a test of respiratory drive (Table 15.3).

# The diagnosis of BSD in special situations

## Paediatric considerations
In children aged over 2 months the criteria for BSD should be the same as in adults. Between a gestational age of 37 weeks and 2 months, the diagnosis of BSD can be difficult to make and below 37 weeks BSD criteria cannot be applied. For anencephalic infants, organ donation can proceed if two clinicians (not in the transplant team) agree that spontaneous respirations have ceased.

## Chronic lung disease
Patients with significant pre-existing chronic lung disease may need greater levels of hypercarbia to produce maximal stimulation of the respiratory centre. These special cases should be managed using an expert in respiratory disease.

## High spinal cord injury
The presence of high spinal cord injury will prevent full BSD testing being performed.

## Presence of long-acting sedative agents
Diagnosing BSD is problematical following sedation. When small doses of short-acting agents are used during resuscitation and evaluation of the patient, clinical judgement alone can be used to time the performance of BSD tests. Due to the unpredictable

**Table 15.3.** BSD tests and the cranial nerves they examine

| BSD test | Cranial nerves |
|---|---|
| **Pupils are fixed and unresponsive to light (direct and consensual)** | II and III |
| *Pupils may be unequal or not fully dilated.* | |
| **Absence of corneal reflex** | III, V and VII |
| *Avoiding corneal injury and stimulation of lash reflex.* | |
| **Absence of vestibulo-ocular reflexes** | III, IV, VI and VIII |
| **Absent eye movements on instillation of >50 mls ice-cold water over 1 minute in to each external auditory meatus in turn.** | |
| **Head flexed to 30° plus access to tympanic membrane is confirmed with an otoscope (removing wax or debris first if needed).** | |
| **Local injury or disease may prevent this test being performed on one or other side, but this does not prevent or invalidate the diagnosis of BSD.** | |
| **Motor responses in the cranial nerve distribution cannot be elicited by stimulation of any somatic area. Absence of limb responses to supra-orbital pressure** | V and VII |
| **Absence of gag reflex** | |
| *Using orange stick or flat spatula to stimulate soft palate and oropharynx* | IX, X |
| **Absence of cough or reflex response to tracheal stimulation with suction catheter** | IX, X |
| **Absence of spontaneous respiratory effort on disconnection from the ventilator** | IX, X |
| *$PaCO_2$ >6.65 kPa* | |
| *Use passive tracheal insufflation of 100% $O_2$ through a catheter* | |
| *Slow onset of hypercapnæa may require the use of 5% $CO_2/O_2$ mixture* | |

pharmacokinetics and pharmacodynamics of sedative agents in the critically ill, more prolonged use causes uncertainty. Indeed considerable variation exists in UK clinical practice for the delay following cessation of sedation of all types and in the use of antagonists (naloxone and flumazenil).[5,6] Measurement of drug levels can be time consuming, is not invariably available and causes further uncertainty in interpretation. This has led to proposals that confirmatory tests should gain clinical and legal acceptance.

## Confirmatory tests

The code of practice states that the safety of BSD testing has been confirmed by 17 years of use and that confirmatory tests (neurophysiological or radiological) are not justified. Uncertainty in diagnosing BSD may arise in the special situations described previously or when local facial, pharyngeal and aural trauma prevents full BSD testing. Using confirmatory tests remains an attractive prospect in uncertain cases and when residual sedation, hypothermia or metabolic disturbances prevent routine BSD diagnosis. It speeds up BSD diagnosis and reduces the duration of futile treatment and the deterioration of multi-organ function that occurs over time following BSD.[7] There is inadequate evidence to recommend one specific confirmatory test over another and more studies are needed to evaluate their precise role.[8] Techniques demonstrating cerebral circulation or brain tissue perfusion offer most promise and the total absence of cerebral circulation may become acceptable for diagnosing BSD. Cerebral arterial blood flow can persist after clinical BSD and repeated tests of the circulation may be needed for individual patients.[9]

Features of various confirmatory tests are detailed in Table 15.4.[10–12]

**Table 15.4.** Features of confirmatory tests for BSD testing

| Confirmatory test | Potential for BSD testing | Availability | Bedside use? | Safety and level of invasiveness |
|---|---|---|---|---|
| Four-vessel angiography | Good | Limited | No | Risks to patient and donor organs |
| Transcranial Doppler ultrasonography[10] | Poor access to posterior circulation | Variable | Yes | Non-invasive |
| Magnetic resonance imaging and angiography | Good | Variable | No | Low risk |
| Radioisotope scintigraphy[11] | Good | Poor | Yes | Low risk |
| Xenon-enhanced computerized tomography (CT) | Good | Poor | No | Low risk |
| CT angiography | Good | Good | Yes | Low risk |
| Positron emission tomography | Good | Very poor | No | Low risk |
| EEG | Not useful for BSD | Variable | Yes | Non-invasive |
| Multimodality evoked potentials[12] | Good | Variable | Yes | Non-invasive |

   Currently, if confounding factors prevent clinical BSD testing, the sole use of confirmatory tests in the UK is not sanctioned in law or by any national guidelines. However, on a case-by-case basis close involvement of the relatives, early referral to HM Coroner, use of second opinions from neurologists or neurosurgeons and legal opinions from hospital legal departments and medical defence organizations may facilitate BSD diagnosis using such tests without ethical or legal risk.

# International variation in diagnosing brain death

Significant international variation exists in BSD testing. A survey has demonstrated differences between guidelines of 80 countries.[13] Marked variation occurs in such fundamental areas as apnoea testing (targeting $PaCO_2$, using ventilator disconnection alone or not even examining for apnoea), the number of physicians mandated (varying from one to three), using confirmatory tests (mandatory, optional or not permissible) and the time between tests (zero to 24 hours). There appear to be no cultural or religious attitudes that influence the variations. In the USA brain death is defined using the concept of whole brain death. Brain death testing in the USA includes use of a negative atropine test (1–2 mg intravenous atropine resulting in a heart rate rise of less than 5 bpm). Confirmatory testing is also permissible in conditions that might confound brain death testing (such as brainstem encephalitis or persistence of sedative agents). There is variation between the states, but most states mandate separation of the sets of tests by 12–24 hours.

# Organ and tissue donation within critical care

The demand for organ transplantation outstrips the supply of donor organs, whether from living donor or cadaveric donation programmes. Cadaveric organ donation can be from brainstem dead (heart-beating) or less commonly from asystolic (non-heart beating) donors.

Currently, the UK employs an opt-in system for cadaveric organ and tissue donation. Potential donors are identified by being on the Organ Donor Register (ODR) or by family or friends knowing their wishes. There is no strict framework over the timing and manner of requesting assent for donation. Most practitioners wait until BSD is confirmed (i.e. after the second set of tests) unless the relatives raise the issue earlier. Very few contraindications to organ donation are absolute and so all potential donors should be referred for consideration.

## Ethical and legal considerations relating to BSD and organ donation

It is argued that BSD testing is flawed by the lack of controlled studies assessing the true prognosis of the clinical signs of BSD. However, series comprising over 1000 BSD patients receiving organ support have been published. Asystole (usually occurring within a few days) was the invariable outcome after BSD. Although the concept of BSD evolved before organ transplantation could occur from cadaveric donors (limited by surgical techniques and immunosuppression), concerns persist about an apparent linkage of BSD to organ donation. Difficulties arise because the withdrawal of futile multiorgan support does not require formal declaration of BSD. It is argued that the only reason to perform the tests is to facilitate organ donation. However, it remains usual practice in the UK not to withdraw ventilatory support of an apnoeic patient without BSD testing.

Cases proceeding to donation that would normally be referred to the coroner should still be referred so that coronial permission can be granted for donation. The coroner will refuse permission for donation of an organ if that organ may have caused death, if the coroner's enquiries might be obstructed by the organ's removal or if the organ may have evidential value. Therefore close co-operation between clinicians, the donor transplant co-ordinator (DTC), the coroner, the police and the pathologist is required for some coroner's cases.

The UK Human Tissue Act 2004 (HTA) regulates storage and use of organs and tissues from living and deceased patients. Consent underpins the Act, which defines a hierarchy of consent with the patient (or a person with parental responsibility for a child) being at the top, above a new status of a nominated representative and lastly a further hierarchy of qualifying relatives. The HTA states that the known wishes of the deceased take precedence (over relatives' objections) for donation, but falls short of making donation obligatory in this situation and retains a case-by-case basis for decision making, involving consultation with the relatives. The HTA states the ODR should always be checked so that registered patients' wishes can be followed.

## Management of the potential donor

Active management of the patient should continue until BSD is confirmed. The emphasis then changes to optimizing organ function in those patients who are to become organ donors or changes to the cessation of ventilatory support and other therapies until asystole inter-venes in those who are not. Consensus guidelines on optimal donor management have been published.[14–16] However, there is little evidence-based medicine to guide clinical practice more precisely. The basic principles of donor management are summarized in Table 15.5.

## Relatives of the potential donor

The family should be supported and kept fully informed throughout their relative's critical illness. As BSD supervenes, this need becomes greater rather than reduces. A senior clinician should inform the relatives of the grave clinical outlook and the clinical reasons for conducting

**Table 15.5.** Optimal donor management

| Management goal | Clinical intervention | Comments |
| --- | --- | --- |
| Organ perfusion | Optimise preload | |
| | Use advanced cardiac monitoring in labile patients | Evidence for choice of monitor remains unclear |
| | Minimise pressor support | Use vasopressin or noradrenaline |
| | Inotropes if indicated | Dopamine <10 mcg/kg per min |
| | Aggressive treatment of diabetes insipidus | Bolus and/or infusion of intravenous 1-desamino-D-arginine vasopressin |
| | Consider diagnosis and treatment of hypoadrenalism | Uncertainty persists over which test to use |
| | Use of thyroid hormone | There is no current evidence-base supporting its routine use |
| Lung function | Maintain normal ABGs | |
| | Minimize PEEP | Target 5 cm $H_2O$ |
| | Minimize peak inspiratory pressure | Target <30 cm $H_2O$ |
| | Frequent pulmonary physiotherapy and endotracheal suction | Recruitment manoeuvres may help |
| Biochemistry | Maintain strict normoglycaemia | Target 4.0–8.0 mmol/l |
| | Maintain potassium levels | Target 4.0–5.0 mmol/l |
| | Maintain sodium levels | Target 130–155 mmol/l |
| Haematology | Treat coagulopathy | |
| | Maintain haemoglobin concentration | >7.0 g/dl in stable patients and 9.0–10.0 g/dl in unstable patients |
| Temperature | Maintain normothermia | |
| Sepsis | Treat infection with appropriate antimicrobials | Keep donor co-ordinator informed |

brainstem death tests. This should occur in calm and quiet surroundings away from the bedspace. Subsequent request for organ donation should be conducted by a senior clinician or a DTC or by both in tandem. Family refusals are minimized when requests are made by staff experienced in requesting. The DTC obtains a fully informed assent from the family explaining the details of the process and collecting information necessary for retrieval to proceed.

# Organ donation after BSD

Organ donation following BSD should proceed without delay to prevent deteriorating organ function. Optimal donor management continues from the critical care unit throughout the operative procedure. The clinical team's aspiration should be to achieve multiorgan donation; however, this is usually limited by organ and recipient suitability. Anaesthetic drugs such as muscle relaxants and volatile anaesthetic agents may be administered during organ retrieval to prevent spinal reflexes and autonomic surges. It is important that all members of staff involved in the procedure are aware of the rationale. The anaesthetist will be required until the aorta is cross-clamped, extra-corporeal organ perfusion is commenced and ventilation is stopped.

**Table 15.6.** Categories of non-heart beating organ donation

| Category | Description of process | Status of potential donor | Location |
|---|---|---|---|
| 1 | Uncontrolled | Dead on arrival | Emergency department |
| 2 | Uncontrolled | Unsuccessful resuscitation | Emergency department |
| 3 | Controlled | Planned withdrawal of futile treatment | Intensive care unit |
| 4 | Controlled | Cardiac arrest after BSD | Intensive care unit |

## Non-heart beating organ donation

Non-heart beating donation is the donation of organs from asystolic patients. In 1994 a workshop in Maastricht categorized the situations when this may occur (Table 15.6).[17] In the UK this is usually in the setting where asystole follows planned withdrawal of multiorgan support on the grounds of futility. This is controlled non-heart beating donation (CNHBD).[18] It requires rapid pronouncement of death (usually 5 minutes after asystole) and immediate transfer of the patient to the operating theatre where a super-rapid laparotomy is performed and organ retrieval is performed after cold perfusion of the organs. Best results are obtained when both cold and warm ischaemic times are minimized. The results of kidney transplantation from CNHBD are excellent and progress has been made with CNHBD of livers and lungs.[19,20]

## Tissue donation

Patients in intensive care units can be tissue and organ donors or be solely tissue donors. The most commonly retrieved tissues are heart valves and corneas. Depending on local transplant programmes, other tissues such as skin, bone, tendons, cartilage and pericardium may also be retrievable. Local DTCs provide any necessary advice.

## Conclusion

Clinical testing to diagnose BSD remains a valid and legally acceptable method to determine death of an individual. It facilitates both a dignified death and organ donation in appropriate patients. Future developments in this challenging field may see a considered increase in the use of confirmatory tests, which will speed up the process and potentially improve donor organ function.

## References

1. Department of Health. *A Code of Practice for the Diagnosis of Brain Stem Death*. London, HMSO, 1998.
2. Mollaret P, Goulon M. Le coma dépassé. *Rev Neurol* 1959; **101**: 3–15.
3. Anon. A definition of irreversible coma. Report of the ad hoc Committee of the Harvard Medical School to examine the definition of brain death. *J Am Med Assoc* 1968; **205**: 337–40.
4. Conference of Medical Royal Colleges and their Faculties (UK). Diagnosis of brain death. *Br Med J* 1976; **2**: 1187–8.
5. Bell MDD, Moss E, Murphy PG. Brainstem death testing in the UK – time for reappraisal? *Br J Anaesth* 2004; **92**:633–40.
6. Pratt OW, Bowles B, Protheroe RT. Brain stem death testing after thiopental use: a survey of UK neuro critical care practice. *Anaesthesia* 2006; **61**: 1075–8.

7. Lopez-Navidad A, Caballero F, Domingo P et al. Early diagnosis of brain death in patients treated with central nervous system depressant drugs. *Transplantation* 2000; **70**: 131–5.

8. Young GB, Shemie SD, Doig CJ. Brief review: The role of ancillary tests in the neurological determination of death. *Can J Anesth* 2006; **53**: 620–7.

9. Flowers WM Jr, Patel BR. Persistence of cerebral blood flow after brain death. *South Med J* 2000; **93**: 364–70.

10. Monteiro LM, Bollen CW, van Huffelen AC et al. Transcranial Doppler ultrasonography to confirm brain death: a meta-analysis. *Intens Care Medi* 2006; **32**: 1937–44.

11. Yatim A, Mercatello A, Coronel B et al. 99 mTc-HMPAO cerebral scintigraphy in the diagnosis of brain death. *Transpl Proc* 1991; **23**: 2491.

12. de Tourtchaninoff M, Hantson P, Mahieu P et al. Brain death diagnosis in misleading conditions. *Quart J Med* 1999; **92**: 407–14.

13. Wijdicks EFM. Brain death worldwide. Accepted fact but no global consensus in diagnostic criteria. *Neurology* 2002; **58**: 20–5.

14. Intensive Care Society. *Guidelines for Adult Organ and Tissue Donation*. London: Intensive Care Society, 2004.

15. Shemie SD, Ross H, Pagliarello J et al. Organ donor management in Canada: recommendations of the forum on medical management to optimise donor organ potential. *Can Med Associ J* 2006; **174**: S13–30.

16. Rosengard BR, Feng S, Alfrey EJ et al. Report of the Crystal City meeting to maximise the use of organs recovered from the cadaver donor. *Am J Transpl* 2002; **2**: 701–11.

17. Koostra G, Daemen JHC, Oomen APA. Categories of non-heart beating donors. *Transpl Proc* 1995; **27**: 2893–4.

18. Brook NR, Waller JR, Nicholson ML. Non heart-beating kidney donation: current practice and future developments. *Kidney Int* 2003; **63**: 1516–29.

19. Egan TM. Non-heart-beating donors in thoracic transplantation. *J Heart Lung Transpl* 2004; **23**: 3–10.

20. Foley DP, Fernandez LA, Leverson G et al. Donation after cardiac death. The University of Wisconsin experience with liver transplantation. *Ann Surg* 2005; **5**: 724–31.

# Chapter 16

# Anaesthesia for emergency neurosurgery

W. Hiu Lam

## Introduction

Emergency anaesthesia for neurosurgery follows an algorithm of rapid initial assessment, resuscitation, stabilization for transfer, investigation of relevant pathology and timely surgical evacuation of compressive lesions. In order to appreciate the rationale and principle of clinical anaesthetic management in brain injured patients, the following areas must be considered:

- the importance of the preservation of concurrent global neurological status of the patient as assessed by Glasgow Coma Score (GCS).[1]
- an insight of the pathophysiology of brain injury is essential
- awareness of the effects of attenuation of cerebral autoregulation caused by the intracranial pathology[2,3]
- the need for target directed management strategies for the prevention of secondary brain injury (SBI) in patients undergoing anaesthesia.[4]

The existence of co-morbidities, for instance, cervical spine injury and involvement of other systems in the context of polytrauma, must be borne in mind when assessing these patients. Successful outcome relies pivotally on multidisciplinary teamwork from all specialties involved.

## Pathophysiology

Neurological deficit caused by primary brain injury (PBI) is dependent on the severity of the initial impact. Brain ischaemia as a result of SBI is, to a certain extent, preventable although it has been demonstrated in 80% of fatal head injuries.[5] The aims of anaesthetic management are to maintain adequate brain perfusion and to avoid, anticipate and aggressively treat intracranial hypertension (IcHTN).

Any expanding lesion (e.g. haematoma /contusion) causing IcHTN may cause cerebral ischaemia if associated with a reduction of cerebral perfusion pressure or direct focal brain compression; the Monro–Kelly Doctrine.[6] The common surgical indications for patients with head injury are illustrated in Table 16.1.

The extracranial causes of SBI are predominantly non-surgical. These factors include disturbances in haemodynamics, respiratory insufficiency, seizures and metabolic imbalance. Cerebral autoregulation is essential in maintaining an adequate coupling of cerebral blood flow (CBF) and cerebral oxygen metabolism ($CMRO_2$).[7] This is impaired in a proportion of head injury patients,[3] and certain anaesthetic agents also affect cerebral autoregulation. Uncoupling of CBF and $CMRO_2$ leads to brain ischaemia.[8] It is therefore essential to control fluctuations in systemic arterial blood pressure during anaesthesia in order to ensure adequate cerebral perfusion.

*Head Injury: A Multidisciplinary Approach*, ed. Peter C. Whitfield, Elfyn O. Thomas, Fiona Summers, Maggie Whyte and Peter J. Hutchinson. Published by Cambridge University Press. © Cambridge University Press 2009.

**Table 16.1.** The common surgical indications for patients with head injury

| Indications | Notes |
|---|---|
| Depressed skull fracture | To reduce risk of infection and damage to underlying structures |
| Acute extradural haematoma | Due to middle meningeal artery (with skull fracture) or venous sinus injury |
| Acute subdural haematoma | Cortical venous injury and underlying brain contusion is common |
| Parenchymal lesion | Haematoma especially urgent in temporal lobe and/or posterior fossa |
| Intracranial hypertension | Refractory IcHTN may benefit from decompressive craniectomy |
| External ventricular drainage | For secondary hydrocephalus and intraventricular pressure monitor |

At a cellular level, it is now evident from animal studies that increased levels of the excitatory amino acid neurotransmitter glutamate are detected in traumatized brain and in human cerebral spinal fluid after head injury.[9-11] The increase in glutamate appears to initiate an excitotoxic cascade by activating the inotropic and metabotropic glutamate receptors. The former include $N$-methyl D-aspartate (NMDA) receptors; the latter are related to G-proteins and modulate intracellular secondary messengers. The end result is an increase in intracellular calcium, which initiates a cascade of neuronal destruction by activation of protein kinases, phospholipases and proteases.[12] There is experimental evidence that suggests NMDA receptor antagonists may have a role in neuroprotection.[13]

# Target-directed strategy

## Haemodynamics

Hypertension, hypotension and hypoxia have all been shown independently to increase morbidity and mortality in both adults and children.[14-16] There is evidence that a single episode of systolic hypotension (<90 mmHg) or hypoxaemia ($PaO_2 < 8$ kPa) could affect outcome of the brain-injured patient.[17]

### Cerebral perfusion pressure (CPP)

CPP is the difference of mean arterial pressure (MAP) and intracranial pressure (ICP). The original guidelines from the Brain Trauma Foundation advocated 70 mmHg as a target CPP for brain injured patient,[18,19] partially based on Rosner's study which demonstrated a low mortality rate of 29% and a good 6-month post-injury recovery rate of 59%.[20] 'Lund therapy' however, utilizing a reduction in microvascular pressure to minimize oedema, reported an impressive 8% mortality rate and 80% recovery rate in their studies.[21,22] Furthermore, a 50% reduction in secondary brain ischaemia was demonstrated by Robertson's study where the CPP threshold was increased from 40 mmHg to 60 mmHg, but this was accompanied by a five-fold increase of adult respiratory distress syndrome (ARDS).[23,24] The third edition of the Brain Trauma Foundation's guidelines, published in 2007, states that 'aggressive attempts to maintain CPP above 70 mmHg with fluids and pressors should be avoided because of the risk of ARDS ... the CPP value to target lies within the range 50–70 mmHg'.[25]

With this evidence, it seems logical that during anaesthesia, CPP should be maintained between 50–70 mmHg in order to optimize adequate cerebral perfusion as well as avoiding complications such as adult respiratory distress syndrome, pulmonary and cerebral oedema related to hypervolaemia and hypertension.

### Intracranial pressure (ICP)

It is generally accepted that the treatment threshold for ICP should be set at 20–25 mmHg.[25–27] If an ICP monitoring device is *in situ* prior to induction of anaesthesia, it is imperative to treat IcHTN above the set threshold and maintain an adequate MAP to generate the appropriate CPP until the dura is surgically incised. Once the brain is exposed to atmospheric pressure, the CPP then required equals MAP (provided central venous pressure is insignificant).

## Perioperative anaesthetic management

### Preoperative assessment and optimization

In patients with significant head injury requiring urgent surgery, history taking often involves rapidly assimilating information from witnesses and emergency services personnel. Further past medical, drug and allergy history can be obtained from relatives and the patient's GP records, time permitting. The clinical examination must be comprehensive and co-existing injuries and co-morbidities sought.

Anaesthetic assessment must include a global neurological assessment of the patient. The reduction in GCS from the scene of injury onwards may indicate a progressive deterioration. An accurate documentation of the pupil size and reactivity is essential. Any preoperative motor, sensory and speech deficit should be recorded as a baseline, enabling comparison in the postoperative period. Bulbar function needs to be specifically elicited. An impairment of bulbar function may have led to aspiration of gastric contents preoperatively. In addition, the patient may not have sufficient airway protection postoperatively. If lung aspiration is suspected, urgent tracheo-bronchial toileting must be considered prior to surgery. Aspiration pneumonitis increases intrathoracic pressure on intermittent positive pressure ventilation (IPPV), which would in turn impede venous return and worsen existing IcHTN. The increase in venous pressure from IPPV may also render surgical haemostasis more arduous. The resulting ventilation-perfusion mismatch could promote hypercapnoea and hypoxaemia, both of which worsen IcHTN.

Arrhythmias and myocardial stunning are well-established complications of spontaneous subarachnoid haemorrhage, although they occur less frequently after trauma. These factors should form the basis of cardiovascular risk assessment during the preoperative visit.[28–31] The preoperative arterial blood pressure and heart rate should be noted and used to guide management once the patient is under anaesthesia, especially when ICP measurement is not available. Fluid balance record, serum and urine electrolytes and osmolality should be examined as complications from head injury such as diabetes insipidus, syndrome of inappropriate antidiuretic hormone secretion and cerebral salt wasting syndrome can cause significant morbidity and mortality.[32] Serum haemoglobin, platelet count, electrolytes, clotting studies and electrocardiograph (ECG) are mandatory investigations. Cross-matched red cells should be readily available. Sedative premedication is rarely indicated and appropriate monitoring and supplementary oxygen therapy must accompany transfer to the operating theatre.

### Induction of anaesthesia

The objective is to achieve smooth 'tramline' anaesthesia from induction through to emergence from anaesthesia. Pre-induction monitoring of the patient with ECG, invasive arterial blood pressure, pulse oximetry, capnography and agent analyser measurements are mandatory. Central venous and urinary catheters and a nasopharyngeal temperature probe may be introduced post-induction if appropriate, but their placement should not delay urgent surgery.[33] Vasopressors such as metaraminol and ephedrine and anticholinergic agents must be readily available to anticipate hypotension and bradycardia with induction of anaesthesia. Anaesthesia is usually induced intravenously with a hypnotic such as propofol; in obtunded patients the requirement is frequently less than 2–3 mg/kg. Thiopental (5–7 mg/kg), a barbiturate, is another well-tolerated induction agent with a reliable end point and remains very much in use worldwide. Opioids have a major role in neuroanaesthesia. In the UK, fentanyl (7–10 μg/kg) has been traditionally one of the drugs used for analgesia and obtunding the pressor response of laryngoscopy. In recent years remifentanil, an ultra short-acting esterase metabolized mu receptor agonist, has gained wide acceptance as the opioid of choice for intracranial surgery. Similar to other opioids, it has no direct effect on the cerebrovasculature and produces rapid intense analgesia and stable, easily adjustable haemodynamics as well as a rapid postoperative recovery for neurological assessment.[34,35] Rapid sequence induction with adequate depth of anaesthesia and optimal muscle relaxation is required to facilitate tracheal intubation in order to avoid bucking on laryngoscopy (which increases ICP) and regurgitation of gastric contents. Muscle relaxants such as suxamethonium (1.5 mg/kg), atracurium (0.5 mg/kg), vecuronium (0.15 mg/kg) and rocuronium (0.6 mg/kg) have all been used satisfactorily. Vocal cords topicalization with 4% lignocaine may reduce the risk of coughing with the endotracheal tube (ETT) *in situ*. The trachea is often intubated with an armoured ETT to ensure its patency throughout the duration of surgery. Particular attention is also needed to ensure the correct length of the ETT and that both lungs are ventilated equally. Mannitol (0.25–1 g/kg) is often administered early prior to dura incision to provide optimal surgical access, especially if the underlying brain is hyperaemic and swollen. It has been shown to reduce ICP and improve CPP.[36] Anti-seizure prophylaxis should be considered for the first 7 days as it has been shown to reduce the incidence of early post-traumatic seizure.[25,37,38] Antibiotic prophylaxis is recommended according to local antimicrobial guidelines.

## Monitoring

In addition to haemodynamic monitoring, arterial $CO_2$ tension should be maintained between 4.5–5 kPa as elective prophylactic hyperventilation has been associated with adverse outcome in head injury patients.[25,39,40] Hyperglycaemia is associated with poor outcome in head injury and it has been shown that tight glycaemic control may be beneficial to critically ill patients.[41,42] Intra-operative pyrexia must be treated aggressively as this is associated with unfavourable outcome in head injury patients.[43]

## Position

The patient should usually be in reverse Trendelenburg position to encourage adequate venous drainage. The head is either on a horseshoe or secured in headpins. The haemodynamic response to pin fixation may be attenuated by a skull block or a 1–2 μg/kg bolus of remifentanil.[44] The arterial and central venous pressure transducers should be level with the tragus and the right atrium, respectively, to reflect the CPP and atrial filling pressure. Eye protection, ETT position/connections, monitoring equipment attachments and accessibility of vascular accesses must be scrutinised again at this point prior to the application of surgical drape. All pressure points must be meticulously padded to avoid skin damage.

**Table 16.2.** Regimen to achieve propofol TIVA

| Regimen of propofol | Time in minutes |
| --- | --- |
| Commence with 1 mg/kg followed by | bolus |
| 10 mg/kg per hour followed by | 10 |
| 8 mg/kg per hour followed by | 10 |
| 6 mg/kg per hour | rest of case |

### Maintenance

Volatile agents or total intravenous anaesthesia (TIVA) with propofol can be used to maintain anaesthesia. Propofol TIVA can be achieved by a manual regimen described in Table 16.2:[45]

Alternatively, a concept of target controlled infusion (TCI) is also currently used, where an infusion pump with a built-in algorithm would infuse propofol and/or remifentanil at a rate needed to achieve the blood level demanded by the anaesthetist.

In order to minimize effects on ICP, CBF and autoregulation, when using inhalational volatile anaesthetics, less than 1 MAC (minimal alveolar concentration) of isoflurane and desflurane and less than 1.5 MAC of sevoflurane should be delivered.[46] Manual infusions of remifentanil or fentanyl are appropriate analgesics of choice. Neuromuscular junction monitoring should be instituted. 0.9% saline (osmolality = 308 mosmol/kg) is the traditional maintenance fluid of choice but colloid solution may be used to replenish intravascular loss.

### Extubation and postoperative care

A significant proportion of patients will require ongoing postoperative support and management in the intensive care setting. If an armoured ETT has been used, this should be replaced with a standard ETT prior to transfer. Smooth extubation of the trachea (in a reverse Trendelenburg or sitting position) must only take place if adequate respiration and stable haemodynamics are combined with a GCS that is better or at least comparable with pre-induction level. Pain relief can be adequately provided by paracetamol and judicious administration of intravenous morphine. Morphine as a postoperative pain relief has been shown to be equally effective as the traditionally used codeine.[47] Non-steroidal anti-inflammatory drugs must only be administered after careful consideration of risk–benefit assessment. Postoperative vomiting following intracranial surgery can cause an increase in ICP, and ondansetron 4 mg given at dura closure has been shown to reduce incidence of vomiting by 60%.[48] Supplementary oxygen therapy must be continued into the postoperative period. Euvolaemic status is the aim throughout the postoperative period as guided by the trend of central venous pressure and hourly urine output. After discharge from the post-anaesthesia care unit, the patient must be transferred to a unit with appropriately trained nurses and equipment for close observation and invasive monitoring.

In summary, anaesthesia for emergency neurosurgical patients relies on multidisciplinary teamwork, attention to detail in all aspects of perioperative anaesthetic care and a good knowledge of pathophysiology and management strategy for these patients.

## References

1. Teasdale G, Jennett B. Assessment of coma and impaired causes: a practical scale. *Lancet* 1974; **ii**: 81–4.

2. Adelson PP, Clyde B, Kochanek PM *et al.* Cerebral blood flow in children after head injury. *Pediatr Neurosurg* 1997; **26**: 200–7.

3. Bouma GJ, Muizelaar JP, Stringer WA *et al.* Ultra-early evaluation of regional cerebral blood flow in severely head-injured patients using xenon-enhanced computerized tomography. *J Neurosurg* 1992; **77**(3): 360–8.

4. Jones PA, Andrews PJD, Midgley S *et al.* Measuring the burden of secondary insults in head-injured patients during intensive care. *J Neurosurg Anesthe* 1994; **6**: 4–14.

5. Graham DI, Ford I, Adams JH *et al.* Ischaemic brain damage is still common in fatal non-missile head injury. *J Neurol Neurosurg Psychiatry* 1989; **52**: 346–50.

6. Prabhu M, Gupta AK. Intracranial pressure. In: Gupta AK, Summors A. eds. *Notes in Neuroanaesthesia and Critical Care.* Greenwich Medical Media Ltd. 2001; Ch. 6: 23–25.

7. Prabhu M, Gupta AK. Cerebral blood flow. In: Gupta AK, Summors A. *Notes in Neuroanaesthesia and Critical Care.* Greenwich Medical Media Ltd. 2001; Ch. 5: 19–22.

8. Coles JP, Fryer TD, Smielewski P *et al.* Incidence and mechanisms of cerebral ischaemia in early head injury. *J Cereb Blood Flow Metab* 2003; **24**: 202–211.

9. Benveniste H, Drejer J, Schousboe A, Diemer H. Elevation of the extracellular concentrations of glutamate and aspartate in rat hippocampus during transient cerebral ischaemia monitored by intracerebral microdialysis. *J Neurochem* 1984; **43**: 1368–74.

10. Katayama Y, Becker DP, Tamura T, Hovda D. Massive increase in extracellular potassium and the indiscriminate release of glutamate following concussive brain injury. *J Neurosurg* 1990; **73**: 889–900.

11. Baker AJ Moulton RJ, MacMillan VH, Shedden PM. Excitatory amino acids in cerebral spinal fluid following traumatic brain injury in humans. *J Neurosurg* 1993; **79**: 369–72.

12. Hudspith MJ. Glutamate: a role in normal brain function, anaesthesia, analgesia and CNS injury. *Br J Anaesth* 1997; **78**: 731–47.

13. Fawcett JW. Novel Strategies for protection and repair of the central nervous system. *Clin Med* 2006; **6**: 598–603.

14. Chesnut RM, Marshall LF, Klauber MR *et al.* The role of secondary brain injury in determining outcome from severe head injury. *J Trauma* 1993; **34**: 216–22.

15. Marmarou A, Anderson RL, Ward JD *et al.* Impact of ICP instability and hypotension on outcome in patients with severe head trauma. *J Neurosurg* 1991; **75**: s59–66.

16. Lam WH, Mackersie A. Paediatric head injury: incidence, aetiology and management. *Paediatr Anaesth* 1999; **9**(5): 377–85.

17. Pingula FA, Wald SL, Shackford SR, Vane DW. The effect of hypotension and hypoxia on children with severe head injuries. *J Pediatr Surg* 1993; **28**(3): 310–16.

18. Brain Trauma Foundation, American Association of Neurological Surgeons, Joint Section on Neurotrauma and Critical Care: Guidelines for the management of severe head injury. *J Neurotrauma* 1996; **13**: 641–734.

19. Bullock RM, Chesnut R, Clifton GL *et al.* Management and prognosis of severe traumatic brain injury, part 1: Guidelines for management of severe traumatic brain injury. *J Neurotrauma* 2000; **17**: 451–553.

20. Rosner MJ, Rosner SD, Johnson AH. Cerebral perfusion pressure: Management protocol and clinical results. *J Neurosurg* 1995; **83**: 949–62.

21. Eker C, Asgeirsson B, Grande PO *et al.* Improved outcome after severe head injury with a new therapy based on principles for brain volume regulation and preserved microcirculation. *Crit Care Med* 1998; **26**: 1881–6.

22. Grande PO, Asgeirsson B, Nordstrom CH. Physiologic principles for volume regulation of a tissue enclosed in a rigid shell with application to the injured brain. *J Trauma* 1997; **42**: S23–31.

23. Robertson CS, Valadka AB, Hannay HJ *et al.* Prevention of secondary insults after severe head injury. *Crit Care Med* 1999; **27**: 2086–95.

24. Robertson CS. Management of cerebral perfusion pressure after traumatic brain injury. *Anesthesiology* 2001; **95**(6): 1513–17.

25. http://www2.braintrauma.org/guidelines/index.php.

26. Marmarou A, Anderson RL, Ward JD *et al.* Impact of ICP instability and hypotension on outcome in patients with severe head trauma. *J Neurosurg* 1991; **75**: s59–66.

27. Saul TG, Ducker TB. Effect of intracranial pressure monitoring and aggressive treatment on mortality in severe head injury. *J Neurosurg* 1982; **56**: 498–503.

28. Marion DW, Segal R, Thompson ME. Subarachnoid hemorrhage and the heart. *Neurosurgery* 1986; **18**: 101–6.

29. Andreoli A, Di PG, Pinelli G *et al.* Subarachnoid hemorrhage: frequency and severity of cardiac arrhythmias. A survey of 70 cases studied in the acute phase. *Stroke* 1987; **18**: 558–64.

30. Schell AR, Shenoy MM, Friedman SA, Patel AR. Pulmonary oedema associated with subarachnoid hemorrhage. Evidence for a cardiogenic origin. *Arch Intern Med* 1987; **147**: 591–2.

31. Smith WS, Matthay MA. Evidence for a hydrostatic mechanism in human neurogenic pulmonary oedema. *Chest* 1997; **111**: 1326–33.

32. Arieff AI, Ayus JC, Fraser CL. Hyponatraemia and death or permanent brain damage in healthy children. *Br Med J* 1992; **304**: 1218–22.

33. Recommendations for the safe transfer of patients with brain injury. The Association of Anaesthetists of Great Britain and Ireland. May 2006.

34. Guy J, Hindman BJ, Naker KZ *et al.* Comparison of remifentanil and fentanyl in patients undergoing craniotomy for supratentorial space occupying lesions. *Anesthesiology* 1997; **86**: 514–24.

35. Coles JP, Leary TS, Monteiro JN *et al.* Propofol anaesthesia for craniotomy: a double-blinded comparison of remifentanil, alfentanil and fentanyl. *J Neurosurg Anesthesiol* 2000; **12**: 15–20.

36. Kirkpatrick PJ, Smielewski P, Piechnik S *et al.* Early effects of mannitol in patients with head injuries assessed using bedside multimodality monitoring. *Neurosurgery* 1996; **39**: 714–20.

37. Penry JK, White BG, Brackett CE. A controlled prospective study of the pharmacologic prophylaxis of posttraumatic epilepsy. *Neurology* 1979; **29**: 600A.

38. Temkin NR, Dikmen SS, Winn HR. Management of head injury. Posttraumatic seizures. *Neurosurg Clin N Am* 1991; **2**: 425–35.

39. Muizelaar JP, Marmarou A, Ward JD *et al.* Adverse effects of prolonged hyperventilation in patients with severe head injury: a randomized clinical trial. *J Neurosurg* 1991; **75**: 731–9.

40. Elias-Jones AC, Punt JA, Turnbull AE *et al.* Management and outcome of severe head injuries in the Trent region 1985–90. *Arch Dis Child* 1992; **67**: 1430–5.

41. Lam AM, Winn HR, Cullen BF *et al.* Hyperglycaemia and neurological outcome in patients with head injury. *J Neurosurg* 1991; **75**: 545–51.

42. Van den Berghe G, Wouters P, Weekers F *et al.* Intensive insulin therapy in critically ill patients. *N Engl J Med* 2001; **345**: 1359–67.

43. Wass CT, Lanier WL, Hofer RE *et al.* Temperature changes of >1°C alter functional neurologic outcome and histopathology in a canine model of complete cerebral ischemia. *Anesthesiology* 1995; **83**: 325–35.

44. Pinosky ML, Fishman RL, Reeves ST *et al.* The effect of bupivacaine skull block on the hemodynamic response to craniotomy. *Anesth Analg* 1996; **83**: 1256–61.

45. Roberts FL, Dixon J, Lewis GTR, Tackley RM, Prys Roberts C. Induction and maintenance of propofol anaesthesia. *Anaesthesia* 1988; **43**(suppl): 14–17.

46. Coles J, Summors A. Inhalational anaesthetic agents. In: Gupta AK, Summors A, eds *Notes in Neuroanaesthesia and Critical Care*. Greenwich Medical Media Ltd. 2001; Ch. 9: 35–7.

47. Goldsack C, Scuplak SM, Smith M. A double-blind comparison of codeine and morphine for postoperative analgesia following intracranial surgery. *Anaesthesia* 1996; **51**: 1029–32.

48. Kathirvel S, Dash HH, Bhatia A *et al.* Effect of prophylactic ondansetron on postoperative nausea and vomiting after elective craniotomy. *J Neurosurg Anesthesiol* 2001; **13**: 207–12.

# Surgical issues in the management of head-injured patients

Puneet Plaha and Peter C. Whitfield

This chapter reviews the indications for surgical intervention and operative nuances that may facilitate neurosurgical procedures. This includes discussion on the surgical management of patients with traumatic intracranial haematomas, depressed skull fractures, the placement of external ventricular drains and the application of decompressive craniectomy.

## Traumatic intracranial haematomas

Acute traumatic intracranial haematomas occur in the extradural space, the subdural space or directly into the parenchyma. The latter are often associated with haemorrhagic cerebral contusions. Although haematomas are frequently apparent within the first few hours after trauma, delayed presentation is well recognized and may present with deterioration in level of consciousness or elevation of intracranial pressure. After identifying an intracranial haematoma, a number of factors are considered. Each of these influences the patient's functional outcome as discussed below (Fig. 17.1).

## Age and pre-existing medical conditions

The incidence of extradural haematomas peaks in the second decade of life and is rare in patients older than 50 years of age.[1-4] Within this population group the probability of a good outcome decreases with increasing patient age.[3] Increasing age is also a strong independent variable associated with poor outcome in both acute subdural haematoma and intraparenchymal haematoma patient groups. In patients with acute subdural haematoma aged 18–30 years with GCS <10 the mortality is < 25% at 2–3 months follow-up compared to 75% in older patients (>50yr).[5,6] In patients > 65 years[7] and especially in the >75yrs age group, the mortality increases exponentially and the chance of survival with good functional outcome is virtually zero.[8,9] Evacuation of acute subdural haematomas in this latter age group is therefore probably not justified except in exceptional circumstances.[10]

Pre-existing medical conditions including cardiovascular and respiratory dysfunction have been shown to be associated with poor outcome presumably due to the interplay among cerebral perfusion, microcirculatory function and tissue hypoxia leading to secondary brain injury in addition to increased susceptibility to the complications of prolonged immobilization.[11,12]

## Neurological status

### Glasgow Coma Scale (GCS)

The GCS at admission or prior to surgery is the single most important predictor of outcome for patients with an extradural haematoma.[13-15] The delay between any deterioration and the timing of surgery is critical in achieving a good outcome for EDH patients. An 8.9% mortality was reported if surgery was performed within 2.4 +/−0.6 h and 33.3% if surgery

*Head Injury: A Multidisciplinary Approach*, ed. Peter C. Whitfield, Elfyn O. Thomas, Fiona Summers, Maggie Whyte and Peter J. Hutchinson. Published by Cambridge University Press. © Cambridge University Press 2009.

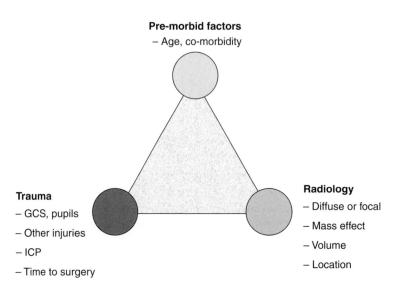

**Pre-morbid factors**
– Age, co-morbidity

**Trauma**
– GCS, pupils
– Other injuries
– ICP
– Time to surgery

**Radiology**
– Diffuse or focal
– Mass effect
– Volume
– Location

**Fig. 17.1.** Factors influencing the outcome following traumatic brain injury.

was delayed by 9.8 +/−6.1 h from the time of deterioration.[16] The GCS also independently prognosticates outcome for patients with subdural haematomas[17,18] and traumatic intra-parenchymal haematomas.[11,19,20]

The timing of surgical evacuation has been reported to correlate with outcome for acute SDH cases with a mortality of 80% if surgery was delayed by >2 h compared with a mortality of 47% if surgery occurred within 2 hours.[21] Other studies have emphasized the need for early surgery (2–4 hours).[7,22] However, this finding is not universal with some series reporting a worse outcome with early surgery, reflecting the effect of associated intracranial injuries rather than isolated SDHs in the majority of patients.[5,23]

Of the three GCS components, the preoperative motor score is the most reliable predictor of functional outcome. In a retrospective analysis of 200 patients with extradural haemato-mas, patients localizing to pain had significantly better outcomes than those with flexion, extension or no motor response ($P < 0.0001$).[15]

### Pupils

In the absence of ocular trauma and mydriatic eye drops, pupil asymmetry is an indicator of mass effect due to compression of the oculomotor nerve. Ipsilateral mydriasis indicates uncal herniation with direct compression of the third cranial nerve. Contralateral mydriasis indicates pressure on the opposite oculomotor nerve at the medial edge of the tentorium. Such pupillary dysfunction is an indicator of brainstem compression and is associated with high mortality.[3,4,24–26] Although bilateral fixed dilated pupils and other brainstem reflexes are associated with a poor outcome,[27] exceptions may occur. In one small retrospective series of extradural haematoma patients with bilateral fixed dilated pupils, rapid surgery was associated with a good outcome or moderate disability in 6/11 (55%) at 1 year. Three cases (27%) had severe disability and two died (18%). All patients with fixed and dilated pupils for longer than 6 hours died.[28] A further retrospective study investigated the latency period between the onset of anisocoria and craniotomy in comatose patients with an EDH. All five patients with a latency period of 70 minutes or less survived and had a good or reasonable outcome. All cases with > 70 minute latency died.[25] A large case series of EDH patients who

**Table 17.1.** The Marshall CT scan classification system[32]. (Reproduced with permission.)

| Categories | Definition |
|---|---|
| Diffuse injury – I (no visible pathology) | no intracranial pathology |
| Diffuse injury – II | cisterns present with midline shift 0–5 mm and/or: <br> (a) no high or mixed density lesion >25 cm$^3$ <br> (b) may include bone fragments and foreign bodies. |
| Diffuse injury – III (swelling) | cisterns compressed or absent with midline shift 0–5 mm, no high- or mixed-density lesion >25 cm$^3$ |
| Diffuse injury – IV(shift) | midline shift >5 mm, no high- or mixed-density lesion >25 cm$^3$ |
| Evacuated mass lesion | Any lesion surgically evacuated |
| Non-evacuated mass lesion | High or mixed density lesion >25 cm$^3$, not surgically evacuated |

underwent craniotomy reported a linear correlation between functional outcome and early surgery following the onset of anisocoria. The combined mortality/severe disability rate in 126 patients who underwent decompressive surgery within 1.5 hours was 7.9% as compared to 22.2% with a latency of 1.5–2.5 hours and 53.8% with a latency of 3.5–4.5 hours between the onset of pupillary asymmetry and surgery.[15]

### Intracranial pressure

The initial management of patients with small subdural haematomas and/or small contusions may be conservative (see below). The peak ICP is a powerful predictor of outcome, especially for frontal lesions.[29] The association between a sustained ICP >30 mmHg and a poor outcome is well established.[30,31]

## Haematoma/CT scan related factors

The severity of the primary injury and the duration and severity of secondary insults determines the prognosis and outcome after traumatic intracranial haematoma evacuation. The CT scan appearance provides a useful guide to the severity of the injury. To enable comparisons of results between studies, a classification scheme is required (Table 17.1).[32] For patients with an EDH, the presence of other intracranial lesions including subdural haematoma, parenchymal lesions[14,15] and traumatic subarachnoid haemorrhage[3,28] is associated with a poor outcome. For patients with focal parenchymal injuries, a single brain contusion was associated with a better outcome than multiple contusions or parenchymal haematomas.[11,26] In this patient group traumatic subarachnoid haemorrhage and thin subdural haematomas reflect a more severe cortical injury and are features associated with a poor outcome.

The volume of focal lesions correlates with outcome. Very large extradural haematomas were reported to be associated with poor outcomes many years ago.[24] Poor outcomes have been associated with extradural haematoma volumes of more than 50 cm$^3$ or 77 ± 63 cm$^3$.[33,15] Other CT scan findings associated with the mass effect of large extradural haematomas (midline shift 5 mm, compression/obliteration of the perimesencephalic cistern or the third ventricle) also correlate with poor outcome.[3,15,24,28] An acute SDH of <10 mm clot thickness was associated with a 10% mortality, while clots thicker than 30 mm resulted in a 90% mortality.[33] Midline shift >15 mm and compression/obliteration of the basal cisterns also

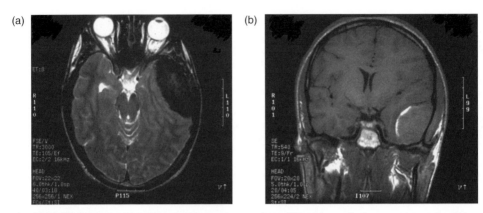

(a)      (b)

**Fig. 17.2.** Most patients with an extradural haematoma undergo CT imaging and subsequent evacuation. This patient presented with headache several days after trauma. The axial T2 (a) and coronal T1-weighted image (b) clearly demonstrate an extra-axial mass lesion causing some brain shift. The patient elected to undergo surgical evacuation of this extradural haematoma and made an uneventful recovery.

correlates with poor outcome.[5,33,34] However, some studies have found no correlation again reflecting the widespread brain injury associated with some acute SDHs.[3,6]

The location of an extradural haematoma appears to be less important at determining outcome than the volume and time delay to theatre.[24,35] However, the location of intracranial haematomas may be of significance in determining outcome. Posterior fossa haematomas are relatively uncommon, but require rapid decompression if they are causing secondary injury. Similarly, the confines of the middle cranial fossa indicate that temporal or temporoparietal parenchymal haematomas are more likely to cause uncal herniation and brainstem compression than a haematoma in other locations.[36] Low attenuation regions within a clot indicate a hyperacute bleed. This may be associated with poor outcome presumably as a consequence of rapid, severe and increasing elevation of intracranial pressure.[15,24]

## Conservative treatment of patients with traumatic intracranial haematomas

Non-comatose patients with small extradural haematomas can be successfully managed conservatively.[1,37] However, most authors would advocate surgery as the safest option if haematoma volume > 30 cm,[3,38,39] clot thickness >15 mm[38–40] and midline shift exceeds 4 or 5 mm.[38–40] (Fig. 17.2). In addition, delayed surgery is common in patients with temporal haematomas initially managed conservatively.

Patients with GCS 13–15 and an acute subdural haematoma <10 mm in thickness can be managed conservatively[41] and those with thickness >10 mm or midline shift greater than 5 mm, irrespective of the GCS, require surgical evacuation.[42] Comatose patients (GCS <9) with clot thickness < 10 mm and midline shift < 5 mm can be managed conservatively with ICP monitoring pressure and evacuation if pressures exceed 20 mmHg.[42]

Parenchymal lesions are dynamic. An increase in size of pre-existing lesions or appearance of new non-contiguous lesions commonly occurs especially within the first 24–48 hours.[43,44] In addition, delayed traumatic intracerebral haematoma (DTICH) or space demanding contusions may develop in patients with diffuse injury on the initial scans.[12,45–47] Clotting abnormalities are associated with this complication.[48] Repeat CT scanning is therefore an important consideration in managing traumatic brain injury patients.[49] If detected early, the high mortality of unrecognized DTICH may be averted.[47,50]

Given the potential for change, conservative management of traumatic intraparenchymal brain injury requires careful supervision. Given this caveat, a conservative approach is sometimes appropriate:

1. Patients with small parenchymal mass lesions, and no radiological signs of significant mass effect (midline shift <5 mm, no basal cistern effacement) who consistently obey commands and harbour no neurological deficits.

2. ICP monitoring is appropriate for patients who do not obey commands when the initial CT scan shows small parenchymal lesions without significant mass effect.

In contrast, a prospective study on 218 patients with intracerebral lesions who did not obey commands within the first 24 hours of the injury concluded that early surgery was indicated for:

(a) Patients with a GCS of > 6 and focal lesion volume > 20 cm$^3$

(b) Temporal contusions with CT scan showing signs of mass effect and GCS >10.[51]

Several factors suggest that surgery is indicated after an initial period of conservative treatment for patients with focal parenchymal lesions. These include a mean hourly ICP > 30 mm Hg [30,31] or a repeat CT scan showing an increase in haematoma/contusion volume with signs of mass effect.[29]

# Surgical techniques

### Extradural and subdural haematomas

Extradural and subdural haematomas are most frequently located in the fronto-temporo-parietal and temporal regions. They are best accessed via a question mark-shaped scalp flap and craniotomy, whose location and size can be adapted according to the site and size of the pathology. Extradural haematomas are often associated with vault fractures. Reconstruction of these needs consideration during elevation of the flap. Suction and irrigation facilitate removal of an extradural haematoma. A glass sucker is particularly effective. The initial burr hole alone can be used to achieve a rapid initial decompression. Bipolar diathermy controls any continuing middle meningeal bleeding, whilst bleeding at the skull base can be controlled by packing the foramen spinosum region with bone wax and oxidized cellulose followed by placement of dural hitch stitches.

A subdural haematoma causes the dura to be tense with a bluish colouration. Although some surgeons advocate making slits in the dura to permit decompression without brain herniation, a wide dural opening is most effective at evacuating the clot and identifying the bleeding source. This is often venous bleeding from contused cortex or bridging veins, although an isolated arterial bleeder is sometimes evident. If brain swelling is evident or anticipated, removal of the bone flap without dural closure affords an effective decompression. For both extradural and subdural haematomas (where bone flap is replaced), routine placement of circumferential dural hitch stitches with a central hitch stitch placed to obliterate the dead space beneath the bone flap help prevent re-accumulation of the haematoma.

### Cerebral contusions and intracerebral haematoma

The location and extent of the contusion/haematoma on the CT scan governs the position of the scalp flap. A large flap provides adequate exposure of contused and haemorrhagic brain and permits an effective decompressive craniectomy if required. Although the head may be positioned on a horseshoe, three-point skull fixation does facilitate intra-operative adjustments of head position and provides a more stable platform for undertaking a craniotomy. Elevation of the head by 20–30° helps to control ICP and reduces venous bleeding. Swollen, contused and haemorrhagic brain is removed using gentle suction and bipolar diathermy. For severe polar injury, a temporal or frontal lobectomy (6 cm from the temporal pole and 7 cm from the frontal pole) may be required to achieve adequate decompression. Bipolar diathermy coagulates larger bleeding vessels. A monolayer of Surgicel™ coated with cottonoids and packed with saline-soaked cotton balls for 5 minutes controls small vessel bleeding from exposed dissected brain. The operating microscope facilitates this potentially tricky stage of the procedure. Any uncertainty about haemostasis leads to re-examination of the cavity. Capillary tube drainage of the cavity reliably helps to prevent secondary clots developing in difficult cases. During closure, prophylactic removal of the bone flap to facilitate the management of post-operative brain swelling is considered. In such cases, subgaleal suction drainage may cause brain shift leading to bradycardia and cardiac arrest. A capillary or non-suction drain is preferred in these circumstances. A standard colostomy bag applied over an exiting capillary drain collects drainage products.

## Depressed skull fractures

Skull fractures are classified by (a) the integrity of the scalp (open or closed), (b) the anatomical location (convexity of skull or basal) and (c) the pattern of fracture (linear, depressed or comminuted). All open fractures require thorough debridement to minimise the risk of infection. In the case of penetrating injury, removal of any accessible debris (e.g. pellets, bullets) minimizes the infection risk. In the absence of any significant intracranial haematoma, the other major indication to elevate a fracture is cosmesis. This is most relevant where the fracture lies on the forehead. Fractures near the major venous sinuses pose special problems due to the risk of bleeding during disimpaction and the risk of thrombotic sinus occlusion if the depressed fragment remains *in situ*.[52,53] Although the removal of impacted fragments from brain is unlikely to improve any neurological deficit, many consider this a relative indication for surgery. Compound depressed fractures in cosmetically unobtrusive sites may be managed with debridement alone, if there is no clinical or radiological evidence of dural violation (exposed brain/CSF leak or pneumocephalus) and if the degree of depression is less than the depth of the skull.[54,55]

The principles for management of compound fractures are well established and to some extent are governed by the cause of injury. For injuries caused by sharp objects such as pencils, screwdrivers and knives, a high index of suspicion is required. Often, a small entry wound bellies a serious penetrating injury and an orbital entry point can obscure the presence of a brain injury. Bullet wounds are subdivided into low velocity injuries (less than 300 ms$^{-1}$) and high velocity trauma. The former are characterized by a track representing the route of potential contamination and injury. High velocity wounds cause intracranial shockwaves and brain cavitation. They are associated with a high early mortality. Aggressive early surgical debridement of entrance and exit wounds, removal of necrotic material and accessible bone and metal fragments is mandatory.[56] It is now accepted that inaccessible in-driven bone and metallic fragments may be safely left *in situ* to minimize collateral brain damage caused by surgery. Although there are no large randomized trials, antimicrobial prophylaxis is recommended for patients with penetrating craniocerebral trauma. The British Society for Antimicrobial Chemotherapy working party recommends 5 days of broad-spectrum cover for such injuries using Co-amoxiclav or a combination of cefuroxime and metronidazole.[57] In the absence of gross wound contamination, bone fragment replacement is appropriate.[56,58–60]

## Surgical techniques

Devitalized or contaminated edges of the scalp require excision and thorough debridement. The impacted depressed fragments usually require placement of an adjacent burr hole to permit disimpaction. Fragments are levered upward sufficient to examine the underlying dura. Visualization of the dura frequently requires removal of the fragments. In the presence of a dural tear the underlying brain requires inspection to permit removal of accessible penetrating bone and fragments of contaminated material. Any cortical bleeding requires attention. A periosteal graft helps repair the dural tear. Bone fragments require thorough irrigation with saline and/or dilute hydrogen peroxide solution. Mini-fixation systems facilitate the re-implantation of large fragments.

## Chronic subdural haematoma (CSDH)

Although small chronic subdural haematomas can be observed, any lesion causing mass effect and neurological features warrants surgical treatment. Patients with these haematomas are often elderly and intolerant of major intervention. Fortunately, the majority of patients can be successfully treated with relatively simple procedures, although an array of surgical approaches exists. This includes burr hole drainage, twist drill drainage, craniotomy and a small craniectomy. Combining each technique with the use of intraoperative irrigation and/or post-operative drainage provides a variety of treatment options.

## Surgical techniques

Two appropriately positioned burr holes placed along the same line as the incision of a trauma flap enable evacuation of most chronic subdural haematomas. Control of dural bleeding is important. A distinctive grey encapsulating membrane usually requires opening to permit drainage of the liquefied haematoma. This is often under considerable initial pressure. Occasionally, conversion to a craniotomy is required if a substantial solid component persists. Irrigation of the subdural space, facilitated by the use of a soft Jacques catheter, facilitates evacuation. Twist drill craniostomy has been advocated in search of a less invasive treatment option with a skull opening usually less than 5 mm. Irrigation through such a small aperture is difficult. A craniotomy permits fluid evacuation and partial removal of the haematoma membrane in patients with recurrent, persistent chronic subdural haematomas.[61] A small craniectomy is an alternative that enables clinical assessment of recurrent collections. A valveless subdural–peritoneal conduit fashioned from a peritoneal catheter with side holes cut for the subdural space and securely anchored to the galea can be useful in the treatment of patients with an atrophic brain where persistence of the subdural collection occurs despite recent drainage.

An analysis of 48 publications from 1981 to 2001 showed a wide range of cure, recurrence and mortality rates for each procedure. There was no overall significant difference in mortality between the techniques with a mortality of up to 11%. Morbidity from a craniotomy was higher than drainage procedures and the recurrence rate was highest for a twist drill craniostomy.[62] Evidence supporting the use of intraoperative irrigation to lower the recurrence rate[63] is not universal.[64–68] Evidence to support the use of closed post-operative subdural drainage is inconclusive with some authors reporting no benefit and others advocating drainage.[61,69–73] Similarly, peri-operative continuous inflow/outflow irrigation after evacuation of the haematoma does not appear to confer significant benefit except in patients undergoing twist drill craniostomy.[74]

# External ventricular drains (EVD)

The reduction of intracranial pressure by placement of a catheter into the frontal horn of the lateral ventricle for cerebrospinal fluid drainage is well established. The technique can be used as an early therapeutic manoeuvre or reserved for patients with refractory intracranial hypertension. In addition, ventricular pressure monitoring is considered the 'gold standard' for ICP measurement. However, the simplicity of intraparenchymal ICP monitoring using robust hardware has superseded ventricular pressure monitoring in many centres.

## Surgical techniques

The patient is positioned with 10° head up tilt. Insertion is usually performed on the right side (non dominant) although, if unilateral hemisphere swelling is evident, ipsilateral placement is advisable to avoid further mid-line shift. A linear incision is performed with a twist drill or burr hole at Kocher's point (1 cm anterior to the coronal suture and in the mid-pupillary line). The catheter, inserted complete with stylet, is directed medially – aiming for the ipsilateral medial canthus – and slightly posteriorly in the sagittal plane – directed at the tragus. A loss of resistance is experienced on entering the ventricle at a depth of 5–6 cm. Withdrawal of the stylet is followed by egress of CSF. If the ventricle is not tapped at a depth of 7 cm, removal and reinsertion in a more medial direction is usually successful. Deeper insertion of the catheter leads to misplacement. Subcutaneous tunnelling for a distance of at least 6 or 7 cm minimizes the risk of infection. A '360° loop' of catheter securely anchored to the scalp in two places effectively reduces the risk of inadvertent catheter removal. The distal end is connected to a manometric EVD drainage system.

### Steps to prevent EVD catheter infection

Coagulase negative Staphylococcal infection is very common after EVD placement. Although prophylactic antibiotics are usually administered, there is no evidence to support the use of prolonged prophylactic antimicrobial administration.[75–79] Tunnelling the distal catheter subcutaneously > 5 cm from the burr hole[80,81] or even further to the chest or upper abdomen[82] has been shown to reduce the infection rate. Silicone catheters are in widespread use. A prospective, randomized, multicentre-controlled trial showed that the colonization of rifampicin and minocycline impregnated catheters was half as likely as the control catheters (17.9 vs. 36.7%, respectively, $P=0.0012$) with a lower incidence of CSF infection in the antibiotic-impregnated catheter group compared with those in the control group (1.3% vs. 9.4%, respectively, $P= 0.002$).[83] Although previously suggested,[75] most authors now agree that prophylactic catheter exchange after 5 days does not reduce the risk of EVD infection [84–86] and may in fact even increase the risk of CSF infection.[87]

# Decompressive craniectomy

Decompressive craniectomy is performed to increase the volume of space available for a post-traumatic swollen brain. It may be performed either as a prophylactic measure after haematoma evacuation when brain swelling is anticipated, or as a therapeutic manoeuvre for the management of raised intracranial pressure. Prophylactic decompressive craniectomy is performed where the brain is considered to be at risk of swelling after evacuation of a mass lesion. In clinical practice this is an effective measure to facilitate post-operative intracranial pressure management. Although much of the early literature showed therapeutic decompressive craniectomy to be associated with a very poor outcome, the technique has increased in popularity in the last 15 years. Early studies reserved craniectomy for patients *in extremis* promulgating the futility of the technique. However, several small studies[88,89] have shown that patients can achieve a favourable outcome following decompression with reduction of intracranial pressure and an improvement in cerebral perfusion pressure and associated parameters.[90,91] Ongoing international clinical trials are currently evaluating decompressive craniectomy as a therapeutic option in the management of patients with refractory intra-cranial hypertension.[92,93]

## Surgical techniques

Therapeutic decompressive craniectomy is most effectively performed as a large bifrontal bone flap, although some recommend a unilateral approach if the CT appearances show swelling of only one hemisphere. A bicoronal skin flap permits exposure of the frontal bone. The craniotomy extends from the supra-orbital ridge to the anterior aspect of the coronal suture. To reduce contamination, entry into the frontal air sinus is avoided by careful study of the pre-operative CT scans. Laterally, the flap extends to the temporal bone. If temporal lobe swelling is evident, the bone flap should extend towards the zygomatic arch. Bleeding from the superior sagittal sinus is not usually problematic and can be controlled with elevation of the head and application of haemostatic sponge. If the dura is opened bilaterally with a medial base on each side, the interhemispheric fissure can be explored to permit division of the falx cerebri and the anterior sagittal sinus. A frontal periosteal flap assists closure, although a watertight approximation is not required. If a favourable outcome is achieved a delayed cranioplasty procedure is performed.

## Clotting abnormalities

Many patients undergoing neurosurgery following trauma have clotting abnormalities. Close discussion with haematologists is necessary to reverse clotting deficiencies in a rapid, timely manner. Warfarin therapy poses specific problems. Historically, warfarin reversal comprised oral or i.v. vitamin K administration supplemented with fresh frozen plasma. Such a process can lead to unacceptable delays in performing emergency surgery while FFP is obtained, thawed, administered and haematological parameters rechecked. Complete and rapid reversal of warfarin over-anticoagulation is better achieved with 5 or 10 mg of intra-venous vitamin K and II, VII, IX and X factor concentrate (Beriplex™).[94,95]

## References

1. Cucciniello B, Martellotta N, Nigro D, Citro E. Conservative management of extradural haematomas. *Acta Neurochir (Wien)* 1993; **120**(1–2): 47–52.

2. Jones NR, Molloy CJ, Kloeden CN, North JB, Simpson DA. Extradural haematoma: trends in outcome over 35 years. *Br J Neurosurg* 1993; 7(5): 465–71.

3. van den Brink WA, Zwienenberg M, Zandee SM, van der Meer L, Maas AI, Avezaat CJ. The prognostic importance of the volume of traumatic epidural and subdural haematomas revisited. *Acta Neurochir (Wien)* 1999; **141**(5): 509–14.

4. Bricolo AP, Pasut LM. Extradural hematoma: toward zero mortality. A prospective study. *Neurosurgery* 1984; **14**(1): 8–12.

5. Kotwica Z, Brzezinski J. Acute subdural haematoma in adults: an analysis of outcome in comatose patients. *Acta Neurochir (Wien)* 1993; **121**(3–4): 95–9.

6. Howard MA, 3rd, Gross AS, Dacey RG, Jr, Winn HR. Acute subdural hematomas: an age-dependent clinical entity. *J Neurosurg* 1989; **71**(6): 858–63.

7. Wilberger JE, Jr, Harris M, Diamond DL. Acute subdural hematoma: morbidity,

mortality, and operative timing. *J Neurosurg* 1991; **74**(2): 212–18.

8. Kotwica Z, Jakubowski JK. Acute head injuries in the elderly. An analysis of 136 consecutive patients. *Acta Neurochir (Wien)* 1992; **118**(3–4): 98–102.

9. Cagetti B, Cossu M, Pau A, Rivano C, Viale G. The outcome from acute subdural and epidural intracranial haematomas in very elderly patients. *Br J Neurosurg* 1992; **6**(3): 227–31.

10. Jamjoom A. Justification for evacuating acute subdural haematomas in patients above the age of 75 years. *Injury* 1992; **23**(8): 518–20.

11. Choksey M, Crockard HA, Sandilands M. Acute traumatic intracerebral haematomas: determinants of outcome in a retrospective series of 202 cases. *Br J Neurosurg* 1993; **7**(6): 611–22.

12. Servadei F, Murray GD, Penny K *et al.* The value of the 'worst' computed tomographic scan in clinical studies of moderate and severe head injury. European Brain Injury Consortium. *Neurosurgery* 2000; **46**(1): 70–5; discussion 75–7.

13. Uzan M, Yentur E, Hanci M *et al.* Is it possible to recover from uncal herniation? Analysis of 71 head injured cases. *J Neurosurg Sci* 1998; **42**(2): 89–94.

14. Kuday C, Uzan M, Hanci M. Statistical analysis of the factors affecting the outcome of extradural haematomas: 115 cases. *Acta Neurochir (Wien)* 1994; **131**(3–4): 203–6.

15. Lee EJ, Hung YC, Wang LC, Chung KC, Chen HH. Factors influencing the functional outcome of patients with acute epidural hematomas: analysis of 200 patients undergoing surgery. *J Trauma* 1998; **45**(5): 946–52.

16. Mendelow AD, Karmi MZ, Paul KS, Fuller GA, Gillingham FJ. Extradural haematoma: effect of delayed treatment. *Br Med J* 1979; **1**(6173): 1240–2.

17. Koc RK, Akdemir H, Oktem IS, Meral M, Menku A. Acute subdural hematoma: outcome and outcome prediction. *Neurosurg Rev* 1997; **20**(4): 239–44.

18. Massaro F, Lanotte M, Faccani G, Triolo C. One hundred and twenty-seven cases of acute subdural haematoma operated on. Correlation between CT scan findings and outcome. *Acta Neurochir (Wien)* 1996; **138**(2): 185–91.

19. Papo I, Caruselli G, Luongo A, Scarpelli M, Pasquini U. Traumatic cerebral mass lesions: correlations between clinical, intracranial pressure, and computed tomographic data. *Neurosurgery* 1980; **7**(4): 337–46.

20. Gennarelli TA, Spielman GM, Langfitt TW *et al.* Influence of the type of intracranial lesion on outcome from severe head injury. *J Neurosurg* 1982; **56**(1): 26–32.

21. Haselsberger K, Pucher R, Auer LM. Prognosis after acute subdural or epidural haemorrhage. *Acta Neurochir (Wien)* 1988; **90**(3–4): 111–16.

22. Seelig JM, Becker DP, Miller JD, Greenberg RP, Ward JD, Choi SC. Traumatic acute subdural hematoma: major mortality reduction in comatose patients treated within four hours. *N Engl J Med* 1981; **304**(25): 1511–18.

23. Dent DL, Croce MA, Menke PG *et al.* Prognostic factors after acute subdural hematoma. *J Trauma* 1995; **39**(1): 36–42; discussion 42–3.

24. Rivas JJ, Lobato RD, Sarabia R, Cordobes F, Cabrera A, Gomez P. Extradural hematoma: analysis of factors influencing the courses of 161 patients. *Neurosurgery* 1988; **23**(1): 44–51.

25. Cohen JE, Montero A, Israel ZH. Prognosis and clinical relevance of anisocoria-craniotomy latency for epidural hematoma in comatose patients. *J Trauma* 1996; **41**(1): 120–2.

26. Lobato RD, Cordobes F, Rivas JJ *et al.* Outcome from severe head injury related to the type of intracranial lesion. A computerized tomography study. *J Neurosurg* 1983; **59**(5): 762–74.

27. Caroli M, Locatelli M, Campanella R, Balbi S, Martinelli F, Arienta C. Multiple intracranial lesions in head injury: clinical considerations, prognostic factors, management, and results in 95 patients. *Surg Neurol* 2001; **56**(2): 82–8.

28. Sakas DE, Bullock MR, Teasdale GM. One-year outcome following craniotomy for traumatic hematoma in patients with fixed dilated pupils. *J Neurosurg* 1995; **82**(6): 961–5.

29. Bullock R, Golek J, Blake G. Traumatic intracerebral hematoma – which patients should undergo surgical evacuation? CT scan features and ICP monitoring as a basis

for decision making. *Surg Neurol* 1989; **32**(3): 181–7.

30. Gallbraith S, Teasdale G. Predicting the need for operation in the patient with an occult traumatic intracranial hematoma. *J Neurosurg* 1981; **55**(1): 75–81.

31. Katayama Y, Tsubokawa T, Miyazaki S, Kawamata T, Yoshino A. Oedema fluid formation within contused brain tissue as a cause of medically uncontrollable elevation of intracranial pressure: the role of surgical therapy. *Acta Neurochir Suppl (Wien)* 1990; **51**: 308–10.

32. Marshall LF, Marshall SB, Klauber MR *et al.* A new classification of head injury based on computerised tomography. *J Neurosurg* 1991; **75**: S14–20.

33. Zumkeller M, Behrmann R, Heissler HE, Dietz H. Computed tomographic criteria and survival rate for patients with acute subdural hematoma. *Neurosurgery* 1996; **39**(4): 708–12; discussion 712–13.

34. Servadei F, Nasi MT, Giuliani G *et al.* CT prognostic factors in acute subdural haematomas: the value of the 'worst' CT scan. *Br J Neurosurg* 2000; **14**(2): 110–16.

35. Seelig JM, Marshall LF, Toutant SM *et al.* Traumatic acute epidural hematoma: unrecognized high lethality in comatose patients. *Neurosurgery* 1984; **15**(5): 617–20.

36. Andrews BT, Chiles BW, 3rd, Olsen WL, Pitts LH. The effect of intracerebral hematoma location on the risk of brain-stem compression and on clinical outcome. *J Neurosurg* 1988; **69**(4): 518–22.

37. Bullock R, Smith RM, van Dellen JR. Nonoperative management of extradural hematoma. *Neurosurgery* 1985; **16**(5): 602–6.

38. Chen N. Traumatic extradural hematoma in the middle cranial fossa base: clinical analysis of 14 cases. *Chin J Traumatol* 2001; **4**(1): 48–50.

39. Bejjani GK, Donahue DJ, Rusin J, Broemeling LD. Radiological and clinical criteria for the management of epidural hematomas in children. *Pediatr Neurosurg* 1996; **25**(6): 302–8.

40. Servadei F, Faccani G, Roccella P *et al.* Asymptomatic extradural haematomas. Results of a multicenter study of 158 cases in minor head injury. *Acta Neurochir (Wien)* 1989; **96**(1–2): 39–45.

41. Mathew P, Oluoch-Olunya DL, Condon BR, Bullock R. Acute subdural haematoma in the conscious patient: outcome with initial non-operative management. *Acta Neurochir (Wien)* 1993; **121**(3–4): 100–8.

42. Servadei F, Nasi MT, Cremonini AM, Giuliani G, Cenni P, Nanni A. Importance of a reliable admission Glasgow Coma Scale score for determining the need for evacuation of posttraumatic subdural hematomas: a prospective study of 65 patients. *J Trauma* 1998; **44**(5): 868–73.

43. Yamaki T, Hirakawa K, Ueguchi T, Tenjin H, Kuboyama T, Nakagawa Y. Chronological evaluation of acute traumatic intracerebral haematoma. *Acta Neurochir (Wien)* 1990; **103**(3–4): 112–15.

44. Servadei F, Nanni A, Nasi MT, Zappi D, Vergoni G, Giuliani G, et al. Evolving brain lesions in the first 12 hours after head injury: analysis of 37 comatose patients. *Neurosurgery* 1995; **37**(5): 899–906; discussion 906–7.

45. Gudeman SK, Kishore PR, Miller JD, Girevendulis AK, Lipper MH, Becker DP. The genesis and significance of delayed traumatic intracerebral hematoma. *Neurosurgery* 1979; **5**(3): 309–13.

46. Gentleman D, Nath F, Macpherson P. Diagnosis and management of delayed traumatic intracerebral haematomas. *Br J Neurosurg* 1989; **3**(3): 367–72.

47. Sprick C, Bettag M, Bock WJ. Delayed traumatic intracranial hematomas – clinical study of seven years. *Neurosurg Rev* 1989; **12** Suppl 1: 228–30.

48. Kaufman HH, Moake JL, Olson JD *et al.* Delayed and recurrent intracranial hematomas related to disseminated intravascular clotting and fibrinolysis in head injury. *Neurosurgery* 1980; **7**(5): 445–9.

49. Durham SR, Liu KC, Selden NR. Utility of serial computed tomography imaging in pediatric patients with head trauma. *J Neurosurg* 2006; **105**(5 Suppl): 365–9.

50. Tseng SH. Delayed traumatic intracerebral hemorrhage: a study of prognostic factors. *J Formos Med Assoc* 1992; **91**(6): 585–9.

51. Mathiesen T, Kakarieka A, Edner G. Traumatic intracerebral lesions without extracerebral haematoma in 218 patients. *Acta Neurochir (Wien)* 1995; **137**(3–4): 155–63, discussion 163.

52. Yokota H, Eguchi T, Nobayashi M, Nishioka T, Nishimura F, Nikaido Y. Persistent

intracranial hypertension caused by superior sagittal sinus stenosis following depressed skull fracture. Case report and review of the literature. *J Neurosurg* 2006; **104**(5): 849–52.

53. Fuentes S, Metellus P, Levrier O, Adetchessi T, Dufour H, Grisoli F. Depressed skull fracture overlying the superior sagittal sinus causing benign intracranial hypertension: description of two cases and review of the literature. *Br J Neurosurg* 2005; **19**(5): 438–42.

54. Heary RF, Hunt CD, Krieger AJ, Schulder M, Vaid C. Nonsurgical treatment of compound depressed skull fractures. *J Trauma* 1993; **35**(3): 441–7.

55. van den Heever CM, van der Merwe DJ. Management of depressed skull fractures: selective conservative management of nonmissile injuries. *J Neurosurg* 1989; **71**(2): 186–90.

56. Jennett B, Miller JD. Infection after depressed fracture of skull: implications for management of nonmissile injuries. *J Neurosurg* 1972; **36**(3): 333–9.

57. Bayston R, de Louvois J, Brown EM, Johnston RA, Lees P, Pople IK. Use of antibiotics in penetrating craniocerebral injuries. "Infection in Neurosurgery" Working Party of British Society for Antimicrobial Chemotherapy. *Lancet* 2000; **355**(9217): 1813–17.

58. Braakman R. Depressed skull fracture: data, treatment, and follow-up in 225 consecutive cases. *J Neurol Neurosurg Psychiatry* 1972; **35**(3): 395–402.

59. Wylen EL, Willis BK, Nanda A. Infection rate with replacement of bone fragment in compound depressed skull fractures. *Surg Neurol* 1999; **51**(4): 452–7.

60. Adeloye A, Shokunbi MT. Immediate bone replacement in compound depressed skull fractures. *Cent Afr J Med* 1993; **39**(4): 70–3.

61. Markwalder TM. Chronic subdural hematomas: a review. *J Neurosurg* 1981; **54**(5): 637–45.

62. Weigel R, Schmiedek P, Krauss JK. Outcome of contemporary surgery for chronic subdural haematoma: evidence based review. *J Neurol Neurosurg Psychiatry* 2003; **74**(7): 937–43.

63. Aoki N. Subdural tapping and irrigation for the treatment of chronic subdural hematoma in adults. *Neurosurgery* 1984; **14**(5): 545–8.

64. Iwadate Y, Ishige N, Hosoi Y. Single burr hole irrigation without drainage in chronic subdural hematoma. *Neurol Med Chir (Tokyo)* 1989; **29**(2): 117–21.

65. Benzel EC, Bridges RM, Jr, Hadden TA, Orrison WW. The single burr hole technique for the evacuation of non-acute subdural hematomas. *J Trauma* 1994; **36**(2): 190–4.

66. Matsumoto K, Akagi K, Abekura M *et al.* Recurrence factors for chronic subdural hematomas after burr-hole craniostomy and closed system drainage. *Neurol Res* 1999; **21**(3): 277–80.

67. Suzuki K, Sugita K, Akai T, Takahata T, Sonobe M, Takahashi S. Treatment of chronic subdural hematoma by closed-system drainage without irrigation. *Surg Neurol* 1998; **50**(3): 231–4.

68. Kuroki T, Katsume M, Harada N, Yamazaki T, Aoki K, Takasu N. Strict closed-system drainage for treating chronic subdural haematoma. *Acta Neurochir (Wien)* 2001; **143**(10): 1041–4.

69. Markwalder TM, Seiler RW. Chronic subdural hematomas: to drain or not to drain? *Neurosurgery* 1985; **16**(2): 185–8.

70. Laumer R, Schramm J, Leykauf K. Implantation of a reservoir for recurrent subdural hematoma drainage. *Neurosurgery* 1989; **25**(6): 991–6.

71. Wakai S, Hashimoto K, Watanabe N, Inoh S, Ochiai C, Nagai M. Efficacy of closed-system drainage in treating chronic subdural hematoma: a prospective comparative study. *Neurosurgery* 1990; **26**(5): 771–3.

72. Nakaguchi H, Tanishima T, Yoshimasu N. Relationship between drainage catheter location and postoperative recurrence of chronic subdural hematoma after burr-hole irrigation and closed-system drainage. *J Neurosurg* 2000; **93**(5): 791–5.

73. Kwon TH, Park YK, Lim DJ *et al.* Chronic subdural hematoma: evaluation of the clinical significance of postoperative drainage volume. *J Neurosurg* 2000; **93**(5): 796–9.

74. Ram Z, Hadani M, Sahar A, Spiegelmann R. Continuous irrigation-drainage of the subdural space for the treatment of chronic subdural haematoma. A prospective clinical trial. *Acta Neurochir (Wien)* 1993; **120**(1–2): 40–3.

75. Mayhall CG, Archer NH, Lamb VA *et al.* Ventriculostomy-related infections: a prospective epidemiologic study. *N Engl J Med* 1984; **310**(9): 553–9.

76. Clark WC, Muhlbauer MS, Lowrey R, Hartman M, Ray MW, Watridge CB. Complications of intracranial pressure monitoring in trauma patients. *Neurosurgery* 1989; **25**(1): 20–4.

77. Alleyne CH, Jr, Hassan M, Zabramski JM. The efficacy and cost of prophylactic and periprocedural antibiotics in patients with external ventricular drains. *Neurosurgery* 2000; **47**(5): 1124–7; discussion 1127–9.

78. Poon WS, Ng S, Wai S. CSF antibiotic prophylaxis for neurosurgical patients with ventriculostomy: a randomised study. *Acta Neurochir Suppl* 1998; **71**: 146–8.

79. Lyke KE, Obasanjo OO, Williams MA, O'Brien M, Chotani R, Perl TM. Ventriculitis complicating use of intraventricular catheters in adult neurosurgical patients. *Clin Infect Dis* 2001; **33**(12): 2028–33.

80. Friedman WA, Vries JK. Percutaneous tunnel ventriculostomy. Summary of 100 procedures. *J Neurosurg* 1980; **53**(5): 662–5.

81. Sandalcioglu IE, Stolke D. Failure of regular external ventricular drain exchange to reduce CSF infection. *J Neurol Neurosurg Psychiatry* 2003; **74**(11): 1598–9; author reply 1599.

82. Khanna RK, Rosenblum ML, Rock JP, Malik GM. Prolonged external ventricular drainage with percutaneous long-tunnel ventriculostomies. *J Neurosurg* 1995; **83**(5): 791–4.

83. Zabramski JM, Whiting D, Darouiche RO *et al.* Efficacy of antimicrobial-impregnated external ventricular drain catheters: a prospective, randomized, controlled trial. *J Neurosurg* 2003; **98**(4): 725–30.

84. Holloway KL, Barnes T, Choi S *et al.* Ventriculostomy infections: the effect of monitoring duration and catheter exchange in 584 patients. *J Neurosurg* 1996; **85**(3): 419–24.

85. Wong GK, Poon WS, Wai S, Yu LM, Lyon D, Lam JM. Failure of regular external ventricular drain exchange to reduce cerebrospinal fluid infection: result of a randomised controlled trial. *J Neurol Neurosurg Psychiatry* 2002; **73**(6): 759–61.

86. Park P, Garton HJ, Kocan MJ, Thompson BG. Risk of infection with prolonged ventricular catheterization. *Neurosurgery* 2004; **55**(3): 594–9; discussion 599–601.

87. Lo CH, Spelman D, Bailey M, Cooper DJ, Rosenfeld JV, Brecknell JE. External ventricular drain infections are independent of drain duration: an argument against elective revision. *J Neurosurg* 2007; **106**(3): 378–83.

88. Polin RS, Shaffrey ME, Bogaev CA *et al.* Decompressive bifrontal craniectomy in the treatment of severe refractory posttraumatic cerebral edema. *Neurosurgery* 1997; **41**(1): 84–92; discussion 92–4.

89. Guerra WK, Piek J, Gaab MR. Decompressive craniectomy to treat intracranial hypertension in head injury patients. *Intens Care Med* 1999; **25**(11): 1327–9.

90. Whitfield PC, Patel H, Hutchinson PJ *et al.* Bifrontal decompressive craniectomy in the management of posttraumatic intracranial hypertension. *Br J Neurosurg* 2001; **15**(6): 500–7.

91. Yoo DS, Kim DS, Cho KS, Huh PW, Park CK, Kang JK. Ventricular pressure monitoring during bilateral decompression with dural expansion. *J Neurosurg* 1999; **91**(6): 953–9.

92. http://clinicaltrials.gov/ct/show/NCT00155987; jsessionid=A383DC8832CBF1969BB0C48C04D4E4C7?order=23.

93. Hutchinson PJ, Corteen E, Czosnyka M *et al.* Decompressive craniectomy in traumatic brain injury: the randomized multicenter RESCUEicp study (www.RESCUEicp.com). *Acta Neurochir Suppl* 2006; **96**: 17–20.

94. Baglin TP, Keeling DM, Watson HG. Guidelines on oral anticoagulation (warfarin): 3rd edition – 2005 update. *Br J Haematol* 2006; **132**(3): 277–85.

95. Evans G, Luddington R, Baglin T. Beriplex P/N reverses severe warfarin-induced overanticoagulation immediately and completely in patients presenting with major bleeding. *Br J Haematol* 2001; **115**(4): 998–1001.

# Craniofacial trauma: injury patterns and management

Paul McArdle

## Introduction

The complexity of management of the patient with a severe craniofacial injury demands multidisciplinary care to deal with neurosurgical, maxillofacial and ophthalmic problems. A dedicated craniofacial service with multiprofessional team working ensures that the long-term issues of neurorehabilitation, psychiatric support and support of the family are met as well as the early challenges of airway threat, hypovolaemia secondary to haemorrhage, head injury and fracture management. Inadequate investigation, planning and management results in missed or inadequately treated injuries and the increased risk of late complications, poor functional and aesthetic results along with the increased need for often unrewarding revision procedures.

## Early management

Craniofacial injuries challenge the surgical team at all stages in their management. The severity of these injuries superimposed on the background of systemic trauma demand a methodical systematic approach to diagnosis and management such as that embodied within the principles of ATLS.[1] At presentation, craniofacial injuries may result in significant airway compromise associated with massive facial bleeding that must be dealt with during the primary survey. Definitive airway management and haemorrhage control minimize the risk of secondary brain injury at a time when autoregulatory control of brain perfusion may be compromised. Hypotension is a common finding in severe head injury occurring in 34% of these patients and is associated with a 150% increase in mortality.[2] Although exsanguination is uncommon as a result of facial injury, intractable bleeding may occur. Usually early fracture reduction along with the placement of anterior and posterior nasal packs is the key to arresting life-threatening haemorrhage. In some cases endovascular treatment may be required to control intractable oronasal bleeding as haemorrhage associated with fractures involving the skull base may be poorly controlled by ligation of the external carotid system owing to retrograde flow from the internal carotid and vertebro-basilar systems.[3] The increased prevalence of cervical spine instability in those with a reduced Glasgow Coma Score compared with those with facial fractures alone further complicates the management of patients following high energy injuries, and demands that in line immobilization is maintained until cervical spine injury is excluded or treated.[4, 5] It is recommended that any patient admitted with a GCS of less than 13, already intubated or who is being scanned for multiregional trauma should have a CT of the spine, as a matter of course.[6]

Cervical spine immobilization may complicate an already difficult intubation and demands high levels of anaesthetic expertise along with the facility to be able to provide an immediate emergency surgical airway if needed at short notice. A well-equipped emergency

*Head Injury: A Multidisciplinary Approach*, ed. Peter C. Whitfield, Elfyn O. Thomas, Fiona Summers, Maggie Whyte and Peter J. Hutchinson. Published by Cambridge University Press. © Cambridge University Press 2009.

room with specialist airway equipment is essential. A trauma team should be available 24 hours a day in specialist trauma centres as part of a receiving team for such specialist cases.[6] Once the patient is adequately stabilized, a full craniofacial assessment, as part of the secondary survey, is made to identify and assess the injuries sustained.

# Craniofacial assessment

The complete assessment of a craniofacial injury requires examination of the head and neck, hard and soft tissues, cranial nerve examination and assessment of orbital injury, supplemented by radiological evaluation. Until neck injury is excluded, cervical spine protection is essential. Although the Glasgow Coma Score will have been evaluated in the primary survey, this is a dynamic score and so will be repeated at a rate determined by the severity of the head injury. Intracranial pressure monitoring may be deemed necessary.

Signs of skull base fractures classically include periorbital ecchymosis, haemotympanum, CSF rhinorrhoea, otorrhoea and Battle's sign (see Fig. 21.1, p. 216). In addition, fractures of the temporal bone may result in hearing loss and facial nerve palsy, whilst fractures of the cribriform plate may result in loss of olfaction. Various syndromes exist with orbital signs that result from trauma, including, superior orbital fissure syndrome, traumatic optic nerve lesions, traumatic mydriasis, caroticocavernous fistula, retrobulbar haemorrhage, traumatic retinal angiopathy and cavernous sinus thrombosis. Visual acuity should be checked with a Snellen chart. Eye movement should be assessed and diplopia ruled out. Visual fields should be checked to confrontation. The globe position should be documented.

When examining the scalp, it is easy to miss lacerations covered by congealed blood matted within the hair. Careful debridement and suture of these areas will help prevent infection and necrosis of skin margins particularly with occipital lacerations. Complex flap reconstruction is only required when large areas of tissue loss are present. Tissue glue for scalp lacerations is rarely successful and often promotes infection. If partial thickness losses occur, these are often best dressed and left to heal with subsequent serial excision if necessary.

The facial soft tissues should be assessed. Lacerations should be dealt with as quickly as possible. Unlike other anatomical areas, it is not necessary to leave open contaminated lacerations since the facial blood supply is so good. Instead, careful debridement followed by layered closure and antibiotic prophylaxis is usually all that is required. If lacerations are complex and require general anaesthesia to enable closure, then these may be lightly tacked, photographed and dressed with betadine soaked packs until definitive surgery. Lacerations crossing vital structures demand special attention including those of the eyelids, overlying the facial nerve and overlying the parotid duct. It should be documented that facial sutures should be removed at 5 days, as in complex cases these are often easy to forget, leaving poor scars.

Fractures of the nasoethmoidal area may result in telecanthus (increased distance between the medial canthi). Associated nasal fractures should be documented. Plain films are of no value in their assessment. Anterior rhinoscopy is performed to rule out a septal haematoma and examine for septal deviation. A septal haematoma usually causes nasal obstruction and is seen as a red soft tissue swelling extending from the septum. It is often bilateral and requires drainage to prevent septal necrosis. A basic clinical assessment of hearing is made and otoscopy should be performed to examine for haemotympanum.

Facial fractures may be indicated by step deformity. In particular, the orbital rims, zygomaticofacial suture and maxilla should be palpated. Anaesthesia of the infraorbital distribution may indicate a fracture of the infraorbital area present in zygomatic and some midfacial fractures. A direct blow to the nerve may also result in anaesthesia secondary to a

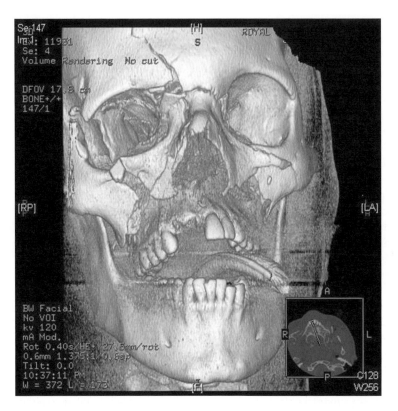

**Fig. 18.1.** Complex craniofacial trauma. Note the frontal bone fracture in the vicinity of the frontal air sinus. In addition there is evidence of complex mid and lateral facial trauma characterized by nasoethmoid fractures, bilateral maxillary fractures, and fractures of the right orbit. The airway has been secured reflecting a systematic approach to the management of the patient.

neuropraxia without a fracture. Similar injuries may occur in the supratrochlear and supra-orbital distributions. Movement at the level of the nasofrontal area on manipulation of the maxilla is indicative of a high Le Fort fracture.

Orotracheal intubation and the presence of a cervical collar make facial fracture assessment difficult, as occlusion cannot be checked. However, careful examination for lacerations within the gingivae, steps in the dentition and the presence of a sublingual haematoma may indicate the presence of an undetected mandibular fracture which may have been missed on the initial radiological evaluation as CT cuts are frequently not continued low enough to include the mandible. Displaced fractures of the central midface above the maxillary alveolus disturb the occlusion resulting in an altered bite. As displaced bony fragments move down the incline of the cranial base, so the posterior teeth occlude resulting in an anterior open bite.

## Imaging in craniofacial injury

Craniofacial injuries are usually best assessed with high resolution CT. Coronal and axial views provide important information regarding the skull base and orbits. Fine cuts facilitate assessment of the likely sites for dural tears in the presence of CSF leaks. Sagittal reformats are helpful in assessment of the anterior skull base and the orbits. Three-dimensional reformatting is helpful for communication with relatives, facilitates teaching and may help identify orientation and size of specific bone fragments such as the mandibular condyles and those carrying the medial canthal ligament (Fig. 18.1).

Multiplanar viewing facilitates greater understanding of the nature and location of fractures. Contrast is not usually required unless intracranial vascular injuries are suspected. In these cases CT or MR angiography may help.

# Classification of craniofacial fractures

Craniofacial fractures are usefully classified into central and lateral injuries.

## Central craniofacial fractures

Those in the central frontobasal region communicate with the paranasal sinuses and so present an increased risk of ascending infection and meningitis in the presence of a dural tear. Type I injuries involve the cribriform plate and may be associated with CSF leak secondary to tears along the dura surrounding the olfactory nerves. Rarely anosmia may result. These injuries can occur following even low energy trauma such as that involved in a simple nasal fracture. In general, however, they result from higher energy injuries. In particular they are involved with the Le Fort II and III fractures which extend to involve the cribriform plate.

Type II injuries are described as involving the frontal or ethmoidal sinuses with associated rhinorrhoea.[7]

## Lateral craniofacial fractures

Lateral craniofacial injuries sited in the frontal area communicate with the orbit. As they lie lateral to the sinuses, the risk of a persistent CSF leak is reduced along with the risk of meningitis. In the absence of a CSF leak the need for the repair will depend on the extent of cosmetic deformity secondary to bony depression and the functional deficit following changes in orbital volume and disturbance of ocular function. Reconstruction is aimed at restoring the orbital volume and contour in the presence of displaced fractures of the orbital walls. To achieve this, bone grafting may be required. Associated midfacial fractures vary according to the amount of energy transferred and the site affected. The orbital rims provide important protection for the eyes whilst the thin bone of the orbital floor and medial wall collapse readily absorbing energy so protecting vital orbital structures. In the same way crumpling of the mid-face may reduce the likelihood of brain injury, although the evidence for this concept in the literature is mixed.[7]

# Facial fractures

Facial fractures frequently accompany craniofacial injuries. High energy craniofacial trauma most frequently results in comminuted facial fracture patterns whilst relatively lower energy impacts may result in the fracture patterns described by Le Fort. Although Le Fort's classification of facial injury is considered by some to be basic and inadequate in describing high energy comminuted fractures, it has stood the test of time and still provides a system of identification of injury which aids communication in relatively low energy injuries. The Le Fort I fracture is a low-level horizontal fracture of the maxilla extending above the maxillary teeth. It passes low down in the maxilla around the level of the nasal floor and maxillary sinus and extends back through the pterygoid plates. It does not involve the skull base. The Le Fort II is a pyramidal fracture that extends from the pterygoid plates across the infraorbital rims and up to the nasofrontal junction. The Le Fort III injury extends from the pterygoid plates up through the zygomatic complex and around the lateral orbit crossing posteriorly to ascend to the nasofrontal suture.[8]

Both the Le Fort II and III fractures may involve the skull base and result in CSF leak in about 30% of cases usually from the cribriform plate.[9] Approximately 60% of midfacial injuries fall into the Le Fort categories.[10] Due to different patterns of injury, this classification is less useful for comminuted injuries.

Reconstruction is planned to restore facial form whilst ensuring isolation and separation of the paranasal sinuses from the brain by repair of the dura and the surrounding bone. Well-planned approaches to the craniofacial skeleton provide access for repair, whilst anticipating the need to minimize brain retraction through incisions that will heal aesthetically.

In both high and low energy trauma, rigid internal fixation using low profile titanium plates stabilizes fractures, restores anatomical form and provides the skeletal framework over which the soft tissues can be redraped. The historical problems of loss of facial height and projection that resulted from closed management of these fractures can now be avoided along with the danger of airway compromise previously associated with wiring of the jaws. Precise replacement of small fragments allows restoration of volume and function in critical areas such as the orbit and enables the anatomical re-establishment of soft tissue form, for example, at the medial canthus. Surgical reconstruction aims to restore height, width and projection of the facial buttresses, which normally absorb and transmit forces from the jaws during eating. Reconstruction of the anterior maxillary buttress (from piriform rim to frontal process of the maxilla) and the zygomaticomaxillary buttress provide the basis for restoration of vertical height. Reconstruction of the zygomatic arch out to length provides the guide to upper mid facial projection and width, providing it is remembered that the arch is essentially straight. If it is plated as a curved arch, the tendency is to reduce anterior projection and widen the face. In a similar fashion reconstruction of the mandible and frontal bone also determine facial width. These reconstructed buttresses provide the base from which reassembly of the facial skeleton can take place. The approaches to the facial skeleton are designed to minimize scarring whilst providing adequate visualization of fractures. These include the sublabial and bicoronal approaches, along with a range of lower lid incisions designed to access the orbit including the subciliary, transconjunctival and mid lid incisions. Using a combination of these approaches allows access to the whole of the facial skeleton.

## Orbital injuries

A fully documented orbital examination is especially important. Periorbital oedema may make examination difficult, but this should only encourage a more rigorous inspection as loss of vision may otherwise go unnoticed.

A formal ophthalmic evaluation is a requirement in the presence of comminuted orbital walls or direct ocular trauma. Assessment of ocular motility, visual acuity and visual fields is needed along with slit lamp examination.

The characteristics of ocular injuries sustained relate to the trauma aetiology. One in five patients with midfacial fractures as a result of a motor vehicle collision and one in ten patients with midfacial fractures secondary to assault sustain severe ocular trauma.[11] In these cases visual acuity, ocular motility, pupillary responses and the presence or absence of diplopia should be documented and a formal ophthalmic opinion sought. Impaired visual acuity is the principal predictor of ocular injury. The presence of a blow out fracture, comminuted zygomatic fractures, double vision and amnesia raise still further the likelihood of severe ocular trauma.[12] When the eyelids are closed by oedema, the perception of light through the lid can only provide limited reassurance, and formal ophthalmic assessment is necessary. The symptoms of pain and proptosis in the presence of decreasing visual acuity, an enlarging pupil, ophthalmoplegia and tense soft tissues raise the likelihood of a retro-bulbar haemorrhage, an ocular emergency. Immediate surgical decompression with can-tholysis via a lateral canthotomy or a medial blepharoplasty may rescue sight, as otherwise central retinal artery ischaemia will result in blindness. Emergency temporisation may be achieved with the use of high-dose steroids (methyl prednisolone or dexamethasone), acete-zolamide 500 mg i.v. followed by 125–250 mg i.v. 4–6 hourly and mannitol 20%, 2 g/kg i.v. over 2 hours until decompression is performed. Surgical decompression would normally be carried out under local anaesthesia, as timely intervention is critical to alleviate the intraorbital pressure rise responsible for this form of compartment syndrome.

Fine cut axial and coronal CT provides the necessary detail to guide diagnosis and reconstruction in orbital trauma. This also allows detailed assessment of the anterior skull base. Coronal reformats should be obtained when injury precludes standard examination. As the most common causes of reduced vision relate to potentially treatable pathologies such as retrobulbar haemorrhage, optic nerve thickening presumably secondary to oedema and surgical emphysema, the importance of early CT scanning is underlined.[13]

Restitution of the orbital tissues aims to provide a fully reconstructed bony orbit with restoration of orbital volume and shape, ocular motility, soft tissue aesthetics, lacrimation and visual function. Early and accurate identification of the nature and extent of injuries, combined with careful surgery, will help prevent the late complications of enophthalmos and of restricted ocular motility with resultant diplopia. Further aspects of management of orbital injuries are outside the remit of this chapter.

## Sequencing in pan-facial injury

In pan-facial injury with severe comminution, the loss of anatomical landmarks complicates reconstruction. As the reconstruction is of a curved structure, minor malpositioning of bone fragments in an area may be amplified and result in significant discrepancies elsewhere. Careful planning and sequencing will help reduce these problems.

Following clinical and radiographic assessment, the incisions required for access are planned. Three-dimensional reconstructions of the CT scans enable full discussion with relatives regarding the nature of the injury and the extent of reconstruction required. The same scans help identify the size and position of bone fragments that will be key in rebuilding the facial skeleton. If possible, study models of the dentition should be made in the dentate patient prior to surgery. The occlusal relationship of the upper and lower teeth may then be used to help guide the positioning of the maxilla to the mandible. Construction of preformed arch bars saves time at surgery.

Using the principles described by Manson, reconstruction is planned dividing the face and cranium into units.[9] The upper and lower units of the face are artificially divided at the Le Fort I level. The sequence in which reconstruction takes place is then determined by the nature of the injury and, in particular, by the non-injured areas, which provide the foundation and reference points from which the rebuilding starts. An example of such a sequence is given below:

- Radiological assessment
- Consent
  This is a difficult area in the management of the unconscious patient or in a patient who may not have the capacity to give consent secondary to head injury. Treatment must be

agreed by the medical team to be in the patient's best interests as in English law one adult cannot give consent for another.[14]

- Secure the airway
  This will usually take the form of a tracheostomy and is discussed in detail below.

- Lower lid incisions
  The approach to the orbit should be made prior to the bicoronal approach as subsequent oedema may prevent accurate identification of the lower lid skin creases.

- Orbital floor exposure
  Although orbital floor exploration may take place at this stage, it will not usually be possible to reconstruct this area until the maxilla has been disimpacted and the orbital rim restored.

- Bicoronal flap
  A well-designed bicoronal incision provides excellent access, is hidden well back in the hair line, preserves the function of the facial nerve and allows a thick pericranial flap to be elevated from the site of the incision (if necessary) extending laterally along the upper margins of the temporalis attachment. Reflection down to, and preservation of, the supra-trochlear and supraorbital vessels provide a long vascularized flap that can be turned intracranially to cover a cranialized sinus and may then be laid along the basal dura to provide additional support against a basal dural repair. If the incision to preserve the temporal branch of the facial nerve is extended to include the heavy deep temporalis fascia, then the detached facial soft tissues can be re-suspended by reattachment of the temporalis fascia at close of play. Further soft tissue support may be provided by suspensory sutures attached to frontal bone plates in a manner similar to that used in open brow lift surgery. The pericranial flap is susceptible to drying during a long procedure and should be protected with a damp swab throughout.

- Exposure of orbits
  The superior aspect of the orbit may now be explored. It may be necessary to osteotomize the foramen surrounding the supra orbital vessels at the orbital rim to mobilize these vessels and allow access to the orbital roof. Access to the lateral wall is made easier once the zygomatic arch is exposed. Dissection in the orbit enables full exposure of the fractures.

- Exposure of zygomas as required.
  When the zygoma is comminuted, the whole of the arch should be exposed and disimpacted.

- Frontal craniotomy
  Pre-plating of frontal fractures prior to frontal craniotomy makes reconstruction much easier providing allowance is made to allow access for placement of the pericranial flap into the anterior cranial fossa at the conclusion of the surgery. The cuts for the craniotomy may be extended laterally to the temporal area to hide the burr holes under the temporalis. The preplated anterior skull vault may now be removed in one piece and stored in a saline soaked swab. The anterior cranial fossa may then be explored.

- Maxillary disimpaction
  Once the zygomas are disimpacted, the maxilla is free for disimpaction. McMahon *et al.* recommend that this should be done with the anterior cranial fossa exposed when the

anterior skull base is fractured.[15] Significant defects in the floor of the anterior fossa may be bone grafted including those of the orbital roof. Plates are not generally placed in the anterior fossa for fear of infection and the difficulty of later removal.

- Frontal sinus management
  The frontal sinus is cranialized or obliterated and sealed with an overlaid pericranial flap. This is discussed in further detail below.

- Orbital roof management
  The orbital roof may be explored subcranially or intracranially. Intracranial exploration is ideal as there is a risk of fractures tearing the dura. Fractures that extend posteriorly across the skull base may defy safe reduction, and mobilization of the frontal area may have to be made via a frontobasal osteotomy to prevent injury.

- Dural repair
  The dura is repaired once the fractures involving the anterior fossa will no longer be manipulated. An intradural repair may be required, particularly for low tears where access is limited by the constraints of brain retraction. Patches of pericranial flap may be inlaid over the defects and sealed with fibrin glue or dural sealants. The brain is then protected with dampened patties, whilst the next stages of repair take place, as the pericranial flap cannot be laid into place until the frontal, orbital and nasal reconstructions are complete.

- Frontonasal reconstruction
  A cantilevered split calvarial bone graft may be needed to restore frontonasal projection.

- Medial orbital margin reconstruction and nasomaxillary reconstruction.
  The reconstruction of the anterior nasoethmoidal area is then completed, ensuring that the nasal bridge width is kept narrow as broadening frequently occurs as a late consequence. Accurate placement of the medial canthal ligament provides a significant challenge. Particular attention is paid to locating it in an overcorrected position behind the level of the anterior projection of the globe superiorly and medially. The medial position is stabilized with transnasal wiring and the superior position by securing it to a plate cantilevered from solid bone in the glabellar region. If broadening of the intercanthal distance occurs, the resulting lid aesthetics are poor. Direct exposure of the canthal ligament may be required to enable its identification.

- Zygomatic disimpaction
  Fractures of the root of the zygoma should be identified and plated. If the temporalis insertion is released cranially and the muscle reflected down, it will allow access to the lateral wall of the orbit. Identification and reduction of the orbital process of the zygoma to the greater wing of the sphenoid at the lateral orbital wall is an excellent guide to the accuracy of fracture reduction and is important in restoring the volume of the orbit. Failure to reduce a fracture at this site may result in enophthalmos.

- Zygomatic plating
  Fractures of the arch and root should be reduced and plated. Frequently, it is necessary to suspend the zygoma at the frontozygomatic suture with a wire or 1.0 mm plate to help support the zygoma whilst allowing it to be rotated as needed as the orbital rim repair is completed, and at a later stage when the zygomatic complex and maxilla are reunited. Once these manoeuvres are complete, it may be necessary to convert this to a weight-bearing plate to prevent relapse during the recovery period.

- Infra-orbital rim reconstruction and restitution of the medial orbit
  Lost bone fragments displaced into the antrum are retrieved and plated into position. Exposure of the orbital floor will help avoid malpositioning of rim fragments that frequently rotate, lifting spurs of orbital floor bone into the orbit. Union across to the medial orbit now completes this horizontal buttress.

- Grafting of the orbital walls
  Orbital shape and volume is restored with split calvarial bone grafts. These may be cantilevered off plates at the orbital rim. Post-operative closure of the periosteum over these plates helps hide them from the palpating finger.

- Exposure of the mandibular condyles and reconstruction to height
  Lower facial height is determined by the occlusion and by the intact mandibular condyle. Reconstruction in cases where bilateral fractures have occurred will prevent loss of facial height and a resulting anterior open bite. High intracapsular fractures cannot be plated successfully and when bilateral will create the need for intermaxillary fixation to be maintained postoperatively to try to prevent this occurrence.

- Mandibular reconstruction
  If the maxillary dentition is intact with no midline palatal split (present in about 8% of maxillary midfacial fractures) and no dentoalveolar fractures, then the mandible can be accurately reconstructed with temporary intermaxillary fixation to locate the fragments. If not, then the palatal split should first be plated anteriorly and across the palate and the mandible used as a guide for width. In cases with a midline mandibular split, then careful assessment should be made at fracture reduction to avoid flaring of the rami.

- Maxillary plating at the Le Fort I level
  The upper and lower facial segments may now be reunited by plating of the vertical buttresses.

- Soft tissue resuspension
  Where dissection is not required across areas of the facial skeleton, then the soft tissues should be left attached to the periosteum. In all other areas, the periosteum should be resuspended with non-resorbable sutures.

## Frontal sinus fracture management

Frontal sinus fractures are reported to occur in 2%–12% of cranial fractures and 5% of facial fractures (Fig. 18.2). One-third involves the anterior wall alone, whilst two-thirds of cases involve a combination of fractures of the frontal recess, posterior and anterior walls. Very rarely is the floor affected alone.[16] Up to one third have an associated CSF leak. Other complications of frontal sinus fractures include mucocoele, pyelocoele, brain abscess, frontal osteomyelitis and meningitis.

The management of the fractured frontal sinus is controversial. The following principles seem clear.

*Undisplaced fractures of the anterior wall* do not require correction. Gross comminution and depression of the anterior wall require correction to avoid aesthetic deformity. The bicoronal incision is best for adequate visualization of the fractures and restoration of form. Overlying lacerations should be used only if extensive and when limited access is required for repair. The bicoronal approach allows disarticulation of the front wall and debridement of the sinus if needed. The pericranial tissues are preserved if needed for repair. Multiple small fragments can be difficult to locate in the presence of severe

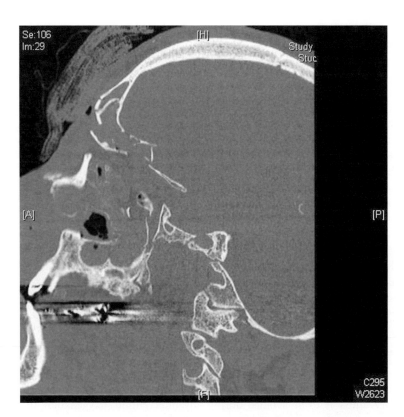

Se:106
Im:29
[H]
Study
Stuc
[A]
[P]
C295
W2623
[F]

**Fig. 18.2.** A sagittal reformat showing complex craniofacial trauma. The anterior cranial fossa floor has been fractured and appears to be in communication with the frontal air sinus.

comminution, when bone grafting with split calvarium may produce a more satisfactory end result. Fractures affecting the anterior wall alone should be rigidly fixed and the sinus mucosa left *in situ* if the frontonasal duct is not affected by the fracture. Plating of comminuted bone fragments held in place by sinus lining may be useful prior to removal of the anterior wall to allow accurate apposition of bone fragments. Simply removing the fragments and hoping to replace them correctly is the province of jigsaw enthusiasts. Early treatment with removal of fragments displaced into the frontal sinus will help prevent infection.[17]

Isolated *fractures of the posterior wall* require treatment when displaced by the thickness of the posterior wall or in the presence of CSF leak. A frontal craniotomy facilitates access and exploration of the posterior wall, the frontal and the basal dura. Burr holes placed laterally under the temporalis reduce the likelihood of cosmetic deformity. A low bone flap provides access to the sinus and minimizes brain retraction when the basal dura is explored, although difficulty may be experienced moving the saw across the sinus. Cranialization is preferred over obliteration as successful obliteration with bone in the presence of all but the smallest sinuses is difficult and the reported rates of infection following placement of fat grafts or allografts is high.[18,19]

Management of fractures of the posterior wall in combination with associated CSF rhinorrhoea which stops within 7 days presents an area of uncertainty. The arrest of the leak may be secondary to brain plugging the dural defect rather than spontaneous repair. The Mayo clinic experience was of 16% of patients presenting with delayed onset of meningitis at an average of 6.5 years following CSF leakage lasting greater than 24 hours.[20] Eljamel and Foy describe a 7.5% CSF leak recurrence rate following spontaneous cessation and a recurrent rate of meningitis of 30.6%.[21] Communication between the brain and paranasal sinuses appears to place the patient at significant risk from ascending infection and supports the case for early intervention. Donald and Bernstein allude to the fact that sinus lining appears to invaginate the bone lining the sinus and that only by drilling out the sinus can it be rendered truly safe.[22] For this reason cranialization of the sinus and inlaying of a vascularized pericranial flap to separate the brain and obturation of the nasofrontal duct is the preferred option.

The evidence for intervention in management of fractures involving the frontonasal duct on the floor of the frontal sinus is difficult to interpret. Intubation of the duct may result in late problems with stenosis. Conservative management may leave the patient susceptible to mucocoele and pyelocoele formation, whilst obliteration may be difficult secondary to extensive pneumatization. Preoperative imaging to determine the presence of a fracture involving the frontonasal duct is not always reliable. This has led some to advocate that all posterior wall fractures with displacement and any fractures involving the frontonasal duct should be treated with removal of the sinus lining and cranialization of the sinus or obliteration with autologous fat. Intervention, of course, may expose the patient to the risks associated with brain retraction and the potential for infection.

These controversies are thrown into light when the adjacent ethmoidal complex may be fractured, but escapes intervention and seems to result in few problems, despite also draining into the nasal cavity.

## Timing of surgical intervention

The timing of reconstruction in the presence of brain injury requires careful planning. Operative intervention in the presence of raised intracranial pressure may result in adverse outcome. If secondary injury is to be avoided during any intervention, oxygenation and blood supply to the brain must be ensured and hypotension secondary to anaesthetic agents and surgical bleeding minimized. Lengthy procedures in physiologically unstable patients may worsen the effects of brain retraction and promote further brain injury by creating oedema. Deferring the definitive management of facial injuries may be necessary to allow a patient to stabilize. On occasion, this may compromise the final soft tissue form as healing and fibrosis may have commenced.

The timing of intervention will therefore depend on:

- Severity of the injury
  Complex treatment is not indicated if survival is very unlikely

- Intracranial pressure
  Wait until intracranial pressure settles. Early aggressive intervention is advocated by some, but this may result in increased morbidity and even mortality.

- Facial swelling
  Massive facial swelling precludes early intervention, as the placement of incisions and the assessment of facial contour are difficult. Furthermore, the soft tissues may be difficult to handle in the presence of oedema.

- Anaesthetic considerations
  Intubation of patients allows definitive airway management and control of intracranial pressure. As the patient improves and is weaned off anaesthesia to allow assessment of neurological function, tolerance of intubation reduces, necessitating extubation or placement of a tracheostomy tube. Otherwise, coughing will further exacerbate

the problems of intracranial pressure rise. This may be the ideal time to proceed to surgery.

To allow satisfactory repair of panfacial fractures, intermaxillary fixation may be required. Under normal circumstances nasal intubation would be ideal but may not be possible because of midfacial and skull base fractures; instead tracheostomy may be the best option.

- Surgical team availability
  Sufficient theatre time and availability of all teams involved in the repair will also influence timing as joint operating will be needed.

  Antibiotic cover during the delay phase is necessary as infection rates following midfacial injuries are high.

## Cerebrospinal fluid leak

Identification of a CSF leak implies a dural tear and the possibility of ascending infection. In the past, management has often centred on whether the CSF leak arrests spontaneously. Opinion varies, as some argue that repair should be based on the extent of the associated fractures accepting that dural tears are present in most cases when explored.

Clearly, some craniofacial fractures demand open fixation by virtue of associated facial deformity, but where the leak stops spontaneously the evidence regarding the need for surgical intervention is less clear. In these cases the leak may have stopped as a result of necrotic brain tissue plugging the defect. The literature does not identify the levels of complications that occur long term when managing these situations conservatively, nor does it quantify the extent of secondary injury resulting from aggressive repair of potential dural tears that occurs secondary to brain retraction.

The first sign of CSF leak may be the tell-tale tramline of CSF mixed with blood extending across the face from the patient's nose. The glucose oxidase test strip test may be falsely positive in nearly half of cases.[22] Beta-2-transferrin analysis of a collected specimen has been demonstrated as the most efficacious way of confirming a CSF leak, but it usually takes time to process a result. High resolution CT has a high sensitivity for identification of the site of CSF leak and this may usefully be supplemented by MR cisternography and intrathecal fluorescein with intraoperative visualisation.[23]

The leak may be managed conservatively, depending on the location and the need for exploration as a result of other injuries. Conservative management includes bed rest, head elevation, avoidance of coughing, sneezing and straining and the use of stool softeners/laxatives. Most effective is the use of lumbar drainage. Bell describes successful conservative management in 85% of cases within 2–10 days.[24]

## Airway considerations

The concept of a shared airway must be followed for craniofacial cases with an understanding of surgical and anaesthetic needs. In the early post-injury phase ventilation may be used to control $CO_2$ and hence intracranial pressure. Intraoperatively, restoration of occlusion may require intermaxillary fixation. This may require placement of a tracheostomy facilitating post-operative airway management by reducing dead space and allowing early weaning of the patient, whilst retaining a definitive airway. Alternatively, submental or nasal intubation may be performed.[25] The establishment of a correct occlusal relationship between the upper and lower jaws is essential to long-term achievement of masticatory function and, in cases of severe midfacial trauma, may be the key step in achieving a base from which to rebuild the

**191**

midface. In the cases where there is a complete dentition, tracheostomy is likely to be required. Where the dentition is not complete, it may be possible to pass an armoured tube between or behind the remaining teeth. If an extended period of recovery is likely, then tracheostomy may be the preferred option to facilitate postoperative management of the respiratory tract.

# References

1. American College of Surgeons. *Advanced Trauma Life Support Manual*. American College of Surgeons committee on trauma. Chicago, 2004.

2. Chesnut RM, Marshall LF, Klauber MR *et al.* The role of secondary brain injury in determining outcome from severe head injury. *J Trauma* 1993; **34**(2): 216–22.

3. Komiyama M, Nishikawa M, Kan M, Shigemoto T, Kaji A. Endovascular treatment of intractable oronasal bleeding associated with severe craniofacial injury. *J Trauma* 1998; **44**(2): 330–4.

4. Williams J, Jehle D, Cottington E, Shufflebarger C. Head, facial, and clavicular trauma as a predictor of cervical-spine injury. *Ann Emerg Med* 1992; **21**(6): 719–22.

5. Hills MW, Deane SA. Head injury and facial injury: is there an increased risk of cervical spine injury? *J Trauma*. 1993; **34**(4): 549–53.

6. Baker NJ, Evans BT, Neil Dwyer G, Lang DA. Guidelines for reviewing participation in the National Confidential Enquiry into patient outcome and Death and Implementing NCEPOD recommendations: frontal sinus fractures. In: Ward Booth P, Eppley BL, Schmelzeisen R, eds. *Maxillofacial Trauma and Esthetic Facial Reconstruction*. Churchill Livingstone, 2003; 200.

7. Martin RC, Spain DA, Richardson JD. Do facial fractures protect the brain or are they a marker for severe head injury? *Am Surg* 2002; **68**(5): 477–81.

8. Stewart MG. *Head, Face and Neck Trauma. Comprehensive Management*. Thième, 2005.

9. Manson PN Maxillofacial injuries *Emerg Med Clin North Am* 1984; **2**(4):168–78.

10. Manson PN, Clarke N, Robertson B *et al.* Subunit principles in midface fractures: the importance of sagittal buttresses, soft tissue reductions and sequencing treatment of segmental fractures. *Plastic Reconstruc Surg* 1999; **103**(4): 1287–307.

11. al-Qurainy IA, Stassen LF, Dutton GN, Moos KF, el-Attar A. The characteristics of midfacial fractures and the association with ocular injury: a prospective study. *Br J Oral Maxillofac Surg* 1991; **29**(5): 291–301.

12. al-Qurainy IA, Titterington DM, Dutton GN, Stassen LF, Moos KF, el-Attar A. Midfacial fractures and the eye: the development of a system for detecting patients at risk of eye injury. *Br J Oral Maxillofac Surg* 1991; **29**(6): 363–7.

13. Lee HJ, Jilani M, Frohman L, Baker S. CT of orbital trauma. *Emerg Radiol* 2004; **10**(4): 168–72.

14. Seeking patients' consent: the ethical guidelines. GMC, 1998.

15. McMahon JD, Koppel DA, Devlin M, Moos KF. Maxillary and panfacial fractures. In: Wardbooth P Epply BL, Schmelzeizen R, eds. *Maxillofacial Trauma and Esthetic Reconstruction*. Churchill Livingstone, 2003; 251.

16. Wallis A, Donald PJ. Frontal sinus fractures: a review of 72 cases. *Laryngoscope* 1988; **98**: 593–598.

17. Gruss JS, Pollock RA, Phillips JH, Antonyshyn O. Combined injuries to the cranium and face. *Br J Plastic Surg* 1999; **42**: 385–98.

18. Wilson BC, Davidson B, Corey JP, Haydon RC 3rd. Comparison of complications following frontal sinus fractures managed with or without obliteration over ten years. *Laryngoscope* 1998; **98**(5): 516–520.

19. Bell RB, Dierks EJ, Brar P, Potter JK, Potter BE. A protocol for the management of frontal sinus fractures emphasising sinus preservation. *J Oral Maxillofac Surg* 2007; **65**(5): 825–39.

20. Friedman JA, Ebersold MJ, Quast LM. Post traumatic cerebrospinal fluid leakage. *World J Surg* 2001; **25**(8): 1062–6.

21. Eljamel MS, Foy PM. Acute traumatic CSF fistulae. The risk of intracranial infection. *Br J Neurosurg* 1990; **4**(6): 479–83

22. Donald PJ, Bernstein L. Compound frontal sinus injuries with intracranial penetration. *Laryngoscope* 1978; **88**: 225–32.

23. Zapalac JS, Marple BF, Schwade ND. Skull base cerebrospinal fistulas: a comprehensive diagnostic algorithm. *Otolaryngol Head Neck Surg* 2002; **126**(6): 669–76.

24. Bell RB, Dierks EJ, Brar P, Potter JK, Potter BE. A protocol for the management of frontal sinus fractures emphasising sinus preservation. *J Oral Maxillofac Surg* 2007; **65**(5): 825–39.

25. Hernandez Altemir F. The submental route for endotracheal intubation: a new technique. *J Maxillofac Surg.* 1986; **14**(1): 64–65.

# Cranioplasty after head injury

Heinke Pülhorn and Robert Redfern

## History

Cranioplasty is the repair of a cranial defect or deformation. Whilst it is well known that trephination was performed as early as 3000 BC by the Incans and Neolithic Stone Age cultures in Europe and Russia,[1] it is not common knowledge that cranioplasty was also carried out in Peru using gold or silver plates and by Celts using ovoid bony 'rondelles'.[2,3]

The first bone graft cranioplasty was reported in 1668 by van Meekeren who described the use of a piece of dog cranium to replace part of the calvarium of a nobleman, who had received a sword blow to the head in Moscow. Apparently, the patient's health was restored, but he was subsequently excommunicated from the Russian church, which could not accept the presence of animal bone on a human skull. Subsequent removal of the graft was not possible due to bony union.[2,3]

In the late nineteenth century MacEwen popularized the repair of skull defects with bone pieces and Müller described an osteoplastic rotational flap using the outer table of the skull.[4] Around the same time Barth (1893) described the dynamic nature of bone implantation referring to the 'creeping substitution' of implanted bone with new viable bone tissue. These historical texts have been elegantly reviewed.[2,5]

## Materials

The ideal material for a cranioplasty should be strong, lightweight and sufficiently malleable to precisely fit complicated cranial defects. The cranioplasty should be easily secured to the cranium, chemically inert, biocompatible, radiolucent, non-ferromagnetic, readily available and inexpensive. Needless to say, no such material exists to date.

### Bone autograft

Bone is the obvious choice of cranioplasty material with the original flap being the simplest solution. This may be contraindicated if the bone is shattered, infiltrated with tumour or infected. In these circumstances bone harvested from elsewhere in the same patient may be used. Most commonly this is membranous bone from the cranium or occasionally endochondral bone, e.g. ribs. Such autografts have the obvious advantage of minimizing immune reaction and cross-infection. Furthermore, autologous bone has viability and the potential to grow. On the other hand, the bone may not readily fit the defect and its use may require a second operative field with associated morbidity. A split calvarial graft can be obtained in two ways: either a section of donor skull is totally removed and then split through the diploe, or the outer table is removed *in situ* using curved osteotomes. This graft is then used to cover the craniotomy defect leaving the inner table to cover the donor site. Split calvarial grafts result in an aesthetically pleasing contour, but are not usually available to cover large defects. Furthermore, both the donor and recipient sites are less biomechanically stable than adjacent skull and resorption of bone mass may occur.

*Head Injury: A Multidisciplinary Approach*, ed. Peter C. Whitfield, Elfyn O. Thomas, Fiona Summers, Maggie Whyte and Peter J. Hutchinson. Published by Cambridge University Press. © Cambridge University Press 2009.

If closure of the craniotomy has to be delayed and the original flap is to be used, storage problems arise. Devascularized bone will eventually die with the exception of some periosteal, endosteal and medullary cells and osteocytes within 0.2 mm of cortical bone surfaces.[6] This complicates all extracorporeal storage systems including autoclaved sterile bone, frozen storage and bone stored in 80% alcohol or 10% formaldehyde leading to a risk of necrosis of reimplanted bone.[7] The UK Human Tissue Act (2004) governs the consent and standard operating procedures required for storage of bone flaps. Storage of the bone flap in a subcutaneous pocket within the abdominal wall or thigh may enhance bone flap viability, but does require an additional procedure with the attendant risks of infection, poor cosmesis and discomfort.[8] In addition, early shrinkage of the flap has been reported, leading to poor apposition at the time of reimplantation.

### Graft consolidation

After bone implantation, graft survival depends on the reaction of the surrounding tissue and upon functional contact between cancellous bone and adjacent resident bone. During the *first week* capillaries from surrounding diploe, dura and scalp infiltrate the transplant bed. During the *second week* fibrous granulation tissue proliferates and osteoplastic activity occurs with primitive mesenchymal cells differentiating into osteoprogenitor cells. These then differentiate into osteoblasts capable of forming new bone to replace the necrosing implanted bone flap. Bone morphogenetic proteins play a central role in this osteoinductive process.[9] Osteoconduction is a parallel process whereby osteoprogenitor cells from the surrounding tissue migrate into the bony–protein matrix consolidating graft incorporation.

## Bone allografts and xenografts

Allografts are obtained as live or cadaveric donations from another individual of the same species and are now commercially available from bone banks. Although they have the advantage of being in good supply, there is the risk of disease transmission and use is limited.[10] Demineralized allogeneic bone matrix is commercially available and has been used with encouraging results.[11] After implantation, multipotent mesenchymal cells begin to proliferate from the recipient site and transform into cartilage. New bone is then formed by ossification of the cartilaginous matrix, osteoid formation and mineralization.[10] Whilst unpredictable bone absorption limits use of the matrix for covering large defects, it has been shown that chaulking the demineralized bone powder with autologous bone paste, obtained by mixing blood and bone dust from the operative site, can enhance the cosmetic results in this situation.[10,12] The use of xenografts taken from a wide range of species including dog, goose, ape, rabbit, calf and eagle and the use of other bone substitutes such as horn and ivory has been abandoned.

## Bone substitutes

Temporalis fascia, fat and cartilage have been used to cover cranial defects. However, these substances lack structural support and lead to an undesirable cosmetic result for many patients. Consequently, a large number of metallic and non-metallic substances have been used for cranioplasty.

### Metals

Gold and silver were the first metals to be used in cranioplasty. Both are soft and prohibitively expensive. Platinum is also too expensive for clinical use. Aluminium irritates the surrounding tissues, slowly disintegrates over time and appears to be epileptogenic. Other discarded materials include lead, the brittle alloy vitallium and ticonium. Stainless steel and tantalum were first successfully used to cover defects during World War II. In 1965, titanium was used for the first time. This metal remains a popular choice for a cranioplasty flap, although it is not easy to mould intraoperatively. It is normally fixed to the skull with mini-plates and screws.

### Non-metals

Due to the radio-opacity of metals and the difficulty with intra-operative moulding, many non-metallic bony substitutes have been used. Methylmethacrylate has stood the test of time since first being used in 1940. It is chemically inert, malleable before it sets, lightweight, non-magnetic and similar to bone in strength.[13] The main drawback is the exothermic reaction produced during setting of the polymer, which reaches temperatures in excess of 100 °C and can damage underlying brain tissue. This is counteracted by washing the implant with cold saline while it sets. Methylmethacrylate is also very brittle and can fracture.[13] To reduce the frequency of plate fractures and resulting complications, methylmethacrylate can be applied over a stainless steel or titanium mesh placed in the extradural plane. Methylmethacrylate can also be preformed using the original flap as a template or by the use of 3D computer reconstruction techniques saving on operative time, avoiding the heat production of the setting and providing a near-perfect fit.

Hydroxyapatite is a calcium-phosphate compound that is found naturally in human bone and teeth. It is now manufactured as a paste, granules and preformed buttons and plates. It can be applied with ease and sets without the exothermic reaction of methymethacrylate.[14] The porosity of the hydroxyapatite framework encourages the ingrowth of fibrovascular tissue, which subsequently ossifies leaving only small areas of cement loss on follow-up scans.[15,16] However, hydroxyapatite does not set when exposed to fluids and it therefore requires a dry surgical field and is, compared with methylmethacrylate, relatively expensive.[16,17]

# Indications, contraindications and timing

Skull defects result from trauma, excision of tumours, infections, necrosis of the skull and congenital absence of portions of the skull. Additionally, cerebral swelling with the subsequent need for decompressive craniectomy can result in a skull defect.

The main indications for undertaking cranioplasty include protection of the cranial contents and aesthetic considerations with their psychosocial implications. Sporadic reports of improvements in craniectomy site pain, scalp pulsation and neurological symptoms such as headaches, epilepsy and speech impairment have been published.[18] It is now generally accepted that the 'syndrome of the trephined' with headache, dizziness, intolerance of vibration and noise, irritability and fatigability is a clinical expression of post-concussion or post-traumatic syndrome and is not reliably helped by cranioplasty. Nevertheless, craniectomy site tenderness and discomfort relating to changes in the environment as an expression of deranged intracranial pressure relationships or collapsed cerebral hemispheres can be improved and should be considered as an indication for cranioplasty.[19] In children, it is important to provide an intact vault for the normal growth and development of the brain.

Cranioplasty is most commonly performed some weeks or months after the primary procedure.[6,9] Infection is the major contraindication to cranioplasty. Compound wounds and exposed paranasal sinuses offer relative contraindications. Closure of the cranial cavity can be problematic if hydrocephalus or cerebral swelling exists. A thin or devitalized scalp may

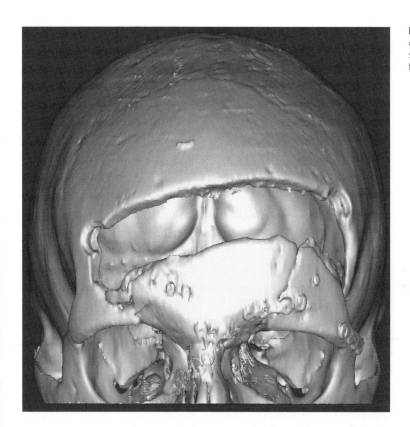

**Fig. 19.1.** Three-dimensional CT showing a large frontal skull defect.

lead to wound breakdown warranting plastic procedures. In elevating the scalp flap, care needs to be taken to prevent damaging the underlying brain. The use of strong curved Mayo scissors usually enables a satisfactory plane of dissection to be achieved. The bony margins then require delineation using a periosteal elevator before securing the cranioplasty flap to the skull.

Modern 3D-reconstructive CT imaging has improved the prefabrication of implants. Commercially available stereolithographic software enables accurate reconstruction of axial images, enabling a resin model of the skull to be manufactured using fused deposition modelling techniques. This model is then used as a template permitting the design and construction of an anatomically shaped cranioplasty plate from the material of choice (Figs. 19.1 to 19.3).

## Complications

Complications occurring from cranioplasty can be broadly divided into those related to the operative procedure in general and those related to the particular material used. In general, mortality from cranioplasty is low at approximately 0.2%.[6] The obvious risk is infection (meningitis, abscess and sinus formation) since most cranioplasty materials are foreign bodies or stored bone. An infected cranioplasty generally has to be removed, and prolonged treatment with antibiotics is necessary. Infection rates are quoted at approximately 5% for methylmethacrylate but less for bone implants.[6] Tissue reactions like fibrous encapsulation with exudate formation, inflammatory reactions, granuloma formation, loosening and

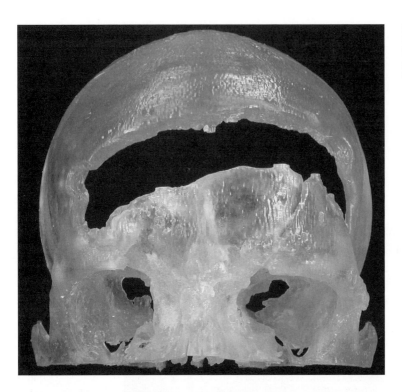

**Fig. 19.2.** Resin model manufactured from three-dimensional reconstructive data.

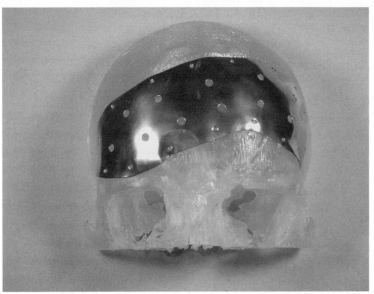

**Fig. 19.3.** Titanium plate manufactured using the resin model as a template. This provides an accurate anatomical cranioplasty to be performed with relative ease.

exposure of the graft through the skin have also been reported. These seem to be more of a problem with bone substitutes, especially acrylic resins, than with bone.[10,16] Alloplastic materials can also result in erosion of the underlying bone, which in turn results in a larger cranial defect.[12]

Unpredictable resorption of cranioplasty material is a complication when using bone, especially autoclaved bone, and it can be as high as 25%–40%.[9,20] Among the factors thought to be responsible for resorption of a bone graft are multiple fractures, age of the patient and shunt operations.[7] Other complications specific to bone relate to its harvest: split calvarial grafts carry the risk of intracranial trauma, while other sources of bone may lead to donor-site morbidity such as pain, infection, unsightly scarring and specific injuries dependent upon the source including nerve injury, hernias, pelvic fractures, tibial fractures, bowel perforation and pneumothorax.

## Future developments

The search for the ideal cranioplasty material continues unabated. Natural corals with their porous structure similar to human bone can undergo ossification and may be of clinical use.[2] Norian bone cement system, a synthetic carbonated calcium phosphate compound, can be reabsorbed and replaced by human bone secondary to osteoconduction.[21] Preformed implants shaped using 3D CT scanning and stereolithography have been widely adopted.[17,22] The application of novel techniques, such as mixing known materials, e.g. acrylic resins and titanium struts,[23] and improving their qualities, e.g. antibiotic coating of preformed plates, continues.[17] Transferring techniques from other operative fields, e.g. distraction osteogenesis with contractile polymers or even bioresorbable dynamic implants that can be applied without transcutaneous pins, may be of use in some patients.[24]

There have been exciting developments in 'tissue engineering' using molecular biology techniques, such as harvesting osteoblasts or bone marrow-derived mesenchymal stem cells, to seed onto the scaffold for the cranioplasty.[25] Bone morphogenesis proteins of the transforming-growth factor-β family and various polypeptide growth factors play a central role in fracture healing. These factors can now be manufactured by recombinant DNA techniques and potentially incorporated into implants to evoke osteoinduction.[25,26] Thus, 'smart biomaterials' are the latest addition to the experimental armamentarium of cranioplasty surgery. Absorption of circulating endogenous or exogenous bone morphogenetic protein leads to secondary induction of bone growth.[27] Also, retroviral transfection of bone morphogenetic protein-7 into periosteal cells, which are then seeded onto cranioplasty matrices, results in increased bone regeneration.[28] Therefore, the prospect of biodegradable implants that can be used to provide immediate cover of the cranial defect, whilst over time releasing bioactive molecules to regenerate the perfectly fitted implant into living bone, may be realized.

## References

1. Haeger K, Harold Starke. *The illustrated History of Surgery*. London, 1989.
2. Sanan A, Haines S. Repairing holes in the head: a history of cranioplasty. *Neurosurgery* 1997; **40**(3): 588–603.
3. Steward T. Stone Age skull surgery: a general review with emphasis on the new world. *Ann Rep Smithson Inst* 1957; **107**: 469–591.
4. MacEwen W. Illustrative cases of cerebral surgery. *Lancet* 1885; **1**: 881–3, 934–6.
5. Woolf JL, Walker AE. Cranioplasty: Collective Review *Int Abst Surg* 1945; **81**: 1–23.
6. Wilkins RH, Rengachary SS, *Neurosurgery*. eds New York, McGraw-Hill, 1996.
7. Iwama T, Yamada J, Imai S, Shinoda J, Funakoshi T, Sakai N. The use of frozen autogenous bone flaps in delayed cranioplasty revisited. *Neurosurgery* 2003; **52**(3): 591–6.
8. Movassaghi K, Ver Halen J, Ganchi P, Amin-Hanjani S, Mesa J, Yaremchuk M. Cranioplasty with subcutaneously preserved autologous bone grafts. *Plast Reconstruc. Surg* 2006; **117**(1): 202–6.
9. Apuzzo MLJ. *Brain Surgery: Complication Avoidance and Management*. New York, Churchill Livingstone, 1993.
10. Chen T, Wang H. Cranioplasty using allogenic perforated demineralized bone

matrix with autogenous bone paste. *Ann Plast Surg* 2002; **49**(3): 272–9.

11. Mulliken JB. Glowacki J. Kaban LB. Folkman J. Murray JE. Use of demineralized allogeneic bone implants for the correction of maxillocraniofacial deformities. *Ann Surg* 1981; **194**(3): 366–72.

12. Arun K, Gosain M. Biomaterials for reconstruction of the cranial vault. *Plast Reconstruc. Surg* 2005; **116**(2): 663–6.

13. Youmans JR. *Neurological Surgery*. 3rd edition, Philadelphia, WB Saunders, 1990.

14. Maniker A, Cantrell S, Vaicys C. Failure of hydroxyapatite cement to set in repair of a cranial defect. Case Rep. *Neurosurgery* 1998; **43**: 953–4.

15. Yamashima, T. Modern cranioplasty with hydroxyapatite ceramic granules buttons and plates. *Neurosurgery* 1993; **33**(5): 939–40.

16. Chen T, Wang H, Chen S, Lin F. Reconstruction of post-traumatic frontal-bone depression using hydroxyapatite cement. *Ann Plas Surgery* 2004; **52**(3): 303–8.

17. Taub P, Rudkin G, Clearihue W. Prefabricated alloplastic implants for cranial defects. *Plast Reconstruc Surg* 2003; **111**(3): 1233–40.

18. Segal D, Oppenheim J, Murovic J. Neurological recovery after cranioplasty (case report). *Neurosurgery* 1994; **34**(4): 729–31.

19. Stula D. Intrakranielle Druckmessung bei großen Schädelkalottendefekten [in German]. *Neurochirurgia* 1985; **28**: 164–9.

20. Manson P, Crawley W, Hoopes J. Frontal cranioplasty: risk factors and choice of cranial vault reconstructive material. *Plast Reconstruc Surg* 1986; **77**(6): 888–904.

21. Baker SB, Weinzweig J, Kirschner RE, Bartlett SP. Applications of a new carbonated calcium phosphate bone cement: early experience in pediatric and adult craniofacial reconstruction. *Plast Reconstruc Surg* 2002; **109**: 1789–96.

22. Eppley B, Kilgo M, Coleman J. Cranial reconstruction with computer-generated hard-tissue replacement patient-matched implants: indications, surgical technique and long-term follow-up. *Plast Reconstruc Surg* 2002; **109**(3): 864–71.

23. Repologle R, Lanzino G, Francel P, Henson S, Lin K, Jane J. Acrylic cranioplasty using miniplate Struts. *Neurosurgery* 1996; **39**(4): 747–9.

24. Guimaraes-Ferreira J, Gewalli F, David L, Maltese G, Heino H, Lauritzen C. Calvarial bone distraction with a contractile bioresorbable polymer. *Plast Reconstruc Surg* 2002; **109**(4): 1325–31.

25. Chim H, Schantz J. New frontiers in calvarial reconstruction: integrating computer-assisted design and tissue engineering in cranioplasty. *Plast Reconstruc Surg* 2005; **116**(6): 1726–41.

26. Wozney J. Bone morphogenetic proteins. *Prog Growth Factor Res* 1989; **1**: 267–80.

27. Ripamonti U. Soluble osteogenic molecular signals and the induction of bone formation. *Biomaterials* 2006; **27**(6): 807–22.

28. Breitbart AS, Grande DA, Mason J, Barcia M, James T, Grant RT. Gene-enhanced tissue engineering: applications for bone healing using cultured periosteal cells transduced retrovirally with the BMP-7 gene. *Ann Plastic Surg* 1999; **43**(6): 632–9.

# Chapter 20

# Neurosurgical complications of head injury

Peter C. Whitfield and Laurence Watkins

## Skull base fracture – CSF leak

CSF rhinorrhoea or otorrhoea indicates that a skull base fracture has breached the dura and formed a communication between the intracranial contents and the external environment. This places the patient at risk of meningitis while the CSF leak continues. Since 90% of cases seal spontaneously within 2 weeks, neurosurgical intervention is not usually considered until this time has elapsed. An exception is a fracture of the posterior wall of the frontal sinus where a persistent leak is likely. Early anterior fossa repair is normally considered in such cases (see Chapter 18).

Sometimes a CSF leak is clinically obvious. If a leak is suspected but not overt, leaning the patient's head forward may provoke a characteristic nasal drip. Further provocation can be sought by laying the patient prone with the head dependant over the end of the couch. However, a small amount of clear nasal fluid can be of doubtful significance. It can be difficult to differentiate between CSF and thin nasal mucus, particularly if the discharge is also stained by blood after trauma. Since CSF and blood both contain glucose, and nasal secretions can contain glucose, the sensitivity and specificity of a positive glucose oxidase strip test are poor.[1] The $\tau$-fraction of transferrin, known as $\tau$-transferrin, $\tau$-protein, $\tau$-globulin, $\beta_2$ transferrin, asialotransferrin or more commonly tau protein, is present in normal CSF and absent from the blood except in patients with sustained alcohol abuse and rare carbohydrate deficient glyco-protein syndromes. If a sample of fluid can be collected, then a relatively quick laboratory test for tau protein can confirm CSF leakage.[2] If the CT scan of the head reveals intracranial air, then a CSF leak can be inferred, even if it is not clinically obvious.

The value of prophylactic antibiotics in patients with CSF leak has been debated for many years. Eljamel reported a retrospective, non-randomized study of 253 patients with CSF leak. Of the 106 cases treated with antibiotics, 6.6% developed meningitis in the first week compared with 9.17% of the 109 cases not administered prophylactic antibiotics. The annual risk of meningitis was 7.6% in the treated and 11.9% in the untreated group. Despite the slightly higher infection rate in the untreated group, this did not reach statistical significance. The author concluded that prophylactic antibiotics did not significantly reduce meningitis in this patient group.[3]

A Cochrane review in 2006 also studied the evidence from several randomized controlled trials of prophylactic antibiotics in patients with basal skull fracture. With only 206 random-ized cases to consider, the authors also undertook a meta-analysis on 2168 non-randomized cases reported in the literature. They concluded that there was no evidence that preventive antibiotic drugs reduced meningitis in patients with skull base fractures with or without accompanying CSF leakage.[4]

In clinical practice, patients may present with a delayed CSF leak, some years after trauma. Management is directed at confirming the presence of a CSF leak followed by identification of the site of leakage. The pathogenesis of such a leak is obscure, although it

*Head Injury: A Multidisciplinary Approach*, ed. Peter C. Whitfield, Elfyn O. Thomas, Fiona Summers, Maggie Whyte and Peter J. Hutchinson. Published by Cambridge University Press. © Cambridge University Press 2009.

is usually surmised that, following trauma, brain tissue effected a plug in a dural breach and that changes over time have led to re-opening of the fistula.

A variety of imaging techniques are used to identify the source of a CSF leak. If the tympanic membrane has been ruptured, CSF otorrhoea secondary to a petrous bone fracture may ensue. If the tympanic membrane is intact, CSF may pass down the Eustachian tube leading to CSF rhinorrhea in association with petrous or mastoid fractures. Anterior fossa fractures, including ethmoidal injuries, commonly cause CSF rhinorrhea. Such injuries are usually accompanied by anosmia. Many patients also report diminished (hypoageusia) or an unpleasant taste, consistent with the contribution of olfaction to the interpretation of taste sensations. A sphenoid bone fracture or frontal sinus injury can also cause CSF to leak through the nose due to the ducts that drain the paranasal sinuses to the nasal cavity. Thin section axial and coronal cranial and facial CT scans with 3-D reconstruction provide useful information on the anatomical sites of skull base fractures and provide strong clues regarding the site of CSF leakage. CT cisternography using water-soluble iodinated intrathecal contrast has commonly been used to identify the active site of leakage. Similarly, intrathecal radio-nucleide studies have been used to localize a CSF leak. More recently, non-invasive MR cisternography has been utilized to identify the site of a fistula. This uses heavily T2-weighted fast spin echo studies with fat suppression to assist identification of the leak. Although it has a high sensitivity, the specificity is relatively low, especially in the presence of paranasal sinus disease.[5] In recent years small studies have established the safety of low-dose intrathecal gadolinium as a contrast agent. This has led to publications demonstrating the utility of invasive MR cisternography in identifying the source of a CSF fistula.[6]

## Skull base fracture – repair techniques for CSF fistula

Surgery is most likely to be successful if the CSF fistula can be identified intra-operatively. A trans-nasal approach is commonly employed enabling an endoscopic extradural repair of anterior fossa leaks. This approach is optimized by injecting a low dose of fluoroscein intrathecally (0.1–0.2 ml of 5% solution mixed with 5–10 ml of CSF) at the onset of anaesthesia. Rapid circulation of fluorescein in the CSF enables the exact location of the fistula to be identified when viewed with the operating microscope or endoscope. A variety of soft tissues (muscle, fat, cartilage, fascia and mucosa) are commonly used to plug the defect. These are usually supplanted with tissue glues and frequently protection of the repair with a transient period of lumbar CSF drainage. The success rate of such procedures exceeds 90% and has led to this being the treatment of choice for the majority of leaks.[7]

Cranial approaches are now only performed if a nasal approach has failed or if CSF is leaking through a fracture of the petrous bone. The latter is actually quite a rare occurrence. In a study of 820 temporal bone fractures treated over a 5-year period, 122 patients had CSF fistulae (97 with otorrhoea, 16 with rhinorrhoea and 8 with both). In 95 cases spontaneous closure occurred within 7 days, a further 21 closed within 2 weeks and only five had persistent drainage over 14 days. In all, seven patients underwent surgery for repair of the CSF leak (middle cranial fossa, transmastoid or combined).[8] A subtemporal approach, coupled with a mastoidectomy, provides good access to temporal bone fistulae. A bicoronal approach is normally used for refractory anterior fossa CSF leaks. An extradural or intradural technique may be adopted. The latter is more invasive but offers better prospects of achieving successful obliteration of the fistula due to the ability to place an inlay graft. Careful attention to placement of the graft (fascia or pericranium) across the contoured floor of the fractured anterior fossa maximises the chances of fistula obliteration. The management of frontal sinus fractures is considered in Chapter 18.

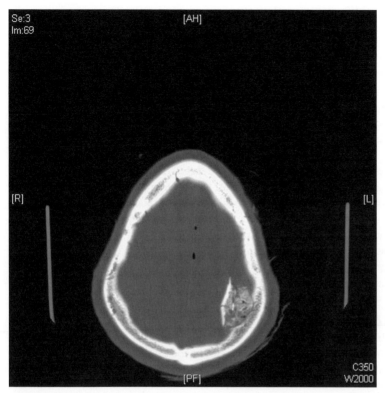

**Fig. 20.1.** This patient was assaulted with a blunt object and presented with right-sided weakness. A depressed parietal fracture is seen. In addition, some intracranial air can be seen consistent with a dural tear. At surgery a burr-hole was placed adjacent to the fracture. Contaminated bone fragments were removed and sent for microbiological analysis. The dural tear was opened further to permit adequate wound toilet. Primary closure of the scalp was performed over the craniectomy defect. Postoperatively the patient experienced focal seizures. A scan 2 weeks postoperatively did not show any signs of abscess formation. A cranioplasty can be performed if required as a second, delayed procedure.

## Depressed skull fractures – infection risk

Meningitis, brain abscess and rarely subdural empyemata can develop following a head injury in which a communication has been made between the environment and the intra-cranial contents. Patients with a CSF leak harbour this risk and their management is discussed above. The other main group of patients at risk of infective complications comprises those with penetrating craniocerebral trauma where comminuted and perhaps contaminated bone fragments and scalp tissues have been forced inwards breaching the dura (Fig. 20.1). With some penetrating injuries (such as a fall on to a sharp object or assault with a pointed weapon), the visible wound may be small and appear insignificant. In such cases the patient may have a deceptively normal level of consciousness, at least initially. This is due to a low velocity mechanism with little in the way of diffuse damage. This potential pitfall in the early assessment of the head trauma patient requires a degree of clinical acumen in the assessment of these injuries. In other cases such as assaults with a blunt object, vehicular trauma and gunshot injuries the fracture is obvious. In such cases the wound should be photographed and then covered with a sterile dressing in the emergency department. Once ATLS care has been implemented to exclude other life-threatening injuries, compound skull

**203**

fracture patients should be transferred to the neurosurgical unit. The wound generally requires early debridement and dural repair to reduce the risk of developing intracranial infection. Where accessible, fragments of bone and contaminated material should be retrieved. Thorough irrigation of the wound with excision of devitalized tissues and primary closure of the scalp is recommended. The role of antibiotics in the management of compound depressed skull fractures has not been studied in randomized controlled trials. The 'Infection in Neurosurgery' working party of the British Society for Antimicrobial Chemotherapy recommended the use of a 5-day course of prophylactic antibiotics in the management of patients with penetrating craniocerebral trauma. Broad spectrum cover with i.v. co-amoxiclav or a i.v. cefuroxime + p.o. or rectal metronidazole was advised.[9]

Particular care must be exercised if a compound depressed fracture overlies the posterior two-thirds of the sagittal sinus or a transverse sinus. Elevation of bone fragments can lead to torrential bleeding, which may prove difficult to control. It is prudent to treat such fractures with wound toilet, cautious decontamination and closure of the scalp. Removal of bone fragments poses risks that outweigh the risk of infection.

A closed depressed fracture does not require surgery except for cosmetic reasons and protection of the intracranial contents. This can be performed within the first week following surgery through a carefully planned, unobtrusive scalp incision.

## Meningitis, brain abscess and subdural empyema

Post-traumatic meningitis typically presents with fever, depressed level of consciousness, photophobia and nuchal rigidity. If infection presents in the early stages, these signs may be masked by the primary brain injury. In severe brain injury a more common scenario is ventriculitis secondary to an external ventricular drain. CSF should be sampled from the ventricular drain and i.v. and intrathecal antibiotics administered according to organism type and sensitivity. If meningitis is suspected, a lumbar puncture should be performed, provided the CT head indicates that there is no intracranial space occupying lesion. The commonest infecting organism is *Strepococcus pneumoniae*. Appropriate intravenous antibiotics should be administered early, giving consideration to CSF penetration and the likely sensitivity of the infecting organisms. Rarely, infection can occur months or even years after trauma due to the presence of an occult CSF fistula.

Brain abscesses and sub-dural empyemata are rare sequelae of penetrating trauma. Both present with symptoms of raised intracranial pressure and focal neurological deficits. Focal or generalized seizures are common. Abscesses are treated by stereotactic aspiration or craniotomy and marsupialisation (or excision) with thorough irrigation of the cavity. Some surgeons advocate instillation of antibiotics (e.g. gentamicin) into the abscess cavity. Empyemas can be difficult to see on a CT scan. Commonly, they lie in the parafalcine region. Treatment is to thoroughly irrigate the subdural space usually via a generous craniotomy. Surveillance CT scans are performed every week or two after surgery for brain abscess or empyema, to ensure that pus does not re-accumulate in the first couple of months.

## Pneumocephalus

Pneumocephalus is the presence of air within the cranial cavity. This is frequently seen as small bubbles of gas on an early CT scan and provides useful evidence of a dural tear in association with either a skull base fracture or a compound depressed calvarial fracture. Small volumes of intracranial air are reabsorbed into the bloodstream without clinical consequence. Rarely, complex skull base fractures may be associated with air in the spinal canal; pneumorachis.

Large amounts of intracranial air can be seen in either low-pressure or high-pressure situations. The low-pressure type is typically seen in an elderly patient with significant cerebral atrophy and therefore a large CSF compartment. If large amounts of CSF are lost through a skull base fracture, the space is filled with incoming air. In an individual patient this may have very little effect but sometimes the atrophic brain can 'slump' when not supported by surrounding CSF. The associated brain distortion can lead to decreased conscious level.

Such circumstances are usually treated conservatively by encouraging the patient to lie flat (tending to re-expand the brain) and by giving high flow oxygen to reduce the partial pressure of nitrogen in the bloodstream and encourage re-absorption of air from the intracranial space.

Intracranial air under high pressure can occur when a soft-tissue flap causes a skull base fracture to act as a 'one-way valve'. This raised intracranial pressure can compromise cerebral blood flow and is sometimes referred to as tension pneumocephalus. This is characterized by an appearance called the 'Mount Fuji' sign on the uppermost axial slices of the CT scan.[10] Occasionally, an urgent burr-hole or twist drill hole with insertion of a drain into the intracranial air space is performed if the clinical situation has rapidly evolved.

## Growing skull fracture

If a young child (< 3 years) sustains a skull fracture with an underlying dural tear, a growing skull fracture can develop. Clinicians should be aware of this rare complication. Growing skull fractures usually present weeks or months after the primary injury, although a small number of cases have presented years after trauma. From a pathological perspective, the brain herniates through the dural tear and keeps the fracture open, preventing healing of the bone. This brain may form a leptomeningeal cyst at the point of herniation. A craniotomy is required to expose the full extent of the dural tear. Dural repair must be achieved to prevent brain herniation. The bone flap is then replaced to achieve maximal cover of the bone defect. The fracture will then usually heal.

## Vascular complications

Vascular lesions can occur after blunt or penetrating traumatic brain injury. Although vascular problems can present immediately after trauma, a delayed presentation is generally more common.

## Occlusive injuries

The arteries supplying the brain are vulnerable to traumatic damage. In clinical practice such lesions are rare but must be considered if a post-traumatic stroke syndrome evolves. Injury most commonly occurs in the extracranial or skull base segments of the carotid arteries.[11] These injuries are usually due to rotational injury, direct blunt neck trauma or skull base fractures. Vertebral artery injury is extremely rare and may be associated with a cervical spine fracture. Carotid and vertebral artery trauma may lead to 'dissection'. Intimal damage occurs and permits a false passage for blood flow within the vessel wall. Such blood reaches a blind end after a variable distance, or may force its way back into the parent vessel lumen. In both cases vessel occlusion occurs either as a result of mural thrombosis or thrombosis within the lumen. This may propagate distally toward the skull base. This complication probably occurs without clinical consequence in many cases due to adequate collateral perfusion. However, clinical presentation may occur due to direct ischaemia in the appropriate vascular territory. In some cases the thrombus may lead to delayed embolic events occasionally with devastating clinical consequences. Occlusive vascular injuries are investigated with several modalities including CT angiography, Doppler ultrasound, MR angiography and invasive cerebral angiography. The treatment of vascular occlusive events is anecdotal. Anticoagulant therapy usually provides the mainstay of care, although endovascular and surgical options, including extracranial-intracranial by-pass, have been reported.

Occlusive events in the smaller intracranial vessels (e.g. middle cerebral artery) have been reported but are even rarer. The principles of management remain the same as for large vessel disease.

## Arteriovenous fistulae

Blunt trauma can also lead to arteriovenous fistulae. These can sometimes be identified clinically. The commonest site for a post-traumatic fistula is in the cavernous segment of the carotid artery, producing a caroticocavernous fistula (CCF). This is usually clinically obvious due to pulsatile proptosis, congestion of the scleral vessels and an obvious bruit. Any skull fracture, however, whether of skull vault or base, can be associated with a small dural fistula which can subsequently lead to subarachnoid haemorrhage or 'spontaneous' subdural haemorrhage. Rarely, a penetrating injury can lead to a parenchymal arteriovenous fistula. Most CCF are treated using endovascular techniques. Convexity fistulae are managed on merit. After careful assessment, it may be appropriate to leave some convexity dural fistulae untreated. However, the presence of cortical venous reflux is associated with a higher risk of intracranial haemorrhage and should be managed by endovascular occlusion or surgical excision.

## Traumatic intracranial aneurysms

Traumatic intracranial aneurysms are rare. Vessel wall damage leads to formation of a false aneurysm or a pseudoaneurysm. About one-third are due to penetrating trauma and two-thirds due to closed injuries. Penetrating injuries usually cause middle cerebral artery aneurysms, whilst closed head injuries more commonly affect the internal carotid arteries. Aneurysms due to closed injuries are not normally detected unless a delayed post-traumatic subarachnoid haemorrhage occurs. There is, of course, doubt whether an aneurysm discovered in a patient who has suffered a head injury is truly traumatic in etiology or, in fact, an incidental finding, since few patients will have had previous vascular investigation. Du Trevou and van Dellen reported a 12% incidence of traumatic aneurysm formation in a series of 181 patients undergoing cerebral angiography at various time points after penetrating cranial stab wounds.[12] Ten per cent of cases with intracerebral haematomas had an underlying traumatic aneurysm. Early angiography was advocated following all cranial stab injuries to detect aneurysm formation before any further intracranial haemorrhage occurred. Although an argument for delayed angiography has been made, this South African study group did not find any evidence to support such an approach, although they concluded that a second delayed angiogram is sometimes required especially if there is vasospasm or a 'cut off' vessel on the initial study.

In addition to occlusive disease, trauma to the neck can lead to extracranial carotid or vertebral artery aneurysm formation. Symptoms may include a pulsatile mass, dysphagia, lower cranial nerve palsies and focal cerebral ischaemia. Treatment is based upon exclusion of the aneurysm from the circulation by an interventional or surgical approach. The literature is replete with studies describing the management of small numbers of cases.

# Traumatic subarachnoid haemorrhage

Around 33% of moderate and severely head-injured patients demonstrate traumatic subarachnoid haemorrhage (tSAH) on an early CT scan. In addition, tSAH is an independent factor predictive of a poor outcome. In a large European study the incidence of a poor outcome was increased two-fold in patients with tSAH.[13] Transcranial Doppler studies have demonstrated increased flow velocities consistent with vasospasm in many of these patients. These observations led to a series of randomized controlled trials of the neuroprotective agent nimodipine in patients with tSAH. A recent evidence-based review concluded that the mortality and poor outcome rates were similar in the treatment and placebo patient groups and therefore did not support the routine use of nimodipine in tSAH.[14]

# Chronic subdural haematoma

A chronic subdural haematoma can occur many weeks after head injury. The injury may have seemed minor; in fact, the patient often does not remember a particular predisposing injury. The most common symptom is headache, which worsens progressively and is eventually accompanied by vomiting. There may also be a focal deficit, which can vary in severity. Sometimes neurological deficits can fluctuate in severity. Even in the absence of focal deficit, increasing ICP may lead to cognitive impairment and eventually a depressed level of consciousness.

A chronic subdural hematoma appears to develop as a complication in patients who have sustained a small acute subdural haematoma. The initial clot becomes surrounded by a membrane. This appears as a thin, glistening grey layer. The clot within then liquefies and expands. This may be due to an osmotic effect or perhaps an inflammatory process caused by the presence of blood breakdown products. Fresh bleeding into the subdural space can also cause further expansion of the haematoma.

Whatever the pathophysiology, the treatment of choice is evacuation of the subdural collection. This is considered in some detail in Chapter 17. Surgery can even be performed under local anaesthetic; therefore age and general fragility should not be taken to contraindicate treatment of this condition.

# Epilepsy

Post-traumatic seizures are classified into immediate (during the first 24 hours after injury), early (within 7 days of injury) and late (more than 7 days after injury). Late seizures are often referred to as 'unprovoked seizures'. Different types of seizure can manifest after TBI. Around 70% of cases lose consciousness and around 40% have some focal component to the seizure.

Several key studies have investigated factors associated with an increased risk of post-traumatic seizures. Annegers et al. conducted a population-based study on 4541 patients (adults and children) who survived TBI between 1935 and 1984 and found a clear correlation with the severity of the primary injury.[15] Following mild injury the standardized incidence ratio (SIR) at 1 year was 3.1. Between 1 and 4 years the SIR remained elevated (2.1), but after 5 years there was no increase in seizure risk. For patients with moderate injuries, the SIR by the end of year 1 was 6.7. The risk remained around 3× that of the normal population for the next 8 years. Even after 10 years the risk was double that of the general population. The risks were even greater for patients with severe brain trauma. The SIR was 95.0 at 1 year. It remained at 16.7 for years 1 to 4. After 5 years the risk was still 12× normal. Even at 10 years and beyond the risk was 4× the normal population risk. The overall risk of seizures at 5 years was 0.7% for mild injuries; 1.2% for moderate injuries and 10% for severe injuries. The 30-year cumulative incidence was 2.1%,

4.2% and 16.7% for these groups, respectively. These data provide convincing evidence that moderate and severe head injury significantly increase the lifetime risk of seizures.

Jennett conducted important studies and found that the risk of late seizures was increased if: (i) an intracranial haematoma had been evacuated; (ii) a depressed fracture was present and (iii) an early seizure had occurred.[16] Evacuated intracerebral haematomas carried a 45% risk of late seizures compared with a 22% risk for an extradural clot. Dural tears, focal signs, early seizures and post-traumatic amnesia (PTA) of >24 hours all increased the risk of late post-traumatic seizures in a synergistic fashion. If only one of these factors was present, the risk of late seizures was 3–10%. If a combination of dural tear, PTA > 24 hours and an early seizure occurred, the risk of late post-traumatic seizure was around 60%. The presence of an early or immediate fit always appears to pose an increased risk of late seizures although this effect is less marked in children.

## Prophylactic anticonvulsants

Seizures can have deleterious effects causing secondary brain injury, metabolic disturbances and sudden death, in addition to psychological deficits related to a diagnosis of epilepsy. Prophylaxis would therefore seem to be a logical step provided drug treatment is effective and well tolerated. Temkin *et al.* conducted a careful, randomized controlled trial with phenytoin and placebo treatment arms in over 400 severe head injury cases. Whilst the risk of early seizures was significantly lower in the phenytoin group (3.6% vs. 14.2%), there were no significant differences in the incidence of late seizures between treatment groups.[17] Early treatment was well tolerated with few side effects. Several other trials (but not all) have reported a reduction in early seizures using anticonvulsants, although improvements in outcome were not associated with this. None of the trials have demonstrated a reduction in the incidence of late seizures or any improvements in outcome.[18,19] Long-term prophylaxis is therefore not recommended. Many neurosurgeons use short-term prophylaxis for high-risk cases.

If seizures occur during the initial phase of post-traumatic hospitalization, intravenous phenytoin is often commenced. Other drugs with lower side effect profiles are often used in preference to phenytoin in later phases of care. These are selected according to seizure type, dosing frequency, route of administration, beneficial effects, teratogenicity, drug interactions and side effects.

Long-term epilepsy significantly restricts prospects for future employment, particularly, since it excludes the patient from driving. In about half of patients with post traumatic epilepsy, it is their only residual physical disability, significantly restricting the lifestyle of a patient who has otherwise made a good recovery. Any patient who has had a seizure, a craniotomy, a depressed skull fracture or a cerebral contusion should be advised not to drive or operate dangerous machinery. They should also contact the appropriate Driving and Vehicle Licensing Authority. If seizures appear to cease, it is appropriate to consider gradual withdrawal of anticonvulsant medication after two years. However, this decision should be made in conjunction with the patient. Some patients prefer to remain on an anticonvulsant rather than take the risk of having a further seizure, particularly if they drive.

## Hydrocephalus

Hydrocephalus occasionally occurs after severe head injury with traumatic subarachnoid or intraventricular haemorrhage. Presentation in the acute stages is rare, although CSF drainage via an external ventricular drain is commonly employed to reduce intracranial pressure.

Clinical features of hydrocephalus may present months or even years after the primary injury. Head injury patients constitute a subset of cases with communicating 'normal pressure hydrocephalus'. Symptoms most commonly include cognitive decline and poor mobility, rather than the headache of raised intracranial pressure. Sometimes movement disorders due to basal ganglia dysfunction occur. These may be secondary to a dilated ventricular system altering blood flow patterns within the periventricular basal ganglia and white matter pathways. Urinary urgency may be evident. If doubt exists regarding the significance of clinical and imaging findings, supplementary tests may be performed to assist in making a diagnosis. These include CSF infusion studies and a period of CSF drainage. If a diagnosis of post-traumatic hydrocephalus is made, the treatment of choice is placement of a ventriculoperitoneal shunt. Flow control devices and programmable valves are commonly used to minimize the risk of CSF overdrainage.

## Cranial nerve trauma

Permanent cranial nerve damage can occur after head injury. An impaired sense of smell is commonly reported. This is often associated with an anterior cranial fossa fracture or occipital impact. In many cases disruption of the olfactory nerves from the olfactory bulbs appears to be causative, although injuries to the orbitofrontal cortex, medial temporal cortex and septal nuclei may also be important in some patients.[20] Most patients have total anosmia, although about 25% have hyposmia (reduced smell) or parosmia (distortion of smells). The sense of smell should be assessed using mild odours such as cloves, coffee and vanilla. If noxious substances are used (e.g. peppermint, ammonia), trigeminal nerve fibres may be stimulated giving false reassurance of sense of smell preservation. A more thorough assessment can be made using a quantitative odour identification test. Using such techniques Doty *et al.* studied a large series of head injured patients with an impaired sense of smell and showed that none of the anosmic cases regained normal olfactory function. However, about one-third of patients with olfactory dysfunction experienced slight objective improvements. This included some cases with anosmia. About 60% of cases with parosmia improved over an 8-year period.[21]

Craniofacial injuries are commonly associated with visual impairment. Injuries to the orbit need to be distinguished from cranial nerve trauma. The optic nerve can be transected leading to visual loss with an afferent pupillary defect. Diplopia may be due to an abducent nerve injury, or less commonly a trochlear or oculomotor deficit. The latter is characterized by ptosis and ipsilateral pupil dilatation. The trigeminal nerve divisions are rarely damaged in isolation. Peripheral branches can be traumatized, particularly if craniofacial fractures are present.

Facial nerve trauma is a common sequela of a petrous bone fracture. Weakness may be partial and can recover. Steroids are sometimes used in this situation, although the clinical evidence to support this approach is questionable. Facial nerve lesions can occur in unison with hearing loss. Hearing deficits need to be characterised as either a conductive loss or a sensorineural impairment. Conductive loss may be due to blockage of the external auditory canal, tympanic membrane disruption, fluid within the middle ear cavity or ossicular chain trauma. Sensorineural injuries are common accompaniments of petrous bone fractures and may be permanent.

Lower cranial nerve palsies (glossopharyngeal, vagal, spinal accessory and hypoglossal) usually present as a complication of an occipital bone fracture extending to the jugular foramen or the hypoglossal canal. Fine-cut CT scans may be necessary to adequately visualize such injuries. The close anatomical relationships of these nerves to the vertebral artery should alert the clinician to ruling out significant vascular trauma.

# Concussion in sport

Concussion is a complex pathophysiological process affecting the brain, induced by traumatic forces. Sportsmen are at a particular risk of concussive injury. Concussion typically results in short-lived impairment of neurological function and is associated with normal neuro-imaging studies. The pathological substrate is unknown. Not all patients with concussion have a history of 'loss of consciousness'. Concussion may be categorized as simple or complex. The former resolves without complication in 7–10 days. Complex concussion is associated with persistent symptoms and prolonged cognitive impairment. It also includes athletes who experience motor convulsive posturing at the time of impact or suffer multiple concussive episodes over time, often with decreasing impact force. Neuropsychological assessment may prove invaluable in evaluating and managing these cases.[22]

The Sports Concussion Assessment Tool (SCAT) is widely used to enable medical personnel and athletes to recognize the features of concussion. These include confusion, amnesia, loss of consciousness, headache, balance impairment, dizziness, vomiting, feeling 'stunned', visual symptoms, tinnitus and irritability. Simple cognitive questions (e.g. list the months backwards, starting with any month other than January or December; recall five nouns; digit recall) help assess whether a sports person is concussed. These tests are more reliable than assessing orientation in time, place and person.[22]

It is well recognized that a patient with a history of recent concussion can sustain severe life-threatening cerebral oedema if a second injury occurs soon after trauma.[23] To prevent this rare 'second impact syndrome', most sporting authorities implement a period of non-participation after a first injury. The International Rugby Board states that 'a player who has suffered concussion shall not participate in any match or training session for a minimum period of three weeks from the time of the injury, and may then only do so when symptom-free and declared fit, after proper medical examination. Such declaration must be recorded in a written report prepared by the person who carried out the medical examination of the player.' The return to play should follow a stepwise progression with an initial period of cognitive and physical rest. This is followed by resumption of non-contact exercise, sports training and then game participation. For cases with complex concussion, the rehabilitation period will be longer.

# Post-traumatic encephalopathy after repeated injury

Boxing may cause an acute severe head injury with intracranial bleeding. The repeated trauma to the brain can also lead to long-term neuropathological sequelae. Many other sports including horse racing, rugby, football and American football may also result in acute and chronic brain injury. Much debate exists regarding the risk associated with boxing. Early reports showed that boxers can develop features of brain degeneration including cognitive, psychiatric and motor disorders.[24] This 'punch drunk syndrome' or 'dementia pugilistica' is a progressive neurodegenerative disorder that has recognized stages including affective disorder, incoordination, dysphasia, apraxia, cognitive decline and Parkinsonism.[25,26] Post-mortem and imaging studies have shown structural changes that appear to correlate with clinical reports. These changes include cerebral atrophy; degeneration of midline or paramedian structures including the fornix, thalamus, hypothalamus, corpus callosum and substantia nigra; cerebellar degeneration with Purkinje cell loss; hemosiderin staining and cortical gliosis; and β-amyloid plaque formation.[27,28] The British Medical Association has voiced much concern about the risks associated with boxing. However, a recent systematic review has shown that, if any harmful effects operate in amateur boxers, the effect is small and of doubtful significance.[29,30] In summary, the evidence appears to show that boxing has a dose–response effect upon the brain. Factors contributing to the dose comprise the numbers of fights, knock-outs and defeats for an individual, coupled with any genetic predisposition risk-factors such as the Apo E alleles.[31]

## Acknowledgements

The authors would like to thank Dr Helen Gooday for her contribution to the epilepsy section of this chapter.

## References

1. Baker EH, Wood DM, Brennan AL, Baines DL, Philips BJ. New insights into the glucose oxidase stick test for cerebrospinal fluid rhinorrhoea. *Emerg Med J* 2005; **22**: 556–7.

2. Porter MJ, Brookes GB, Zeman AZJ, Keir, G. Use of protein electrophoresis in the diagnosis of cerebrospinal fluid rhinorrhoea. *J Laryng Otol* 1992; **106**: 504–6.

3. Eljamel MS. Antibiotic prophylaxis in unrepaired CSF fistulae. *Br J Neurosurg* 1993; 7(5): 501–5.

4. Ratilal B, Costa J, Sampaio C. Antibiotic prophylaxis for preventing meningitis in patients with basilar skull fractures. *Cochrane Database of Systematic Reviews* 2006, Issue 1. Art. No.: CD004884. DOI: 10.1002/14651858.CD004884.pub2

5. Gammal TE, Sobol W, Wadlington VR *et al.* Cerebrospinal fluid fistula: detection with MR cisternography. *Am J Neuroradiol* 1998; **19**: 627–31.

6. Jinkins JR, Rudwan M, Krumina G, Tali ET. Intrathecal gadolinium-enhanced MR cisternography in the evaluation of clinically suspected cerebrospinal fluid rhinorrhea in humans: early experience. *Radiology* 2002; **222**: 555–9.

7. Hegazy HM, Carrau RL, Snyderman CH, Kassam A, Zweig J. Transnasal endoscopic repair of cerebrospinal fluid rhinorrhoea: a meta-analysis. *Laryngoscopy* 2000; **110**: 1166–72.

8. Brodie HA, Thompson TC. Management of complications from 820 temporal bone fractures. *Am J Otol* 1997; **18**: 188–97.

9. Bayston R, de Louvois J, Brown EM, Johnston RA, Lees P, Pople IK. Use of antibiotics in penetrating craniocerebral injuries. *Lancet* 2000; **355**: 1813–17.

10. Michel SJ. The Mount Fuji sign. *Radiology* 2004; **232**: 449–50.

11. Stringer WL, Kelly DL. Traumatic dissection of the extracranial internal carotid artery. *Neurosurgery* 1980; **6**: 123–30.

12. du Trevou MD, van Dellen JR. Penetrating stab wounds to the brain: the timing of angiography in patients presenting with the weapon already removed. *Neurosurgery* 1992; **31**: 905–11; discussion 911–12.

13. The European Study Group on Nimodipine in Severe Head Injury. A multicenter trial of the efficacy of nimodipine on outcome after severe head injury. *J Neurosurg* 1994; **80**: 797–804.

14. Vergouwen MDI, Vermeulen M, Roos YBWEM. Effect of nimodipine on outcome in patients with traumatic subarachnoid haemorrhage: a systematic review. *Lancet Neurology* 2006; **5**: 1029–32.

15. Annegers JF, Hauser A, Coan SP, Rocca WA. A population-based study of seizures after traumatic brain injuries. *N Engl J Med* 1998; **338**: 20–4.

16. Jennett B. *Epilepsy After Non-missile Head Injury.* London, Heinemann, 1975.

17. Temkin NR, Dikmen SS, Wilensky AJ, Keihm J, Chabal S, Winn HR. A randomized, double-blind study of phenytoin for the prevention of post-traumatic seizures. *N Engl J Med* 1990; **323**: 497–502.

18. Schierhout G, Roberts I. Prophylactic antiepileptic agents after head injury: a systematic review. *J Neurol Neurosurg Psychiatry* 1998; **64**: 108–12.

19. Brain Trauma Foundation. Guidelines for the management of severe traumatic brain injury, 3rd edition. XIII. Antiseizure prophylaxis. *J Neurotrauma* 2007; **24** (Suppl 1): S83–6.

20. Yousem DM, Geckle RJ, Bilker WB, McKeown DA, Doty RL. Post-traumatic olfactory dysfunction: MR and clinical evaluation. *Am J Neuroradiol* 1996; **17**: 1171–9.

21. Doty RL, Yousem DM, Pham LT, Kreshak AA, Geckle R, Lee WW. Olfactory dysfunction in patients with head trauma. *Arch Neurol* 1997; **54**: 1131–40.

22. McCrory P, Johnston K, Meeuwisse W *et al.* Summary and agreement statement of the 2nd International conference on concussion in sport, Prague 2004. *Clin J Sport Med* 2005; **15**: 48–57.

23. Saunders RL, Harbaugh RE. The second impact in catastrophic contact-sports head trauma. *J Am Med Assoc* 1984; **252**: 538–9.

24. Martland HS. Punch drunk. *J Am Med Assoc* 1928; **9**a: 1103–7.

25. Millspaugh JA. Dementia pugilistica. *US Naval Bull* 1937; **35**: 297–302.

26. *The Boxing Debate. British Medical Association.* London, Chameleon Press Ltd; 96.

27. Corsellis JAN. Boxing and the brain. *Br Med J* 1989; **298**: 105–9.

28. Roberts AH. *Brain Damage in Boxers. A Study of the Prevalence of Traumatic Encephalopathy Among Ex-professional Boxers.* London, Pitman, 1969.

29. Loosemore M, Knowles CH, Whyte GP. Amateur boxing and risk of chronic traumatic brain injury: systematic review of observational studies. *Br Med J* 2007; **335**: 809–12.

30. McCrory P. Boxing and the risk of chronic brain injury. *Br Med J* 2007; **335**: 781–2.

31. Jordan BD, Relkin NR, Ravdin LD, Jacobs AR, Bennett A, Gandy S. Apolipoprotein E epsilon4 associated with chronic traumatic brain injury in boxing. *J Am Med Assoc* 1997; **278**: 136–40.

# Paediatric head injury management

Patrick Mitchell

Many treatment decisions in the management of acute head injuries are not well supported by reliable evidence. This is especially true in children. There are good reasons for this which will continue to apply, so it is anticipated that this situation will not change rapidly. The head-injured child is one of the most distressing of clinical situations. High-quality data collection requires informed consent for participation in research studies and such discussions often may not be appropriate. It is not an area that lends itself to randomized controlled trials and very few have been conducted. As a result, treatments tend to fall into two groups: those that are thought to be effective on mechanistic grounds and have been standard for many years, such as protecting the airway as early as possible, maintaining blood pressure and surgical removal of significant extra-axial (outside the central nervous system but inside the head) mass lesions; and treatments that are not associated with compelling mechanistic justification. These have generally been the subject of case series and comparative studies with a few notable cases being the subject of randomized controlled trials.

Recent advances in the management of head injury have evolved around three areas: screening of minor head injuries for the early detection of treatable complications, improving communication and logistics to allow early surgical intervention to be carried out when needed, and developing medical treatment of severe brain injury. More significant than these has been a steady fall in incidence of head injury in children over recent decades in the Western world.[1-3] This may be contributed to by a range of environmental improvements, including improved motor vehicle design, improved road safety measures and use of cycle helmets.[4,5]

## Mild head injury

Between 0.5 and 1% of all children in the Western world attend accident and emergency departments each year with head injuries of which only a small minority are severe.[6-8] The mildest injuries do not cause loss of consciousness. Isolated episodes carry extremely low risks of developing later complications and are thought to be largely benign.[9,10] Of some concern is the cumulative effect of repeated very mild head injuries as may occur during sports such as soccer.[11] There are reports of elevated biochemical markers of brain injury after games involving heading of balls though other studies have found no effect.[12-14]

Definitions are not absolute but head injuries that result in loss of consciousness are referred to as concussive and those with a Glasgow Coma Score (GCS) of nine or more on arrival at an accident and emergency department are generally described as mild or moderate. The overwhelming majority will make a complete and uncomplicated recovery.[8] There is no specific acute phase treatment that will assist in this recovery and management revolves around counselling and screening for the early detection of rare but grievous complications. As such, the management of this group of patients becomes routine but it should be remembered that the condition is not trivial.

*Head Injury: A Multidisciplinary Approach*, ed. Peter C. Whitfield, Elfyn O. Thomas, Fiona Summers, Maggie Whyte and Peter J. Hutchinson. Published by Cambridge University Press. © Cambridge University Press 2009.

The natural history of a concussive mild to moderate head injury is of sudden onset of profound coma immediately after the injury. The child becomes totally unresponsive to pain with fixed dilated pupils, floppy areflexic limbs and quite frequently transient apnoea. This picture causes profound distress in anyone witnessing it, and would be grave indeed if it persisted until the child was brought to accident and emergency, however it is fleeting and within seconds, or at most minutes, signs of responsiveness return. The child then goes through phases of improving responsiveness from confused to increasingly lucid communication but persisting disorientation to full recovery. During recovery, the conscious level may appear to fluctuate because of changing levels of alertness. To avoid potential confusion, the child should be actively stimulated fully to wake them up before formally assessing their level of consciousness. In general, the last function to recover is the ability to lay down new memories and there is a phase when a child appears to be fully alert on cursory examination but on closer questioning cannot remember the recent past. Specifically, a clinician may review a child and ask if they can remember seeing the clinician previously. If the child has seen them but cannot remember, it is likely that they are still in the post-traumatic amnesic period.

Following recovery of full orientation and new memory formation, a post-concussional syndrome often persists, slowly recovering over weeks or months depending on the severity of the injury. This syndrome consists of irritability, fears, sleep disorders, learning difficulties, poor concentration, poor short-term memory, short attention span, easy fatigability, and headache on physical exertion.[15] This has significant implications for children of school age, especially if they are facing important exams in the near future. Isolated mild head injuries appear to be relatively benign with full recovery being expected eventually.[15,16] Repeated concussive injuries carry a risk of cumulative neurological deficit, first noted in the sport of boxing and also found in other sports.[17,18] There is evidence suggesting that exposure to repeated minor head injuries leads to an earlier onset of symptoms of degenerative dementia in later life.[19] A further issue pertaining to mild to moderate head injuries is the second impact syndrome. Some evidence suggests that, if a second injury occurs before the first has fully recovered, it carries a greater neurological morbidity and risk of haemorrhagic complications possibly because of impaired cerebral blood flow autoregulation following the first injury.[20] Furthermore, children who have presented with one injury are at increased risk of further injuries.[21] Because of these concerns, it is important that clinicians treating sports-related head injuries require that children are not exposed to further risk of injury until the symptoms of post-concussive syndrome following the first have fully recovered.[22]

## Screening minor head injuries

Around 100 000 children present each year in the UK with head injuries. Of these, the overwhelming majority will make an uneventful recovery. Less than 500 are severe enough to require admission to intensive care units.[23] Those presenting with a GCS of 8 or less are generally stabilized and scanned with further management being decided on progress and scan findings. Of those who present with an apparently minor head injury, a small minority will later develop complications which can threaten permanent neurological deficit or death.[9,10] This population has caused particular concern as many of the deficits and deaths resulting from late complications in the past could, in principle, have been prevented had they been detected earlier. This has prompted a series of guidelines to be developed. In many Western countries there is an ongoing system of guideline review and audit aimed at accurate screening of minor injuries. In the past, screening involved skull X-rays and admission for

**Table 21.1.** Paediatric version of the GCS

| Best eye opening | Best verbal response | Best motor response |
|---|---|---|
| 1 – none | 1 – none | 1 – none |
| 2 – to pain | 2 – occasional moans/ whimpers | 2 – extends to pain |
| 3 – to command | 3 – inappropriate crying | 3 – flexes to pain |
| 4 – spontaneous | 4 – less than normal/ irritable crying | 4 – localizes to pain |
| | 5 – normal | 5 – obeys command |

From Morray JP *et al.* Coma scale for use in brain-injured children. *Critical Care Medicine* 12:1018, 1984. Reproduced with permission from Lippincott, Williams & Wilkins 1984. All rights reserved.

in-hospital observation until the child has recovered orientation and new memory formation, and this latter is still important, both to protect the child while they are vulnerable and to detect deterioration early. The principal screening tool now is computed tomography (CT), which involves some exposure to X-rays. Widespread use of CT in screening programmes therefore, involves exposing the population to a significant radiation dose. A balance must be struck between indiscriminate CT scanning in children who have an exceedingly low chance of developing complications and reluctance to scan, leading to late diagnoses and avoidable adverse outcome. The current standard in the UK is detailed in the NICE guidelines, which are summarized below.[24]

One of the limitations of current guidelines is the rather ambiguous nature of impaired consciousness in children. The GCS is not fully applicable to children, particularly before they learn to speak, usually by the age of 3 years. Assessment of consciousness in children is less objective and more dependent on experience of children in general and the individual child in particular, than it is in adults. Alternative scales have been developed for children but there is no universal standard comparable with the adult GCS.[25–28] The UK NICE guidelines assume the following paediatric version of the GCS where the verbal score differs from that recorded in adults (Table 21.1).

The NICE criteria for a CT head scan within 1 hour of assessment are:

- GCS under 14 on presentation or under 15 2 hours after the injury
- vomiting three or more times
- seizures (unless a known epileptic)
- evidence of a skull fracture (bruising behind the ear – see Fig. 21.1; CSF leak)
- focal neurological deficits
- amnesia for the injury
- unconsciousness lasting 5 minutes or more.

If the child is under the age of 1 year, additional criteria are:

- a bruise or laceration over 5 cm long
- GCS under 15 when assessed.

In addition suspicion of non-accidental injury, 'abnormal' drowsiness or a 'dangerous mechanism of injury' prompt a scan.

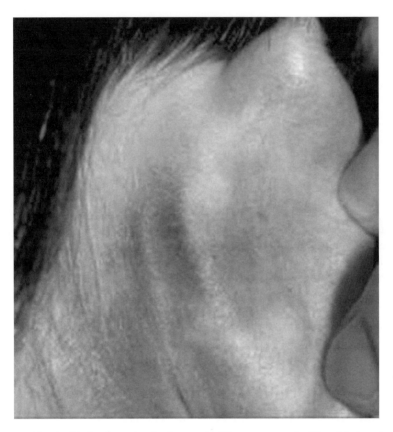

**Fig. 21.1.** Battle's sign. Bruising behind the ear without direct trauma to the area after a head injury is diagnostic of a basal skull fracture. The bruising may not appear for hours to days.

Cervical spine imaging is also part of the assessment of head-injured children. The NICE criteria for a CT of the cervical spine with the head scan are:

- GCS less than 13
- the child is intubated
- plain X-rays are inadequate or suspicious of a fracture
- a CT for multiple injuries is being done

In children under 10 the risk of radiation exposure, especially to the thyroid, is greater and plain X-rays are easier, so the criteria for a CT of the neck are more stringent:

- GCS 8 or less
- Plain X-rays suspicious or inadequate.

## Severe head injury

Head injuries presenting with a GCS of 8 or less or CT evidence of a haemorrhagic complication are referred to as severe. In these, CT is performed as a diagnostic investigation rather than as a screening tool and so with a greater degree of urgency, but it is not the highest priority when dealing with a trauma victim. Only when the child has a protected airway with stable gas exchange and haemodynamics can a CT safely be undertaken. These priorities are now widely followed, but some judgement is necessary as to the degree of stability and level of monitoring necessary before scanning. In those rare cases with a deteriorating conscious level, there is time pressure to scan and treat, delays beyond the minimum necessary may result in significantly poorer outcomes. Rapidly developing brain compression may cause haemodynamic instability that can only be satisfactorily treated by surgical decompression.

## Trauma systems

There is some evidence to suggest that children with severe head injuries fare better if treated in dedicated paediatric trauma units or dedicated trauma units with some paediatric experience. In a retrospective study in Pennsylvania between 1993 and 1997, it appeared that survival was improved if injured children were treated in either a dedicated paediatric, or adult with specific paediatric interest, trauma centres as opposed to purely adult trauma centres.[29] A further study in Washington, DC, spanning 1985 to 1988, compared patients transferred directly from the accident scene to a paediatric trauma centre with those transferred to a non-paediatric hospital first and then transferred onto the trauma centre. The chance of survival following severe head injury appeared better in the directly transferred group, but there was no significant difference for mild to moderate head injuries.[30] Not all studies reached the same conclusion, however. Hulka conducted a population-based study in Washington and Oregon from 1985 to 1987 and from 1991 to 1993.[31] Between 1987 and 1991 trauma systems were introduced in both states allowing historical comparison of outcomes before and after their introduction. This found no improvement in survival and in Washington survival was poorer after the introduction of the trauma system than it was beforehand. Ambiguous as the evidence is the trend is now towards treatment at dedicated paediatric centres.

## Extra-axial haematomas

The treatment of extra-axial haematomas illustrates the point that effective treatments introduced long ago may be widely accepted though not supported by high-quality evidence. There is no class I evidence pertaining to the treatment of acute extra-axial clots, but it is universally accepted that when significant they should be removed as quickly as possible. There are two types: subdural and extradural.

In children, extradural haematomas are commoner than subdurals occurring in 1.4% of children admitted with head injury in one series.[32,33] They are not a complication of a brain injury. Rather, they are generally a complication of a skull fracture.[34,35] The main dural arteries run in grooves on the inner table of the skull. The anatomy of these arteries and grooves is variable and, in some cases, the grooves are deep or even completely enclosed to form tunnels. If the bone adjacent to an artery is fractured, there is a risk that the artery will be torn or branches avulsed. This leads to bleeding from the artery outside the dura and the formation of an extradural haematoma. The majority of cases occur in the distribution of the middle meningeal artery on the side of the head.[35] Meningeal arteries can be of a substantial size, leading to rapid expansion of an extradural haematoma, especially in children where the dura is not as tightly adherent to the skull as it is in adults. As an extradural haematoma is not a complication of a brain injury, it is frequently associated with minimal or no primary brain damage. Because of this, outcome following prompt removal is usually excellent; there is a lot to lose by delay.[35,36] Furthermore, the diagnosis of an extradural haematoma is fairly straightforward. There may be a palpable boggy scalp swelling on the affected side. If there has been no significant brain injury, the onset of neurological deficits will be delayed. If there has been an injury sufficient to cause concussion, the child may recover in a few minutes only to later deteriorate because of the expanding extradural haematoma. This leads to the classic 'lucid interval' that is seen in a minority of cases. Surgery to deal with an extradural is more straightforward than for a subdural and this means that, in very remote areas, it may be appropriate to drain an extradural haematoma outwith a neurosurgery department and even without a CT diagnosis. It is reasonable to incise the scalp where a sub-galeal haematoma may be found. The periosteum is then scraped off the bone, at which point a fracture is likely to be visible. It is also likely that blood will be seen emanating from the fracture. The next step is to remove bone around where the blood is coming from using ronguers. A burr hole will facilitate this manoeuvre. Clot found immediately underneath the bone indicates an extradural collection. This is removed to reveal the white dura. Control of bleeding is normally possible with pressure, diathermy, wax and ligating sutures, although difficulties may be encountered.

Subdural haematomas are less common than extradurals in children, occurring in 0.4% of admitted head injuries in the series mentioned above.[32] In those under 3 years old they are more common than extradurals and are often associated with non-accidental injury especially if bilateral, interhemispheric or tentorial.[37-39] They are usually a complication of a brain injury. They result from bleeding veins or cortical vessels torn in association with brain movements. Recovery from a subdural haematoma is often incomplete, even if they are promptly evacuated. Furthermore, the vessels responsible for the haemorrhage are usually veins or fairly small arteries; hence subdurals tend to evolve more slowly than extradurals in children. Operating on subdurals is technically more difficult due to the presence of swollen, haemorrhagic brain tissue. Subdural haematomas tend to be more laterally extensive for a given volume than extradurals. For these reasons, removal of a subdural haematoma lies in the hands of a neurosurgeon.

## Severe head injury without extra-axial clots

The treatment of severe traumatic brain injury has been the subject of intense research over several decades but, as yet, the applicable results of this effort are disappointing. There have been three major avenues of inquiry: a search for neuroprotective agents, the development and assessment of monitoring modalities and developing treatments aimed at surrogate endpoints, most notably intracranial pressure (ICP). Neuroprotective agents are loosely described as those that improve the outcome following an acute brain insult, with or without an effect on surrogate markers such as ICP. Despite encouraging results in animals and an extensive search spanning adult and paediatric patients with a wide range of brain insults, none has yet been found. The Brain Trauma Foundation guidelines for the management of severe head injury and head injury in children are particularly recommended synopses.[40,41]

## Intracranial pressure monitoring

Intracranial pressure has become the single most important surrogate endpoint of treatment efficacy in head-injured children and monitoring has been an integral part of many of the protocols used for the treatment of severe head injury in the last two decades (Fig. 21.2). Raised intracranial pressure is closely *associated* with a poor outcome but whether this is because it contributes to a poor outcome *per se* or because both are linked with injury severity is not so clear.[42] Many of the treatments discussed below are used as they are known to reduce ICP rather than because they are known to improve outcomes. They are subject to the uncertainty of relationship between the two.

Children presenting with a GCS of 8 or less will generally be sedated and intubated to secure the airway for transfer between hospitals or for scanning. If the scan shows no

**Typical protocol for the management of paediatric traumatic intracranial hypertension**

**Fig. 21.2.** The management of severe head injury with raised ICP is often driven by protocols of which this is an example.

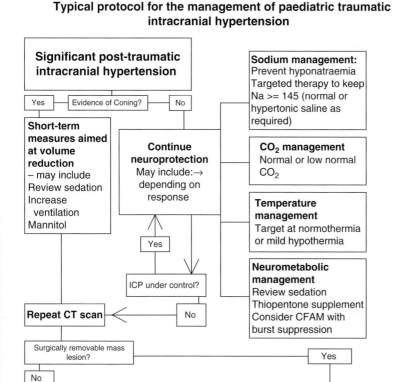

significant contusion or evidence of raised ICP, most clinicians would discontinue sedation and see if the child wakes up. If not, or if there is significant evidence of contusion or raised ICP, many clinicians insert an ICP monitor and wake the child up if the pressure remains within normal limits. If the ICP is elevated for more than a few minutes, various treatment options are available discussed in turn below.

Intracranial pressure monitoring is a diagnostic modality and not a treatment. We would not expect monitoring alone to have any impact on outcome other than by virtue of the risks of haemorrhage and infection that it involves. Clinically, significant risks have been reported to be as low as 0.6% but when haemorrhages that are not surgically removed are included, reported rates are 10 and 14%.[43–45] With these risks and uncertain benefits, should we monitor? If a clinician believes that there are treatments which are both effective at improving outcome following head injury and whose administration is dependent on a knowledge of ICP, then they should monitor. There is currently no treatment with class I evidence of benefit at improving outcome, so the issue remains controversial. The treatment under current consideration that is most likely to fit this criterion is decompressive craniectomy. If a clinician does not believe in such a treatment, they could still justifiably monitor in the context of research. Large-scale randomized trials of monitoring *per se* are difficult to justify because they would become immediately outdated by the development of such treatments.

The purpose of monitoring is to maintain ICP below a specific value by treating excursions beyond it. This raises the question of what the target value should be. At the time of writing, there is insufficient evidence to make this strategy a standard of care and the evidence available to guide a target pressure is weaker still. Receiver operating characteristic (ROC) analysis of intracranial pressure as a predictor of poor outcome after head injury in children and adults suggest that prolonged excursions of ICP over 35–40 mmHg should be treated.[46,47] This is still significantly above the normal intracranial pressure which in children remains below 20 mmHg except for transient higher excursions lasting a few seconds only.[48] Most clinicians who employ ICP-directed treatment use targets between these values.

Related to ICP is cerebral perfusion pressure (CPP). This is calculated as the difference between mean arterial blood pressure and mean intracranial pressure. Mean arterial pressure can crudely be calculated as the diastolic blood pressure plus a third of the pulse pressure. In practice, modern equipment calculates perfusion pressure by high time resolution integration of the arterial and intracranial pressure waveforms. Intracranial pressure-based management protocols can be divided into those that aim to minimize ICP and those that aim to keep CPP up. The latter have the disadvantage that CPP is a more indirect measurement, however ROC analysis suggests it is slightly more predictive of a poor outcome.[47] Normal blood pressure rises significantly with age in children, as do CPP thresholds below which a poor outcome is predicted by ROCs.[46] Suggested targets are perfusion pressure of $\geqslant 48$ mmHg in children between 2 and 6 years old, $\geqslant 54$ in children from 7 to 10 and $\geqslant 58$ in children over 10.[49] Both ICP- and CPP-guided protocols use treatment to control ICP as a first line. Cerebral perfusion pressure-guided protocols use hypertensive treatment as a second line.

## CSF drainage

One means of measuring intracranial pressure is to place an intraventricular catheter and measure CSF pressure. This has a higher complication rate than intraparenchymal pressure monitoring but permits CSF drainage.[45] A series of 22 patients including adults and children found that CSF drainage reduced ICP more than mannitol or hyperventilation.[50] In another series of 22 children with severe head injury ventricular drainage was similarly effective at reducing ICP; two deaths occurred, which was relatively few for the severity of injury.[51] Lumbar drainage has also been used. In five children in whom ventricular drainage and barbiturate coma did not control raised ICP, three responded to lumbar drainage and two made a good recovery with one moderate disability. The other two had no response to lumbar drainage and both died.[52] In a further report involving simultaneous lumbar and ventricular drainage in 16 patients with severe head injury, ICP was reduced in 14 who survived and not in 2 who died.[53] In a prospective non-randomized comparative study patients received either ventricular drainage or not, depending on the admitting physician. Mortality was 12% in those who received drainage and 53% of those who did not. A similar difference in the rates of good outcome was reported.[54] These results have brought CSF drainage into many management protocols but high-class evidence for benefit is lacking.

## Hypocapnoea

During the 1960s and 1970s it was believed that raised intracranial pressure associated with head injury in children was in large part due to hyperaemia and associated swelling. To counter this, hyperventilation-induced hypocapnoea was used as a treatment. In an uncontrolled series dating from the 1970s Bruce found remarkably good results from a protocol based management system that included hyperventilation.[55] Since then, several studies have been published examining the relationship between hyperventilation and two surrogate endpoints: intracranial pressure and cerebral blood flow. These showed that hyperventilation does reduce intracranial pressure, but this is not generally in cases associated with traumatic hyperaemia. The reduction in cerebral blood flow caused by low $CO_2$ is considered more likely to increase cerebral ischaemia than to normalize hyperaemia.[56] In the light of this, opinion has moved away from the use of hyperventilation. Current recommendations are that $CO_2$ should generally be maintained within normal limits.[57] Hyperventilation can be used as a means of controlling intracranial pressure if other medical methods have failed, but it is recommended that monitoring be instituted to assess cerebral blood flow or ischaemia when this is done. Although clinical practice has moved away from the use of hyperventilation, it should be noted that no study has compared the clinical outcome of patients receiving hyperventilation with those receiving normal ventilation. The results reported by Bruce in 1979 were very good, especially for their historical period, and have not been consistently bettered.[55]

## Osmotic management

The principal osmotic agents currently in use for treating raised ICP in children are mannitol and hypertonic saline. Mannitol is a long-established treatment, introduced when the standards of medical evidence were less rigorous than they are today. The evidence base for the use of hypertonic saline is stronger than for mannitol. This is not because hypertonic saline is necessarily better, but because it was introduced at a time when the fashions of evidence gathering were different.[58] A further problem specific to high-dose mannitol is that three randomized trials reported in adults suggested a significant benefit but they were later questioned as possibly fraudulent.[59–62]

Mannitol reduces ICP by two mechanisms.[63] It reduces blood viscosity thereby reducing blood vessel diameter, while maintaining cerebral blood flow mediated by autoregulation.[64–67] This effect has a rapid onset but a duration lasting less than 75 minutes.[65] The other effect is osmotic, causing tissue shrinkage by increasing the osmotic pressure of the vascular compartment. The osmotic effect is slower in onset taking 15 to 30 minutes but lasts up to 6 hours. It requires an intact blood–brain barrier. There has been some concern that mannitol may cross a compromised blood–brain barrier in areas of injured brain causing a reverse osmotic swelling when the intravascular mannitol levels fall.[63,68,69] This effect may be most pronounced with sustained levels of mannitol and minimized if intermittent boluses are given.[70]

Although hypertonic saline has received a lot of recent attention, it has a longer history than mannitol. Its effect on ICP was first described in 1919.[71] It has recently been investigated for the treatment of haemorrhagic shock and brain injury.[72] It shares mannitol's two mechanisms of action and has other theoretical advantages, including stimulation of atrial natriuretic peptide release and inhibition of inflammation.[72,73] Possible side effects include central pontine myelinolysis. Hypertonic saline has been the subject of several studies, the results of which show it to be effective at reducing ICP. In one small randomized pilot study in 32 children it was associated with shorter length of stay on ITU and fewer complications than isotonic Ringer's lactate; however, no study has addressed the question of long-term outcome.[74–77]

# Metabolic management

A variety of treatments can be grouped under a general heading of metabolic management. These include prophylactic steroids, anticonvulsants and barbiturates.

## Steroids

There have been two randomized controlled trials of dexamethasone as a treatment for head injury in children and one that included children.[78–80] These have not shown any efficacy in terms of ICP, CPP or outcome, but they were relatively small with a total fewer than 100 cases randomized between them. The issue is dominated by extrapolation from the large adult CRASH trial, which was stopped early after randomizing 10 008 cases to methylprednisolone or placebo because of a significant excess of deaths in the methylprednisolone group.[81] Follow-up analysis showed that both death and severe disability were more likely in the treatment group. Steroids are not therefore recommended except to correct adrenocortical insufficiency.

## Anticonvulsants

Infants and children have a greater incidence of early post-traumatic seizures than adults varying from 7 to 10% of children admitted and rising to 16% in those under 2.[82–84] Ninety-five per cent of these seizures developed within 24 hours of the injury. When they occur, they are treated with anticonvulsants but should prophylactic anticonvulsants be used? There are three questions at issue. If given early, do prophylactic anticonvulsants prevent early seizures? If given early, do they prevent late seizures and if given late do they prevent late seizures? To date, there is no good evidence that they do any of these things! One randomized trial of early phenytoin prophylaxis with 18 month follow-up found no reduction in seizure incidence early or late.[85] Routine prophylaxis is therefore not recommended but the evidence remains limited.

## Barbiturates

The barbiturates thiopentone and phenobarbitone have been used to treat head injury for several decades. They reduce intracranial pressure and animal studies suggest two mechanisms: reduced cerebral metabolic rate and altered vascular tone. Several case series have been reported but as yet there are no randomized trials on their use. Because of side effects of hypotension, reduced cardiac output and arrhythmias they are only used in refractory cases of raised ICP, if at all.[58,86,87]

# Hypothermia

The use of hypothermia to treat head injuries has a history dating back over 50 years. Interest was stimulated because accidents involving hypothermia and experience from cardiac surgery showed that a cold brain is considerably more tolerant of low blood flow than a warm one. Furthermore, evidence from clinical studies suggest that fever in head injury is associated with poor outcome.[88] A retrospective series of 18 severely head injured children dating from 1959 suggests that moderate hypothermia is effective at improving outcome.[89] A randomized trial from 1973 compared hypothermia with and without dexamethasone.[90] The overall survival rate was exceptionally good but there was no normothermic group for comparison. Data from two small randomized trials totalling 75 cases suggest that hypothermia appears to be safe and may improve outcome.[91] A phase III trial of 24 hours of

(a) (b)

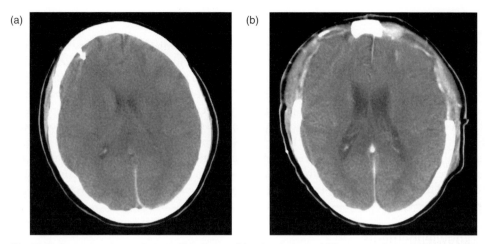

**Fig. 21.3.** Decompressive craniectomy. This 15-year-old patient had raised ICP unresponsive to medical treatment after a head injury. (a) The pre-operative scan shows the ICP monitoring device. (b) The post-operative scan shows the areas of skull removed allowing brain expansion.

moderate hypothermia versus normothermia is currently recruiting patients (hypothermia paediatric head injury trial).[92]

## Decompressive craniectomy

Post-traumatic intracranial hypertension occurs because the brain swells within the confined space of the cranium. Decompressive craniectomy opens the confined space (Fig. 21.3). There is little doubt that this is effective at reducing ICP or that it saves lives.[93] The problem is that many of the lives saved in the past have been of poor quality. Decompressive craniectomy will not improve the outcome unless the ICP is raised and it is likely to be more effective with greater degrees of raised pressure. Furthermore it tends to be reserved for cases where pressure cannot be controlled by other means. This means that it has its greatest effect in patients who are the most severely injured and this, in turn, means that the operation may be more effective at saving the lives of those with ongoing severe disability than at improving the quality of life of patients who would have survived without it. There was interest in the 1970s but reception was mixed because the morbidity among the survivors was severe.[94,95] Interest has been stimulated in the past 15 years by the wide availability of reliable intracranial pressure monitoring devices. These have allowed recognition of changes in ICP before signs of neurological deterioration develop. Consequently, there has been interest in performing decompressive craniectomy in a putative window of opportunity after the ICP rises but before irreversible brain damage occurs. Several series have been published since 1996 totalling 101 children.[96–102] They appear to show a substantial advantage from decompressive craniectomy in both survival and good recovery with no long-term severely disabled survivors reported. A randomized controlled trial in children showed a substantial benefit, but it was stopped before reaching significance.[103] There is a need for better evidence and trials in children (SUDEN) and in adults including children over 10 years old (RescueICP) are currently recruiting.[104,105]

## Non-accidental head injury

This topic is discussed in Chapters 2 (neuropathology) and 4 (clinical presentation).

# Conclusions

The most significant progress made in recent decades in paediatric head injury has been in public safety measures that have resulted in a falling incidence across the western world. Medical management has seen a trend in recent years to replace plain skull X-rays with CT scans and to concentrate the more severely head-injured children into specialist paediatric centres. There have been some changes in the management of raised intracranial pressure. The use of steroids and prophylactic anticonvulsants is not recommended routinely. Hyperventilation was popular in the 1970s but has become unfashionable because of reduced cerebral blood flow. Both hypothermia and hypertonic saline are under investigation. An extensive search for neuroprotective drugs has not been successful. Surgical decompression for raised intracranial pressure is receiving increasing attention and is the subject of ongoing trials.

# Acknowledgements

NICE guidelines reproduced with kind permission from National Institute for Health and Clinical Excellence (2007) CG56 Head injury: triage, assessment, investigation and early management of head injury in infants, children and adults. London: NICE. Available from www.nice.org.uk/CG056.

# References

1. Baldo V, Marcolongo A, Floreani A *et al.* Epidemiological aspect of traumatic brain injury in Northeast Italy. *Eur J Epidemiol* 2003: **18**(11): 1059–63.

2. Thurman D, Guerrero J. Trends in hospitalization associated with traumatic brain injury. *J Am Med Assoc* 1999; **282**(10): 954–7.

3. Sosin DM, Sacks JJ, Smith SM. Head injury-associated deaths in the United States from 1979 to 1986. *J Am Med Assoc* 1989; **262**(16): 2251–5.

4. MacKella A. Head injuries in children and implications for their prevention. *J Pediatr Surg* 1989; **24**(6): 577–9.

5. Macpherson A, Spinks A. Bicycle helmet legislation for the uptake of helmet use and prevention of head injuries. *Cochrane Database Syst Rev* 2007: CD005401.

6. Falk AC, Klang B, Paavonen EJ, von Wendt L. Current incidence and management of children with traumatic head injuries: the Stockholm experience. *Dev Neurorehabil* 2007; **10**(1): 49–55.

7. Schneier AJ, Shields BJ, Hostetler SG, Xiang H, Smith GA. Incidence of pediatric traumatic brain injury and associated hospital resource utilization in the United States. *Pediatrics* 2006; **118**(2): 483–92.

8. Gordon KE. Pediatric minor traumatic brain injury. *Semin Pediatr Neurol* 2006; **13**(4): 243–55.

9. Teasdale GM, Murray G, Anderson E. Risks of acute traumatic intracranial haematoma in children and adults: implications for managing head injuries. *Br Med J* 1990; **300**: 363–7.

10. Valovich McLeod TC. The prediction of intracranial injury after minor head trauma in the pediatric population. *J Athl Train* 2005; **40**(2): 123–5.

11. Duma SM, Maoogian SJ, Bussone WR *et al.* Analysis of real-time head accelerations in collegiate football players. *Clin J Sport Med* 2005; **15**(1): 3–8.

12. Stalnacke BM, Ohlsson A, Tegner Y, Sojka P. Serum concentrations of two biochemical markers of brain tissue damage S-100B and neurone specific enolase are increased in elite female soccer players after a competitive game. *Br J Sports Med* 2006; **40**(4): 313–16.

13. Stalnacke BM, Tegner Y, Sojka P. Playing ice hockey and basketball increases serum levels of S-100B in elite players: a pilot study. *Clin J Sport Med* 2003; **13**(5): 292–302.

14. Zetterberg H, Jonnson M, Rasulzada A *et al.* No neurochemical evidence for brain injury caused by heading in soccer. *Br J Sports Med* 2007; **41**(9): 574–7.

15. Necajauskaite O, Endziniene M, Jureniene K. The prevalence, course and clinical features of post-concussion syndrome in children. *Medicina (Kaunas)* 2005; **41**(6): 457–64.

16. Nacajauskaite O, Endziniene M, Jureniene K, Schrader H. The validity of post-concussion syndrome in children: a controlled historical cohort study. *Brain Dev* 2006; **28**(8): 507–14.

17. McCrory P, Zazryn T, Cameron P. The evidence for chronic traumatic encephalopathy in boxing. *Sports Med* 2007; **37**(6): 467–76.

18. Rabadi MH, Jordan BD. The cumulative effect of repetitive concussion in sports. *Clin J Sport Med* 2001; **11**(3): 194–8.

19. Guskiewicz KM, Marshall SW, Bailes J *et al.* Association between recurrent concussion and late-life cognitive impairment in retired professional football players. *Neurosurgery* 2005; **57**(4): 719–26.

20. Mori T, Katayama Y, Kawamata T. Acute hemispheric swelling associated with thin subdural hematomas: pathophysiology of repetitive head injury in sports. *Acta Neurochir Suppl* 2006; **96**: 40–3.

21. Swaine BR, Tremblay C, Platt RW, Grimard G, Zhang X, Pless IB. Previous head injury is a risk factor for subsequent head injury in children: a longitudinal cohort study. *Pediatrics* 2007; **119**(4): 749–58.

22. Asthagiri AR, Dumont AS, Sheehan AM. Acute and long-term management of sports-related closed head injuries. *Clin Sports Med* 2003; **22**(3): 559–76.

23. Tasker RC, Morris KP, Forsyth RJ, Hawley CA, Parslow RC. Severe head injury in children: emergency access to neurosurgery in the United Kingdom. *Emerg Med J* 2006; **23**(7): 519–22.

24. NICE. Head Injury: triage, assessment, investigation and early management of head injury in infants, children and adults. in *Clinical Guidance 56*, N.I.f.H.a.C. Excellence, Editor. 2007, National Collaborating Centre for Acute Care at The Royal College of Surgeons of England: London.

25. Cuff S, DiRusso S, Sullivan T *et al.* Validation of a relative head injury severity scale for pediatric trauma. *J Trauma* 2007; **63**(1): 172–7; discussion 177–8.

26. Westbrook A. The use of a paediatric coma scale for monitoring infants and young children with head injuries. *Nurs Crit Care* 1997; **2**(2): 72–5.

27. Tatman A, Warren A, Williams A, Powell JE, Whitehouse W. Development of a modified paediatric coma scale in intensive care clinical practice. *Arch Dis Child* 1997; **77**(6): 519–21.

28. Durham SR, Clancy R, Leuthardt E, *et al.* CHOP Infant Coma Scale ('Infant Face Scale'): a novel coma scale for children less than two years of age. *J Neurotrauma* 2000; **17**(9): 729–37.

29. Potoka DA, Schall LC, Gardner MJ, Stafford PW, Peitzman AB, Ford HR. Impact of pediatric trauma centers on mortality in a statewide system. *J Trauma* 2000; **49**(2): 237–45.

30. Johnson DL, Krishnamurthy S. Send severely head-injured children to a pediatric trauma center. *Pediatr Neurosurg* 1996; **25**(6): 309–14.

31. Hulka F, Mullins RJ, Mann NC *et al.* Influence of a statewide trauma system on pediatric hospitalization and outcome. *J Trauma* 1997; **42**(3): 514–19.

32. Berney J, Favier J, Froidevaux AC. Paediatric head trauma: influence of age and sex. I. Epidemiology. *Childs Nerv Syst* 1994; **10**(8): 509–16.

33. Godano U, Serracchioli A, Servadei F, Donati R, Piazza G. Intracranial lesions of surgical interest in minor head injuries in paediatric patients. *Childs Nerv Syst* 1992; **8**(3): 136–8.

34. Leggate JR, Lopez-Ramos N, Genitori L, Lena G, Choux M. Extradural haematoma in infants. *Br J Neurosurg* 1989; **3**(5): 533–9.

35. Pillay R, Peter JC. Extradural haematomas in children. *S Afr Med J* 1995; **85**(7): 672–4.

36. Molloy CJ, McCaul KA, McLean AJ, North JB, Simpson DA. Extradural haemorrhage in infancy and childhood. A review of 35 years' experience in South Australia. *Childs Nerv Syst* 1990; **6**(7): 383–7.

37. Hobbs C, Childs A-M, Wynne J, Livingston J, Seal A. Subdural haematoma and effusion in infancy: an epidemiological study. *Arch Dis Child* 2005; **90**(9): 952–5.

38. Datta S, Stoodley N, Jayawant S, Renowden S, Kemp A. Neuroradiological aspects of subdural haemorrhages. *Arch Dis Child* 2005; **90**(9): 947–51.

39. Hoskote A, Richards P, Anslow P, McShane T. Subdural haematoma and non-accidental head injury in children. *Childs Nerv Syst* 2002; **18**(6–7): 311–17.

40. Guidelines for the management of severe traumatic brain injury. *J Neurotrauma*, 2007; **24**, Suppl 1.

41. Adelson PD, Bratton SL, Carney NA *et al.* Guidelines for the acute medical management of severe traumatic brain injury in infants, children, and adolescents. *Pediatr Crit Care Med* 2003; **4**(3 Suppl).

42. Chambers IR, Stobbart L, Jones PA *et al.* Age-related differences in intracranial pressure and cerebral perfusion pressure in the first 6 hours of monitoring after children's head injury: association with outcome. *Childs Nerv Syst* 2005; **21**(3): 195–9.

43. Pople IK, Muhlbauer MS, Sanford RA, Kirk E. Results and complications of intracranial pressure monitoring in 303 children. *Pediatr Neurosurg* 1995; **23**(2): 64–7.

44. Blaha M, Lazar D, Winn RH, Ghatan S. Hemorrhagic complications of intracranial pressure monitors in children. *Pediatr Neurosurg* 2003; **39**(1): 27–31.

45. Anderson RC, Kan P, Klimo P, Brockmeyer DL, Walker ML, Kestle JR. Complications of intracranial pressure monitoring in children with head trauma. *J Neurosurg* 2004; **101**(1 Suppl): 53–8.

46. Carter BG, Butt W, Taylor A. ICP and CPP: excellent predictors of long term outcome in severely brain injured children. *Childs Nerv Syst* 2007; Aug 22: E Pub ahead of print 17712566.

47. Chambers IR, Treadwell L, Mendelow AD,. Determination of threshold levels of cerebral perfusion pressure and intracranial pressure in severe head injury by using receiver-operating characteristic curves: an observational study in 291 patients. *J Neurosurg* 2001; **94**(3): 412–16.

48. Cinalli G, Spennato P, Ruggiero C *et al.* Intracranial pressure monitoring and lumbar puncture after endoscopic third ventriculostomy in children. *Neurosurgery* 2006; **58**(1): 126–36; discussion 126–36.

49. Chambers IR, Jones PA, Lo TYM *et al.* Critical thresholds of intracranial pressure and cerebral perfusion pressure related to age in paediatric head injury. *J Neurol Neurosurg Psychiatry* 2006; **77**(2): 234–40.

50. Fortune JB, Feustel PJ, Graca L, Hasselbarth J, Kuehler DH. Effect of hyperventilation, mannitol, and ventriculostomy drainage on cerebral blood flow after head injury. *J Trauma* 1995; **39**(6): 1091–7; discussion 1097–9.

51. Shapiro K, Marmarou A. Clinical applications of the pressure-volume index in treatment of pediatric head injuries. *J Neurosurg* 1982; **56**(6): 819–25.

52. Baldwin HZ, Rekate HL. Preliminary experience with controlled external lumbar drainage in diffuse pediatric head injury. *Pediatr Neurosurg* 1991; **17**(3): 115–20.

53. Levy DI, Rekate HL, Cherny WB, Manwaring K, Moss SD, Baldwin HZ. Controlled lumbar drainage in pediatric head injury. *J Neurosurg* 1995; **83**(3): 453–60.

54. Ghajar J, Hariri R, Patterson R. Improved outcome from traumatic coma using only ventricular CSF drainage for ICP control. *Adv in Neurosurg* 1993; **21**: 173–7.

55. Bruce DA, Raphaely RC, Goldberg AI *et al.* Pathophysiology, treatment and outcome following severe head injury in children. *Childs Brain* 1979; **5**(3): 174–91.

56. Skippen P, Seear M, Poskitt K *et al.* Effect of hyperventilation on regional cerebral blood flow in head-injured children. *Crit Care Med* 1997; **25**(8): 1402–9.

57. Adelson PD, Bratton SL, Carney NA *et al.* Guidelines for the acute medical management of severe traumatic brain injury in infants, children, and adolescents. Chapter 12. Use of hyperventilation in the acute management of severe pediatric traumatic brain injury. *Pediatr Crit Care Med* 2003; **4**(3 Suppl): S45–8.

58. Adelson PD, Bratton SL, Carney NA *et al.* Guidelines for the acute medical management of severe traumatic brain injury in infants, children, and adolescents. Chapter 11. Use of hyperosmolar therapy in the management of severe pediatric traumatic brain injury. *Pediatr Crit Care Med* 2003; **4**(3 Suppl): S40–44.

59. Cruz J, Minoja G, Okuchi K, Facco E. Successful use of the new high-dose mannitol treatment in patients with Glasgow Coma Scale scores of 3 and bilateral abnormal pupillary widening: a randomized trial. *J Neurosurg* 2004; **100**(3): 376–83.

60. Cruz J, Minoja G, Okuchi K. Major clinical and physiological benefits of early high doses

of mannitol for intraparenchymal temporal lobe hemorrhages with abnormal pupillary widening: a randomized trial. *Neurosurgery* 2002; **51**(3): 628–37; discussion 637–8.

61. Cruz J, Minoja G, Okuchi K. Improving clinical outcomes from acute subdural hematomas with the emergency preoperative administration of high doses of mannitol: a randomized trial. *Neurosurgery* 2001; **49**(4): 864–71.

62. Roberts I, Smith R, Evans S. Doubts over head injury studies. *Br Med J* 2007; **334**: 392–4.

63. James HE. Methodology for the control of intracranial pressure with hypertonic mannitol. *Acta Neurochir (Wien)* 1980; **51**(3–4): 161–72.

64. Levin AB, Duff TA, Javid MJ. Treatment of increased intracranial pressure: a comparison of different hyperosmotic agents and the use of thiopental. *Neurosurgery* 1979; **5**(5): 570–5.

65. Muizelaar JP, Lutz HA 3rd Becker DP. Effect of mannitol on ICP and CBF and correlation with pressure autoregulation in severely head-injured patients. *J Neurosurg* 1984; **61**(4): 700–6.

66. Muizelaar JP, Wei EP, Kontos HA, Becker DP. Mannitol causes compensatory cerebral vasoconstriction and vasodilation in response to blood viscosity changes. *J Neurosurg* 1983; **59**(5): 822–8.

67. Muizelaar JP, Wei EP, Kontos HA, Becker DP. Cerebral blood flow is regulated by changes in blood pressure and in blood viscosity alike. *Stroke* 1986; **17**(1): 44–8.

68. Bouma GJ, Muizelaar JP. Cerebral blood flow, cerebral blood volume, and cerebrovascular reactivity after severe head injury. *J Neurotrauma* 1992; **9** Suppl 1: S333–48.

69. Kaieda R, Todd MM, Cook LN, Warner DS. Acute effects of changing plasma osmolality and colloid oncotic pressure on the formation of brain edema after cryogenic injury. *Neurosurgery* 1989; **24**(5): 671–8.

70. Kaufmann AM, Cardoso ER. Aggravation of vasogenic cerebral edema by multiple-dose mannitol. *J Neurosurg* 1992; **77**(4): 584–9.

71. Weed B, McKibben P. Pressure changes in the cerebrospinal fluid following intravenous injection of solutions of various concentrations. *Am J Physiol* 1919; **48**: 512–53.

72. Qureshi AI, Suarez JI. Use of hypertonic saline solutions in treatment of cerebral edema and intracranial hypertension. *Crit Care Med* 2000; **28**(9): 3301–13.

73. Arjamaa O, Karlqvist K, Kanervo A, Vainiopaa V, Vuolteenaho O, Leppaluoto J. Plasma ANP during hypertonic NaCl infusion in man. *Acta Physiol Scand* 1992; **144**(2): 113–19.

74. Fisher B, Thomas D, Peterson B. Hypertonic saline lowers raised intracranial pressure in children after head trauma. *J Neurosurg Anesthesiol* 1992; **4**(1): 4–10.

75. Peterson B, Khanna S, Fisher B, Marshall L. Prolonged hypernatremia controls elevated intracranial pressure in head-injured pediatric patients. *Crit Care Med* 2000; **28**(4): 1136–43.

76. Khanna S, Davis D, Peterson B, Fisher B, Tung H. Use of hypertonic saline in the treatment of severe refractory posttraumatic intracranial hypertension in pediatric traumatic brain injury. *Crit Care Med* 2000; **28**(4): 1144–51.

77. Simma B, Burger R, Falk M, Sacher P, Fanconi S. A prospective, randomized, and controlled study of fluid management in children with severe head injury: lactated Ringer's solution versus hypertonic saline. *Crit Care Med* 1998; **26**(7): 1265–70.

78. Fanconi S, Klöti J, Meuli M, Zaugg H, Zachmann M. Dexamethasone therapy and endogenous cortisol production in severe pediatric head injury. *Intens Care Med* 1988; **14**(2): 163–6.

79. Kloti J, Fanconi S, Zachmann M, Zaugg H. Dexamethasone therapy and cortisol excretion in severe pediatric head injury. *Childs Nerv Syst* 1987; **3**(2): 103–5.

80. Cooper PR, Moody S, Clark WK et al. Dexamethasone and severe head injury: a prospective double-blind study. *J Neurosurg* 1979; **51**(3): 307–16.

81. Edwards P, Arango M, Balica L et al. Final results of MRC CRASH, a randomised placebo-controlled trial of intravenous corticosteroid in adults with head injury: outcomes at 6 months. *Lancet* 2005; **365**: 1957–9.

82. Annegers JF, Grabow JD, Groover RV, Laws ER, Elveback LR, Kurland LT. Seizures after head trauma: a population study. *Neurology* 1980; **30**: 683–9.

83. Hahn YS, Fuchs S, Flannery AM, Barthel MJ, McLone DG. Factors influencing posttraumatic seizures in children. *Neurosurgery* 1988; **22**(5): 864–7.

84. Hahn YS, Chyung C, Barthel MJ, Bailes J, Flannery AM, McLone DG. Head injuries in children under 36 months of age. Demography and outcome. *Childs Nerv Syst* 1988; **4**(1): 34–40.

85. Young B, Rapp RP, Norton JA, Haack D, Tibbs PA, Bean JR. Failure of prophylactically administered phenytoin to prevent post-traumatic seizures in children. *Childs Brain* 1983; **10**(3): 185–92.

86. Kasoff SS, Lansen TA, Holder D, San Filippo J. Aggressive physiologic monitoring of pediatric head trauma patients with elevated intracranial pressure. *Pediatr Neurosci* 1988; **14**(5): 241–9.

87. Wilberger JE, Cantella D. High-dose barbiturates for intracranial pressure control. *New Horiz* 1995; **3**(3): 469–73.

88. Jones PA, Andrews PJ, Midgley S *et al.* Measuring the burden of secondary insults in head-injured patients during intensive care. *J Neurosurg Anesthesiol* 1994; **6**(1): 4–14.

89. Hendrick EB. The use of hypothermia in severe head injuries in childhood. *Arch Surg* 1959; **79**: 362–4.

90. Gruszkiewicz J, Doron Y, Peyser P. Recovery from severe craniocerebral injury with brain stem lesions in childhood. *Surg Neurol* 1973; **1**(4): 197–201.

91. Adelson PD, Ragheb J, Muizelaar JP *et al.* Phase II clinical trial of moderate hypothermia after severe traumatic brain injury in children. *Neurosurgery* 2005; **56**(4): 740–54.

92. Hutchison J, Ward R, Lacroix J *et al.* Hypothermia pediatric head injury trial: the value of a pretrial clinical evaluation phase. *Dev Neurosci* 2006; **28**(4–5): 291–301.

93. Yoo DS, Kim DS, Cho KS, Huh PW, Park CK, Kang JK. Ventricular pressure monitoring during bilateral decompression with dural expansion. *J Neurosurg* 1999; **91**(6): 953–9.

94. Venes JL, Collins WF. Bifrontal decompressive craniectomy in the management of head trauma. *J Neurosurg* 1975; **42**(4): 429–33.

95. Makino H, Yamaura A. Assessment of outcome following large decompressive craniectomy in management of serious cerebral contusion. A review of 207 cases. *Acta Neurochir Suppl (Wien)* 1979; **28**(1): 193–4.

96. Figaji AA, Fieggen AG, Argent A, Peter JC. Surgical treatment for 'brain compartment syndrome' in children with severe head injury. *S Afr Med J* 2006; **96**: 969–75.

97. Kan P, Amini A, Hansen K *et al.* Outcomes after decompressive craniectomy for severe traumatic brain injury in children. *J Neurosurg* 2006; **105**(5 Suppl): 337–42.

98. Jagannathan J, Okonkwo DO, Dumont AS *et al.* Outcome following decompressive craniectomy in children with severe traumatic brain injury: a 10-year single-center experience with long-term follow up. *J Neurosurg* 2007; **106**(4 Suppl): 268–75.

99. Ruf B, Heckmann M, Schroth I *et al.* Early decompressive craniectomy and duraplasty for refractory intracranial hypertension in children: results of a pilot study. *Crit Care* 2003; **7**(6): R133–8.

100. Figaji AA, Fieggen AG, Peter JC. Early decompressive craniotomy in children with severe traumatic brain injury. *Childs Nerv Syst* 2003; **19**(9): 666–73.

101. Hejazi N, Witzmann A, Fae P. Unilateral decompressive craniectomy for children with severe brain injury. Report of seven cases and review of the relevant literature. *Eur J Pediatr* 2002; **161**(2): 99–104.

102. Dam Hieu P, Sizun J, Person H, Besson G. The place of decompressive surgery in the treatment of uncontrollable post-traumatic intracranial hypertension in children. *Childs Nerv Syst* 1996; **12**(5): 270–5.

103. Taylor A, Butt W, Rosenfeld J *et al.* A randomized trial of very early decompressive craniectomy in children with traumatic brain injury and sustained intracranial hypertension. *Childs Nerv Syst* 2001; **17**(3): 154–62.

104. Mitchell P. *SUDEN trial protocol.* 2006; Available from: http://www.sudentrial. ukpics.org/.

105. Hutchinson P. *Randomised Evaluation of Surgery with Craniectomy for Uncontrollable Elevation of Intra-Cranial Pressure.* 2007; Available from: http://www.rescueicp.com/.

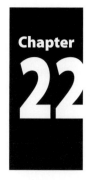

# Chapter 22

# The principles of rehabilitation after head injury

Jonathan J. Evans and Maggie Whyte

Rehabilitation has been defined in many ways, but in the broadest sense, is concerned with maximizing quality of life after injury or illness.[1] More specifically, rehabilitation is about maximizing the ability and opportunity of the head-injured person to participate in those activities of daily living, work, education, leisure and relationships that are valued by that person. Wade discusses the importance of models of illness (and health) and highlights the value of the World Health Organization International Classification of Functioning, Disability and Health (ICF) as a framework for understanding the process of rehabilitation.[2] The ICF emphasizes that health (or illness) and functioning can be considered at the level of (i) body structure (pathology), (ii) body function (impairment) and (iii) participation in activities. As a simple example, someone who has a head injury with frontal and temporal lobe damage (the pathology) may have impaired memory functioning and so not be able to carry out activities that are essential for his job (e.g. remembering task instructions) and hence not be able to return to (participate in) work. The value of the ICF is that it reminds us that rehabilitation should ultimately be concerned with maximizing participation in valued activities, within the limitations imposed by impairments of physical, cognitive or emotional functioning. Rehabilitation is not synonymous with *restoration* of normal functioning. To use another simple example, the person who, despite extensive physiotherapy, cannot walk as a result of hemiplegia, cannot go to the local shop in the usual way, but nevertheless with a wheelchair can complete the activity of shopping independently. The wheelchair compensates for physical impairment, allowing participation in activities of daily living.

Rehabilitation treatments or interventions can be applied at all levels of the ICF, with the nature and focus of the rehabilitation process changing over time. The first minutes, hours or days after the injury are concerned with minimizing the level of secondary damage that would otherwise occur, and maximizing the physical integrity of the brain. Rehabilitation is then concerned with restoring impaired physical or cognitive skills. Finally, as the extent of the permanent level of physical, cognitive and emotional impairment becomes clear, so rehabilitation interventions are aimed at enabling the head-injured person to compensate for impairments or with modifying the environment to minimize demands on impaired functions.

## Models of service

Rehabilitation is a complex process because patients have different needs at different times. Furthermore, head injury can result in a huge range of possible consequences, with outcome dependent upon many factors including the severity of brain injury, the specific areas of brain damage, along with factors such as pre-morbid intellectual ability, psychological coping style and levels of social support. Given the range of possible immediate and longer-term outcomes of head injury, a range of services is required to meet the needs of

*Head Injury: A Multidisciplinary Approach*, ed. Peter C. Whitfield, Elfyn O. Thomas, Fiona Summers, Maggie Whyte and Peter J. Hutchinson. Published by Cambridge University Press. © Cambridge University Press 2009.

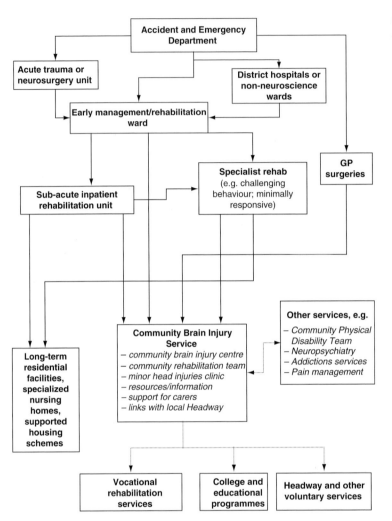

**Fig. 22.1.** The Acquired Brain Injury Service Network. Reproduced with kind permission of the British Psychological Society.

patients at different times post-injury and with different levels of impairment. This is reflected in recent models of service provision (Fig. 22.1).[3,4,5]

Patients should be transferred to rehabilitation facilities as soon as they are medically stable.[6] Failure to do so can result in inappropriate management, which may lead to physical and behavioural complications.[7] McMillan suggests that, for those people with acquired brain injury (ABI) admitted for more than 48 hours, an early management/rehabilitation ward is needed.[3] The functions of this ward are to monitor prolonged coma and recovery, provide a safe environment, prevent contractures and sores developing, maintain posture, offer active rehabilitation for those who are able, taking account of fatigue, and, as soon as appropriate, discharge to the next step in rehabilitation. Beyond this acute stage, several onward routes exist. Some patients will have physical disability and need to transfer to an environment with expertise in the management of physical disability. A small sub-group of patients require long-term coma care. These patients remain in an unresponsive state for several months, or longer. They require specialized medical, nursing and therapy care in order to maintain their physical well-being. An important minority of patients develop challenging behaviour. Appropriate care in the acute stage of recovery can reduce the incidence of this, but the incidence of challenging behaviour increases rather than decreases following discharge from hospital.[7] Evidence has accumulated that appropriate management, intervention and environmental control can significantly reduce the severity of challenging behaviour and allow individuals to lead more independent lives. All brain injury services should be able to successfully manage mild and moderate degrees of challenging behaviour. However there is a continuing need for residential challenging behaviour units that use neurobehavioural models of rehabilitation.[8]

At the hub of the service network, there should be a Community Brain Injury Rehabilitation Centre, providing a number of services that meet the rehabilitation needs of the majority of people who suffer a brain injury and of their families. The centre should provide services such as day-patient rehabilitation programmes, outreach/community rehabilitation, a minor head injuries clinic, a resource and information centre, and a source of support for carers. Such a centre would also promote strong links with voluntary groups such as Headway. Furthermore, the centre should link with vocational rehabilitation services, as well as college education programmes. Very few regions have such a comprehensive community brain injury service, though there is evidence for the effectiveness of the key elements of this service.[9,10]

## Critical features of a rehabilitation service

Two other features are critical to a rehabilitation service – an interdisciplinary team and a goal-setting process.[11] The needs of head-injured patients are complex and cannot be met by one clinical discipline alone. The disciplines involved in rehabilitation include rehabilitation medicine, nursing, occupational therapy, speech and language therapy, clinical psychology/neuropsychology, physiotherapy, social work and psychiatry. The precise composition of the team will vary according to the nature of the service. In recent years the term 'interdisciplinary team' has been adopted to describe those teams who genuinely provide an integrated rehabilitation programme for patients. What defines an integrated programme most clearly is the operation of a patient-centred goal-setting system.[11,12] This means that goals for the rehabilitation programme are set collectively by the team, in conjunction with the patient and/or his or her advocate, rather than by individual disciplines in isolation. Whilst some goals may require input from only one discipline, for many goals the interventions of several team members will be necessary. Goals should be specific and measurable, with the time period for achievement clearly identified. The majority of goals should be written with reference to the activities/participation level of the ICF framework. Recent evidence highlights the value of patient-centred goal setting in improving patients' satisfaction with the rehabilitation process.[13]

## The rehabilitation process

The precise content of a rehabilitation programme varies according to individual need. However, the process always begins with an assessment, to determine the nature of any impairment in cognitive, emotional, behavioural or physical functioning and identify the functional consequences in terms of the ability to participate in activities of daily living, work, education, social and leisure activities. The task then is to formulate or map the relationship between the pathology, the impairments and the functional consequences. It is possible to do this in summary form (e.g. on a flipchart in a rehabilitation team meeting)

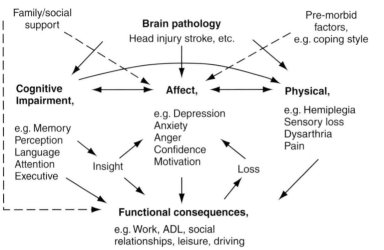

**Fig. 22.2.** A summary of assessment template.

where all elements of the assessment are listed, and a preliminary formulation of the causal relationships between impairment and functional elements can be drawn out. One example of a template used for this purpose at the Oliver Zangwill Centre for Neuropsychological Rehabilitation is provided in Fig. 22.2.[14]

Linked to this assessment process is the setting of the rehabilitation goals. This should, wherever possible, directly involve the patient and his or her advocate. Long-term (i.e. end of programme) goals are identified along with a series of short-term goals that are the stepping stones to the achievement of the long-term goals. At regular goal-review meetings, plans of action relating to achieving short-term goals are set, with each plan of action describing clearly who will do what and by when. It is within these plans of actions that the various interventions to be applied by particular team members can be documented. Progress towards achievement of the short-term goals is recorded at each meeting. This can be done by noting whether a goal is achieved, partially achieved (some progress made, but goal not achieved as defined) or not achieved (no substantial progress made). Alternatively, a more detailed rating of progress can be made using Goal Attainment Scaling system whereby a more detailed record of progress is made with reference to a scale using points relating to degrees of achievement (below or above the anticipated level).[15]

## Cost effectiveness in rehabilitation

Neurosurgical advances mean that increasing numbers of people are surviving brain injury. The costs of brain injury are wide ranging, beginning with the hospitalization and medical care in the acute stages, and often extend into the community. On leaving hospital, a person may need supervision and care or, in some cases, placement in residential supported living. Medical costs may extend to treatment in the community and further hospitalizations may be required. The person may not be able to return to previous employment and therefore cease to contribute taxes and may need to claim disability benefits. Families may suffer financial loss initially during hospitalization, which may include travel and parking costs, loss of earnings and child care. Family members may reduce their tax contributions through reducing working hours or giving up work to care for the person with a brain injury.

Increased family stress as a result of brain injury is recognized and this can increase costs through absence from work or treatment for mental health problems. People with brain injury are significantly more at risk from mental health problems and alcoholism furthering the cost to health services.

Rehabilitation can address many of the above problems and reduce costs. However, in order to fund rehabilitation, authorities need to be convinced not only of its effectiveness *per se* but of the cost effectiveness.

Many of the existing studies attempting to measure cost effectiveness in rehabilitation are methodologically flawed; however, services offering brain injury rehabilitation particularly in Britain are in their infancy.[16] Designing randomized controlled trials (RCTs) to examine the cost effectiveness of rehabilitation poses a number of problems when studying a brain injured population. These include the ethical considerations of excluding those who could benefit from treatment groups, identification of appropriate sample numbers and the consideration that, in rehabilitation, it is difficult to administer treatment in such a way that those involved in the trials are blind to inclusion in the trials.[16] Research in brain injury is complicated by the vast differences between patients and cannot hope to take account of every difference in injury or individual difference including family influences, pre-morbid functioning and behaviour, medical history, demographics, personality and coping styles to name a few. In addition, different types of economic analysis may be appropriate for different rehabilitation. For example, vocational programmes might use a cost–benefit analysis using losses and gains in earnings as a measure, whereas for care and services, cost-effective analysis may include measures of functional outcome, quality of life and economic savings.

Despite these difficulties, some studies have attempted to measure cost-effectiveness in brain injury rehabilitation. Wood in 1999 showed that post-acute community rehabilitation within the first 2 years can reduce costs by over £20 000 per year (nearly £2 million in a lifetime) and for rehabilitation beginning more than 2 years after injury, over £10 000 per year.[17] Turner-Stokes *et al.* present evidence that rehabilitation reduced dependency and care costs by up to £639 per week and that the highest reductions in care could be made in high dependency groups.[18] Khan *et al.* introduced a traumatic brain injury programme during initial treatment in hospital, which included rehabilitation from the acute stages, education and involvement of the families and management by a TBI multi-disciplinary team in sub-acute rehabilitation. The programme resulted in a reduction in average length of hospital stay from 30.5 to 12 days and amounted to savings of over $21.8 million over a period of 6 years.[19]

The high cost of TBI can be reduced through reductions in care, successful return to employment, reduced need for residential care and reduced need for benefits. However, rehabilitation services are costly and unfortunately there is a dearth of research providing good evidence for these gains. More evidence is needed in order to persuade the budget holders of the economic benefits of rehabilitation.

In summary, rehabilitation is a collaborative process whereby the patient and his or her family work with an interdisciplinary team to maximize the patient's ability and opportunity to participate in those activities of everyday life that are valued by the patient. In the following chapters, the contributions of key members of the rehabilitation team are described, along with accounts of how specific cognitive impairments and behavioural problems should be treated. One of the most important outcomes after rehabilitation is return to work and this topic is therefore discussed specifically.

# References

1. Ward CD, McIntosh S. The rehabilitation process: a neurological perspective. In: Greenwood, RJ, Barnes, MP, McMillan TM, Ward, CD, eds. *Handbook of Neurological Rehabilitation*. Hove: Psychology Press, 2003; 15–28.

2. Wade D. Applying the WHO ICF framework to the rehabilitation of patients with cognitive deficits. In: Halligan P, Wade D, eds. *The Effectiveness of Rehabilitation for Cognitive Deficits*. Oxford, Oxford University Press, 2005; 31–42.

3. McMillan TM. Neurorehabilitation services and their delivery. In: Wilson BA, ed. *Neuropsychological Rehabilitation*. Lisse, Swets & Zeitlinger, 2003; 271–91.

4. Herbert C. Planning, delivering and evaluating services. In: Goldstein LH, McNeil JE, eds. *Clinical Neuropsychology: a Practical Guide to Assessment and Management for Clinicians*. Chichester, Wiley, 2004; 367–83.

5. British Psychological Society. *Division of Neuropsychology report on clinical neuropsychology and rehabilitation services for adults with acquired brain injury*. Leicester: BPS, 2005. available online – www. bps.org.uk.

6. Royal College of Surgeons. *Working party on the management of patients with head injury*. London: RCS, 1999.

7. Johnson R, Balleny H. 'Behaviour problems after brain injury: incidence and need for treatment.' *Clin Rehabil* 1996; **10**: 173–81.

8. Wood RL, Worthington AD Neurobehavioural rehabilitation in practice. In: Wood RL, McMillan TM, eds. *Neurobehavioural Disability and Social Handicap Following Traumatic Brain Injury*. Hove: Psychology Press, 2001; 133–55.

9. Powell J, Helsin J, Greenwood R. Community based rehabilitation after severe traumatic brain injury: a randomized controlled trial. *J Neurol, Neurosurg Psychiatry* 2003; **72**: 193–202.

10. Svendsen HA, Teasdale TW. The influence of neuropsychological rehabilitation on symptomatology and quality of life following brain injury: a controlled long-term follow-up. *Brain Injury* 2006; **20**: 1295–306.

11. Barnes MP. Organisation of neurological rehabilitation services. In: Greenwood RJ, Barnes MP, McMillan TM, Ward CD. *Handbook of Neurological Rehabilitation*. Hove: Psychology Press, 2003; 29–40.

12. Hart T, Evans JJ. Self-regulation and goal theories in brain injury rehabilitation. *J Head Trauma Rehabil* 2006; **21**: 142–55.

13. Holliday R, Cano S, Freeman JA, Playford, ED. Should patients participate in clinical decision making? An optimised balance block design controlled study of goal setting in a rehabilitation setting. *J Neurol, Neurosurg Psychiatry* 2007; **78**: 576–80.

14. Wilson BA, Evans JJ, Brentnall S, Bremner S, Keohane C, Williams H. The Oliver Zangwill Centre for Neuropsychological Rehabilitation: a partnership between health care and rehabilitation research. In: Christensen AL, Uzzell BP, eds. *International Handbook of Neuropsychological Rehabilitation* New York, Kluwer Academic/Plenum, 2000; 231–46.

15. Hurn J, Kneebone I, Cropley, M. Goal setting as an outcome measure: a systematic review. *Clin Rehabil* 2006; **20**: 756–72.

16. McGregor K, Pentland B. Head injury rehabilitation in the UK: an economic perspective. *Soc Sci Med* 1997; **45**: 295–303.

17. Wood RL, McCrea JD, Wood LM, Merriman RN. Clinical and cost effectiveness of post-acute neurobehavioural rehabilitation. *Brain Inj* 1999; **13**: 69–88.

18. Turner-Stokes L, Paul S, Williams H. Efficiency of specialist rehabilitation in reducing dependency and costs of continuing care for adults with complex acquired brain injuries. *J Neurol, Neurosurg Psychiatry* 2006; **77**: 634–9.

19. Khan S, Khan A, Feyz M. Decreased length of stay, cost savings and descriptive findings of enhanced patient care resulting from an integrated traumatic brain injury programme. *Brain Inj* 2002; **16**: 537–54.

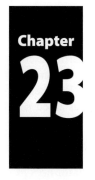

# Chapter 23

# Acute rehabilitation of the head-injured patient

Bruce Downey, Thérèse Jackson, Judith Fewings and Ann-Marie Pringle

The focus of acute inpatient care is often on the medical condition of the patient. It is important, however, that a holistic approach is taken in order to effectively address difficulties with motor abilities, cognition, communication, functional skills, emotion, general psychological well-being and quality of life. The following chapter describes the role of the physiotherapist, speech and language therapist, occupational therapist and neuropsychologist in the care of the acute patient with head injury.

## Physiotherapy

Early physiotherapy intervention aims to maintain optimal respiratory function, thereby limiting secondary brain damage, avoid weaning delay, preserve the integrity of the musculoskeletal system and start the process of regaining motor control. For therapists to manage patients with TBI, they must have an understanding of neural and muscle physiology, pathophysiology of brain injury, a working knowledge of all rehabilitation concepts and clinical experience. An accurate assessment needs to be made. A problem list and individual treatment plan is then constructed; no two head-injured patients will have the same deficits/ medical problems.[1,2]

Advances in medical technology allow patients with extensive neural injuries (who in the past would most certainly have died) to live and be maintained for indefinite periods of time, irrespective of the ultimate neurological outcome. The severity of the primary injury directly relates to the period of unconsciousness, during which time they are more susceptible to secondary adaptations of the musculoskeletal system, and thus poorer functional outcomes.[3,4]

## Respiratory care

Physiotherapeutic interventions facilitate the maintenance of parameters to optimize cerebral oxygenation in the presence of raised intracranial pressure (ICP). The physiotherapist must monitor ICP throughout their treatment provision as the injured brain loses autoregulation and the cerebral perfusion pressure (CPP) becomes directly related to the systemic mean arterial blood pressure (MAP) and the ICP.

$$CPP = MAP - ICP$$

Hypercarbia can result in cerebral vasodilatation, increasing cerebral blood volume, thereby raising ICP. Respiratory physiotherapy must therefore facilitate adequate oxygenation and avoid hypercarbia without precipitating any sustained rise in ICP or fall in MAP.

In the non-intubated TBI patient, supplemental oxygen must be administered to ensure adequate cerebral oxygenation. The decision whether or not to administer respiratory care to the intubated patient is multifactorial and multidisciplinary. Assessment

*Head Injury: A Multidisciplinary Approach*, ed. Peter C. Whitfield, Elfyn O. Thomas, Fiona Summers, Maggie Whyte and Peter J. Hutchinson. Published by Cambridge University Press. © Cambridge University Press 2009.

should aim to establish whether the respiratory status will improve with physiotherapy intervention and also to ascertain the patient's stability in terms of their cardiovascular and intracranial parameters. Consideration must be given to the increased oxygen consumption and poor peripheral oxygen extraction present in the critically ill[5]. Rest periods have been shown to be essential in the care of the TBI patient to prevent sustained rises in ICP.[6,7]

## Positioning

The optimum position, with respect to cerebral perfusion, is head up 15–30° with the neck in a neutral position; venous drainage is facilitated without compromise to systolic blood pressure thereby maximizing CPP.[8,9] Critically ill patients frequently have decreased pulmonary functional reserve; this must be borne in mind when performing routine positional changes. There may be an increase in oxygen consumption of up to 50% following turning patients onto their side.[5,10] The traditional head down postural drainage positions are contraindicated in TBI patients as this increases ICP.[11] Caution is also required in positioning patients with bone flap defects, ensuring that no long-term pressure is applied to the affected area in a side-lying position. When ICP is uncontrolled by sedation alone, muscle relaxants may be used to reduce the metabolic demand, prevent the cough reflex and allow full control of the $PaCO_2$. However, the use of paralysis may contribute to other potential hazards; namely, early changes in skeletal muscle structure and potentially an increased risk of pneumonia.[12–14]

Where clinical assessment of the TBI patient indicates retained secretions, sputum clearance should be undertaken. Patients should be pre-oxygenated prior to positional changes, negating the increase in oxygen consumption, and the secretions removed.[15] If the change in position is tolerated with no detrimental effects on CPP or ICP, it can be repeated on a 2–4-hourly basis if deemed necessary. If these simple manoeuvres do not result in improved oxygenation owing to tenacious/retained secretions, then active humidification and bronchoscopy by the medical staff should be considered.

## Manual hyper-inflation

Manual hyper-inflation (MHI), along with manual chest techniques, quickly and effectively remove sputum and reverse atelectasis. During MHI the therapist must ensure that MAP should be >80 mmHg and that the expiratory phase should be longer than the inspiratory phase.[5,16] MHI consists of short periods of bagging, maintaining ventilatory tidal volumes, followed by five or six breaths of MHI with manual chest shaking and vibrations, repeated as necessary until secretions are loosened.[7] The following parameters are recommended to avoid detrimental effects[16–19]:

- Periods of hyperinflation to be brief <3.5 minutes
- Flow rate of 15 l of 100% $O_2$ to a 2-litre bag
- Tidal volume 1.5 times the ventilator volume up to a maximum of 1000 ml
- Peak inflation pressure less than or equal to 40 mmHg.

In combination with other techniques, MHI can dramatically reduce treatment times. Patients have to be observed carefully during MHI as ICP can be raised secondary to increased intrathoracic pressure. However, hyperventilation can assist in reducing ICP by decreasing $PaCO_2$.[20,21] Manometers should therefore be included in the respiratory circuit. Concerns regarding the detrimental effects of MHI on ICP have not been demonstrated.[22]

# Manual chest techniques – shaking, vibrations and percussion

Manual chest techniques (MCT) are frequently performed physiotherapeutic manoeuvres that, along with the other methods described, aid sputum clearance. The evidence for benefit, however, is sparse, controversial and sometimes conflicting. Some studies show that simple interventions, such as lateral positioning and passive movements, have a significant impact on oxygen consumption whether or not the patient is mechanically ventilated.[5,23] Others, however, have not shown any difference in oxygen consumption or cardiac index with MCT, – the resultant physiological stress being less than turning a patient into the side-lying position.[10,21,24]

Percussion in sedated, ventilated patients results in a fall in ICP. Its effect is greater if the patient is also paralysed.[24] Vibrations during expiration on a ventilated breath have no effect on ICP but shaking during a MHI breath and MHI alone does increase ICP.[17]

# Suction

In ventilated TBI patients, suction is commonly regarded as a treatment that increases ICP; however, it is also viewed as a necessary procedure that is required with a frequency sufficient to maintain a patent airway.[15] The following recommendations have been made to minimize potential hypoxaemia[25]:

- Duration of catheter insertion 10–15 seconds

- Hyperoxygenate pre- and post-suctions using 100% $O_2$ or 20% above baseline.

The American Association of Respiratory Care Guidelines recommends 100% oxygen for 1 minute post-suction.[15] The effectiveness of suction is dependent on adequate patient hydration, humidification and warming of inspired gases.[16] Heat and moisture exchangers usually provide adequate humidification for ventilated patients initially. However, if secretions become thick, purulent or the patient's past medical history and mechanism of injury suggest a potential risk, then the role of active humidification should be considered. The practice of instilling 5 ml sodium chloride 0.9% aseptically and slowly prior to suctioning is widely used, but remains contentious.[26]

In the early stages following TBI, patients have a limited ability to tolerate even the most simple of interventions. Maintaining optimal conditions for brain recovery and avoiding secondary brain damage are the prime treatment maxims. An accurate, functional and respiratory assessment and multidisciplinary treatment approach are vital. Improving and shortening ITU stays ultimately reduces mortality, improves functional outcome and reduces costs.[27–30]

# Speech and language therapy

In the acute stages of recovery of the head-injured patient, speech and language therapists are key in the assessment and intervention of difficulties with swallowing (dysphagia).

The consequences of dysphagia (difficulties with swallowing) can be devastating and include malnutrition, aspiration and aspiration-associated pneumonia, choking, and death. The incidence of swallowing disorders following traumatic brain injury is unknown, although one study identified dysphagia in 61% of patients admitted to an acute rehabilitation unit.[31] The main risk factors for dysphagia are: impaired level of consciousness, severe cognitive impairment, presence of a tracheostomy, and a period of ventilation in excess of 2 weeks.[32,33]

Continuing cognitive and behavioural impairments influence the management of dysphagia and frequently delay the possibility of safe oral intake.[34,32]

The normal swallow has oral, pharyngeal and oesophageal stages.[34,35] These can be disrupted in a number of ways following TBI, including; reduced lip closure; reduced range of tongue movement or reduced co-ordination of tongue movement (creating poor bolus control, slow oral transit times and inefficient oral clearance); delay in triggering the pharyngeal swallow (which may cause aspiration); reduced laryngeal elevation (resulting in residual food in the pyriform sinuses and at the laryngeal entrance) reduced laryngeal closure or absent swallow reflex (resulting in aspiration of food and liquid and cricopharyngeal dysfunction (obstructing the passage of food into the oesophagus and resulting in solids or liquids collecting in the pharyngeal/laryngeal area).[32,33] Additional swallowing disorders can be caused by prolonged endotracheal intubation or emergency tracheostomy.[32]

The main clinical signs, which should prompt a swallowing assessment, are coughing during meals, gurgly voice quality, copious oral or pulmonary secretions, chest infection, obvious difficulty managing food orally and perceived delay in triggering the pharyngeal swallow.[32] Approximately 10% to 15% of dysphagic people with TBI are silent aspirators, however, and do not present with obvious signs.

Early evaluation of swallowing ability and aspiration risk is essential.[36,37] The speech and language therapist will usually undertake a bedside assessment of oral, pharyngeal and laryngeal function, and will evaluate the patient's communication status. Videofluoroscopy (VF), or modified barium swallow, is also often carried out in order to view what can only be assumed at the bedside assessment. Fibreoptic Endoscopic Evaluation of Swallowing (FEES) is available in many acute hospitals and will also provide an objective assessment of swallowing ability.[38] In both cases, patient compliance is essential.

The efficacy of dysphagia therapy after TBI is not well documented.[39,37] Thermal stimulation, where a cold stimulus is applied to the anterior faucial pillars, is commonly used to improve the swallow reflex.[35,40] Other dysphagia treatments in which the patient is an active participant are described elsewhere, but there is little evidence available as to how effective they are or how extensively they are used in patients with TBI.[35] The usual practice from early rehabilitation onwards is to encourage safe eating and drinking by modifying the patient's diet and the immediate environment. A supervised and regularly monitored regime involving practice amounts of thick puree is begun when considered safe to do so, with enteral feeding, usually via percutaneous endoscopic gastrostomy (PEG), meeting the main nutritional needs. With progress, the food gradually becomes more textured and amounts larger, with decreasing reliance on alternative methods of nutrition. Similarly, liquids can be thickened to varying degrees. The patient's seating position can be altered for maximal safety while eating, as can head position. Risk is minimized further by staff supervising and, if necessary, assisting dysphagic patients at mealtimes. It is important for family members and friends to understand the risks and the safe limits and to become involved in the rehabilitation process as early as possible.

## Occupational therapy in the acute phase

In the acute phase and in early stages of recovery the occupational therapist will focus on the reduction of impairment and the prevention of secondary complications to maximize longer-term functional outcome. Continual re-evaluation of performance skills (motor, sensory, cognitive, psychological and social capacities) establishes levels of function, identifying meaningful and achievable goals. Intervention will assist the individual to participate in activities and engage in relevant and meaningful occupations.

During periods of reduced arousal (e.g. coma, minimally conscious state) the occupational therapist will work with colleagues and the person's family and friends to establish a better understanding of the patient's cognitive ability, level and pattern of arousal. Reactions to a variety of stimuli are assessed in order to determine any consistent or meaningful responses and to establish an appropriate treatment programme. Sensory stimulation programmes may be initiated to improve arousal and awareness, thus maximizing a patient's potential for interacting with their environment in an appropriate way. In the acute care setting this may be administered through structured observation of behaviours and responses to stimuli, or via formal standardized assessments more commonly used in the rehabilitation setting such as the Sensory Modality Assessment and Rehabilitation Technique (SMART).[41]

Occupational therapists use activities such as treatment media to increase alertness and awareness and to facilitate appropriate interaction with people and the environment. They may adapt the environment and provide external aids, such as call systems or TV controls, which are adjusted to suit individual functional capacity to aid an independent means of controlling the environment. Other means of therapeutic support may be introduced, such as diaries to be used as memory aids. These measures can also serve to increase participation in the individual's recovery by family and friends who can guide an individualized treatment programme.

Functional recovery is aided by the therapeutic application of activities. These include facilitated practice of daily living skills such as feeding and personal care tasks in order to enhance motor, sensory, psychological, social and cognitive functions. A daily routine may be established, balancing activity and rest according to individual needs and tolerances in order to maximize periods of alertness and to reduce fatigue. The environment will be managed to ensure appropriate levels of sensory input and avoiding over-stimulation in some cases.

The occupational therapist also plays an important role as part of the multidisciplinary team in assessing and monitoring levels of post-traumatic amnesia and providing appropriate interventions.

Ascertaining the patient's level of cognitive ability is essential to anticipate long-term problems. For people with mild brain injury, the occupational therapist will be interested in any cognitive impairment, which is not immediately obvious in the acute care setting but which may present the person with longer-term problems. Screening assessments may highlight these issues and the person is then provided with contacts and information about support services in the community if they are to be discharged home from the acute care setting. Referral for specialized community monitoring and rehabilitation may be appropriate in this case and a more detailed cognitive assessment from a neuropsychologist may be recommended.

For those with moderate or severe brain injury, recommendations for appropriate ongoing rehabilitation will be made by the occupational therapist and the multidisciplinary team. Options range from specialist in-patient brain injury rehabilitation services to community teams and case management services.

Motor and sensory function is assessed using a range of standardized assessments and structured observational methods in order to establish a baseline of abilities and to determine the impact on functional ability (occupational performance). It is essential that a coordinated multidisciplinary approach to the assessment and management of motor and sensory deficits is established to maximise outcome and minimize long-term complications such as contractures and pressure sores. These problems can be addressed through the implementation of a postural management programme in all aspects of the person's daily routines, and through the provision of equipment such as splints, specialized seating, wheelchairs, pressure relieving cushions and positioning aids. Splints or orthoses are made and or fitted to achieve and maintain normal alignment of the limb and muscle length, and to reduce the development of secondary complications. This, in turn, facilitates optimal physical function depending on the level of motor recovery.

Preparation for transfer of care to home or further rehabilitation requires careful planning. The occupational therapist may carry out home assessments to determine any ongoing support or equipment needs for a safe and effective discharge, and will ensure appropriate handover of the treatment plan to rehabilitation colleagues. A key worker system is used successfully (with full participation of the team) in some acute care settings for information transfer in a seamless manner.

The occupational therapist also provides education and support for families, carers and friends throughout the acute phase to ensure appropriate and consistent input for the person with brain injury in all aspects of daily living and for their own support needs.

## Acute neuropsychological intervention

Neuropsychological deficits apparent during the acute phase of care are generally viewed as low priority for intervention, unless their presence is severely interfering with the patient's treatment. Thus, it is evident (and in many ways appropriate) that the interventions introduced at this stage of the patient's recovery commonly follow a medical perspective to rehabilitation. There is a dearth of literature currently available detailing specific neuropsychological rehabilitation interventions for patients in the acute stage of recovery, perhaps reflecting the overriding focus on medical models of treatment and a general under-resourcing of neuropsychological intervention during acute rehabilitation. However, there are a number of ways in which the clinical neuropsychologist can contribute to the patient's rehabilitation during the acute phase of recovery.

## Rehabilitation of patients in a reduced state of consciousness

The past 10 to 15 years has witnessed mounting interest in the rehabilitation of patients in a reduced state of consciousness and, regardless of whether the patient is in a coma, in the vegetative state, in the minimally conscious state or in post-traumatic amnesia (PTA), the neuropsychologist can play an important role in the patient's rehabilitation during this period of recovery. For instance, the neuropsychologist might collaborate with members of the multidisciplinary team in the process of devising an appropriate sensory stimulation programme that attempts to increase arousal of the patient who is in a coma or in a vegetative state. Although there is a lack of controlled studies measuring the efficacy of sensory stimulation programmes, some promising results are beginning to emerge, with many specialists in the area emphasizing the importance of early intervention.[42,43]

As well as providing input on early sensory stimulation programmes, the neuropsychologist can also use their observational skills to help monitor the patient's recovery, determine his or her level of consciousness and assist with setting realistic short-term rehabilitation goals.[44] As the patient's level of awareness continues to improve, the goals of rehabilitation will continue to change. For instance, orientating the person to their environment (time, place and person) and improving day-to-day memory may become rehabilitation priorities. In such circumstances, the neuropsychologist may provide the rehabilitation team with advice on particular strategies that might be useful in terms of reducing disorientation and improving the patient's day-to-day memory. Once the patient has become fully conscious, neuropsychological rehabilitation techniques can be adapted to meet the patient's needs.

## Behavioural management

Changes in a patient's behaviour are one of the most commonly reported consequences of traumatic brain injury. As the person being cared for in the acute medical setting regains consciousness, problem behaviours may become evident. Aggression, disinhibition, wandering, showing limited awareness for personal safety and other socially inappropriate behaviours are just some of the behavioural challenges that ward staff may find difficult to manage. When confronted with such behaviours, seeking neuropsychological advice on managing the patient's behaviour should be considered. The neuropsychologist will apply principles of behaviour analysis in order to understand the behaviour. Following this, an appropriate intervention based on behaviour or learning theory may be suggested.[45] This could involve making changes to the patient's environment, introducing a simple behavioural management programme designed to modify the patient's behaviour and/or encouraging staff to modify their approach when they are working with the patient. Importantly, effective management of challenging behaviour can enable patients to participate more fully in the rehabilitation process. In terms of their efficacy, behavioural interventions introduced in acute medical environments have been shown to help staff manage behavioural changes associated with neurological dysfunction.[45] These interventions are described in more detail in Chapter 24.

## Assessment of capacity

Questions regarding a patient's capacity to make decisions about their treatment are frequently raised during acute medical care. This may arise as a query over capacity to consent to treatment or capacity to refuse treatment. Neuropsychological assessment may be important at this stage to determine the cognitive and emotional effects of the patient's brain injury and the consequential impact on their decision-making abilities. The process and neuropsychological considerations involved in assessment of capacity are outlined in more detail in Chapter 25.

## Assessing cognitive functioning in the acute in-patient environment

A detailed and comprehensive assessment of the patient's cognitive functioning is generally conducted in the post-acute rehabilitation environment. However, on occasion, a request might be made to assess a patient's cognitive abilities while they are receiving acute medical treatment.[46] Even if the patient is in PTA, it may be possible to do some brief cognitive assessments. Although fluctuations in the patient's level of consciousness during the acute period of recovery may devalue the results of any such assessment, Bishop et al. report that, when undertaken, the results and recommendations made in the neuropsychological report often have a significant bearing on the patient's placement at discharge.[46]

Furthermore, documenting the patient's cognitive strengths and weaknesses at the acute stage of recovery can helpfully be utilized by the multidisciplinary team when it comes to planning a rehabilitation programme. The neuropsychologist can make recommendations to other health professionals about ways of modifying their therapeutic approach in order to provide the patient with the optimum environment in which to realize their rehabilitation potential. Regular multidisciplinary consultation and review can be helpful in assessing the potential benefits and disadvantages of a particular intervention. This process of review also allows alternative interventions to be considered according to the patient's changing presentation and stage of recovery.

## Prognosticating

Bearing in mind factors such as aetiology and diagnosis, the neuropsychologist can use the results of any assessment conducted in the acute stage of the patient's recovery to draw conclusions about likely prognosis. This too can influence future management decisions.[47]

## Educating the family and providing family support

Early neuropsychological interventions may also involve providing education to a patient's family and close friends. Discussing the nature of TBI (including its effects, its possible consequences and practical strategies for coping with cognitive and behavioural changes) could help significant others better understand their loved one's behaviour and enable them to develop a realistic perception of their abilities.[48] Increased understanding could help preserve relationships and prevent a decline in family functioning. A recent study conducted by Ponsford *et al.* suggested that providing a brain injury information booklet to children with a mild TBI within 1 week of their injury has a beneficial effect in terms of the child's behaviour and reported symptoms, as well as the family members' level of stress.[49]

Finally, it is important to remember that neuropsychological impairments, medical problems and disabilities not only affect the individual with TBI, but also members of their family. Bearing this in mind, the clinical neuropsychologist may perform a valuable role in providing psychological support for the patient's family during the acute care phase.

In summary, there are a number of ways in which clinical neuropsychology can meaningfully contribute to a patient's rehabilitation during the acute phase of recovery following TBI. However, the potential benefits of such interventions have yet to be fully delineated. It has been suggested that the earlier patients are exposed to neuro-rehabilitation the greater their recovery.[50] Indeed, it seems intuitive to reason that early intervention and timely access to rehabilitation will influence speed of progress and eventual functional outcome, but without appropriate controlled studies measuring the short- and long-term impact of these interventions, questions regarding how much of which interventions are most beneficial will remain unanswered.

## References

1. Clini E, Ambrosino N. Early physiotherapy in the respiratory intensive care unit. *Resp Med* 2005; **99**: 1096–104.

2. Campbell. M. Rehabilitation for traumatic brain injury. In: *Physical Therapy Practice in Context*. Edinburgh, Churchill Livingstone, 2000; 169–205.

3. Ada L, Canning C, Paratz. J. Care of the unconscious Head-injured patient. In Ada L̀, Canning C, Eds. *Key Issues in Neurological Physiotherapy [Physiotherapy: Foundations for Practice]*. Oxford, Butterworth-Heinemann, 1990; 249–89.

4. Stucki G, Steir-Jarmer M, Grill E, Melvin J. Rationale and principles of early rehabilitation after an acute injury or illness. *Disabil Rehabil* 2005; **27**: 353–9.

5. Horiuchi K, Jordan D, Cohen D, Kemper M C, Weissman C. Insights into the increased oxygen demand during chest physiotherapy. *Crit Care Med* 1997; **25**(8): 1347–51.

6. Hough A. *Physiotherapy in Respiratory Care: A Problem Solving Approach to Respiratory and Cardiac Management*. 2nd edn. Cheltenham, Stanley Thornes, 1996.

7. Innocenti D. Handling the critically ill patient. *Physiotherapy* 1986; **73**: 125–8.

8. Chudley S. The effect of nursing activities on intracranial pressure. *Br J Nurs* 1994; **3**(9): 454–5.

9. Feldman Z, Kanter MJ, Robertson CS et al. Effect of head elevation on intracranial pressure, cerebral perfusion pressure and cerebral blood flow in head-injured patients. *J Neurosurg* 1992; **76**: 207–11.

10. Berney S, Denehy. L. The effect of physiotherapy treatment on oxygen consumption and haemodynamics in patients who are critically ill. *Aust J Physiother* 2003; **49**: 99–105.

11. Lee ST. Intracranial pressure changes during positioning of patients with severe head injury. *Heart and Lung* 1989; **18**: 411–14.

12. Williams PE. Use of intermittent stretch in the prevention of serial sarcomere loss in immobilised muscles. *Ann Rheum Dis* 1990; **49**: 316–17.

13. Gossman MR, Sahrmann SA, Rose SJ. Review of length-associated changes in muscle: experimental evidence and clinical implications. *Phys Ther* 1982; **62**: 1799–808.

14. Hsiang JK, Chesnut KM, Crisp CB, Klauber MR, Blunt BA, Marshall LF. Early, routine paralysis for intracranial pressure control in severe head injury: is it necessary? *Crit Care Med* 1994; **22**: 1471–6.

15. American Association of Respiratory Care (AARC) Clinical Practice Guideline: Endotracheal suctioning of mechanically ventilated adults and children with artificial airways. *Respir Care* 1993; **38**: 500–4.

16. Roberts S. Respiratory management of a patient with traumatic head injury. In: Partridge C, ed. *Bases of Evidence for Practice: Neurological Physiotherapy*. London and Philadelphia, Whurr Publishers Ltd, 2005; 63–76.

17. Garradd J, Bullock M. The effect of respiratory therapy on intracranial pressure in ventilated neurosurgical patients. *Aust J Physiother* 1986; **32**: 107–11.

18. Clapham L, Harrison J, Raybold T. A multidisciplinary audit of manual hyperinflation technique (sigh breath) in a neurosurgical intensive care unit. *Intensive Crit Care Nurs* 1995; **11**: 265–71.

19. Rothen HU, Sporre B, Engberg G, Wegenius G, Hedenstierna G. Re-expansion of atelectasis during general anaesthesia: a computed tomography study. *Br J Anaesth* 1993; **71**: 788–95.

20. Robb J. Physiological changes occurring with positive pressure ventilation: Part one. *Intens Crit Care Nurs* 1997; **13**: 293–307.

21. Enright S. Cardio-respiratory effects of chest physiotherapy. *Intensive Care Britain*, London, Greycoat Publishing, 1992: 118–23.

22. McGuire G, Crossley D, Richards J, Wong D. Effects of varying levels of positive end-expiratory pressure on intracranial pressure and cerebral perfusion pressure. *Crit Care Med* 1977; **25**: 1059–62.

23. Dallimore K, Jenkins S, Tucker B. Respiratory and cardiovascular responses to manual chest percussion in normal subjects. *Aust J Physiother* 1998; **44**: 267–73.

24. Paratz J, Burns Y. The effect of respiratory physiotherapy on intracranial pressure, mean arterial pressure, cerebral perfusion pressure and end carbon dioxide in ventilated neurosurgical patients. *Physiother Theory Pract* 1993; **9**: 3–11.

25. Wood C. Endotracheal suctioning: a literature review. *Intensive Crit Care Nurs* 1998; **14**: 124–36.

26. Raymond SJ. Normal saline instillation before suction: helpful or harmful? A review of the literature. *Am J Crit Care* 1995; **4**: 267–71.

27. Audit Commission; Critical to success. The place of Efficient and Effective Critical Care Services within the Acute Hospital. Audit Commission, London, 1999: www.audit-commission.gov.uk.

28. Department of Health: Quality Critical Care. Beyond 'Comprehensive Critical Care'. Critical Care Stakeholder Forum;2005: www.publications.doh.gov.uk.

29. Department of Health: Neuroscience Critical Care Report: Progress in Developing Services; 2004: www.publications.doh.gov.uk.

30. Department of Health: The National Service Framework for Long Term Conditions; 2005: www.publications.doh.gov.uk.

31. Halper AS, Cherney LR, Cichowski K, Zhang M. Dysphagia after head trauma: the effect of cognitive-communicative impairments on functional outcomes. *J Head Trauma Rehabil* 1999; **14** (5): 486–96.

32. Mackay LE, Morgan AS, Bernstein BA. Swallowing disorders in severe brain injury: risk factors affecting return to oral intake. *Arch Phys Medi Rehabil* 1999; **80**: 365–71.

33. Logemann JA, Pepe J, Mackay LE. Disorders of nutrition and swallowing: intervention strategies in the trauma center. *J Head Trauma Rehabil* 1994; **9**(1): 43–56.

34. Mayer V. The challenges of managing dysphagia in brain-injured patients. *Br J Commun Nurs* 2004; **9**(2): 67–73.

35. Logemann J. *Evaluation and Treatment of Swallowing Disorders*. Austin, Texas: Pro-Ed, 1998.

36. Mackay LE, Morgan AS, Bernstein BA. Factors affecting oral feeding with severe traumatic brain injury. *J Head Trauma Rehabil* 1999; **14**(5): 435–47.

37. Ward EC, Green K, Morton A-L. Patterns and predictors of swallowing resolution following adult traumatic brain injury. *J Head Trauma Rehabil*, 2007; **22**(3): 184–91.

38. Kelly AM, Hydes K, McLaughlin C, Wallace S. Fibreoptic Endoscopic Evaluation of Swallowing (FEES): the role of speech and language therapy. Royal College of Speech and Language Therapists Policy Statement, 2007.

39. Schurr MJ, Ebner KA, Maser AL, Sperling KB, Helgerson RB, Harms B. Formal swallowing evaluation and therapy after traumatic brain injury improves dysphagia outcomes. *J Trauma* 1999; **46**(5): 817–23.

40. Hamdy S, Jilani S, Price V, Parker C, Hall N, Power M. Modulation of human swallowing behaviour by thermal and chemical stimulation in health and after brain injury. *Neurogastroenterol Motili* 2003; **15**: 69–77.

41. Gill-Thwaites H, Munday R. The Sensory Modality Assessment and Rehabilitation Technique (SMART). A comprehensive and integrated assessment and treatment protocol for the vegetative state and minimally responsive patient. *Neuropsych Rehabili* 1999; **9** (3–4): 305–20.

42. Hyunsoo O, Whasook S. Sensory stimulation programme to improve recovery in comatose patients. *J Clin Nurs*, 2003; **12**(3): 394–404.

43. Gerber CS. Understanding and managing coma stimulation: are we doing everything we can? *Crit Care Nurs Quart* 2005; **28**(2): 94–108.

44. Shiel A. Rehabilitation of people in reduced states of awareness. In: Wilson B, ed. *Neuropsychological Rehabilitation: Theory and Practice*. Lisse, Swets & Zeitlinger, 2003.

45. Wilson B, Herbert C, Shiel A. *Behavioural Approaches in Neuropsychological Rehabilitation*. Hove, Psychology Press, 2003.

46. Bishop LC, Temple RO, Tremont G, Westervelt HJ, Stern RA. Utility of the neuropsychological evaluation in an acute medical hospital. *Clin Neuropsychol*, 2003; **17**(4): 468–73.

47. Beaumont JG. The aims of neuropsychological assessment. In: Harding L, Beech JR. *Assessment in Neuropsychology*. London, Routledge, 1996.

48. Melchers P, Maluck A, Suhr L, Scholten S, Lehmkuhl G. An early onset rehabilitation program for children and adolescents after traumatic brain injury (TBI): methods and first results. *Restor Neurol Neurosci* 1999; **14**: 153–160.

49. Ponsford J, Willmott C, Rothwell A *et al*. Impact of early intervention on outcome after mild traumatic brain injury in children. *Pediatrics* 2001; **108**(6): 1297–303.

50. Mackay LE, Bernstein BA, Morgan PE, Milazzo LS. Early intervention in severe head injury: long-term benefits of a formalized program. *Arch Phys Med* 1992; **73**(7): 635–41.

# Post-acute and community rehabilitation of the head-injured patient

Jonathan J. Evans, Maggie Whyte, Fiona Summers, Lorna Torrens,
William W. McKinlay, Susan Dutch, Thérèse Jackson, Judith Fewings,
Ann-Marie Pringle, Bruce Downey and Jane V. Russell

## Neuropsychological rehabilitation for cognitive impairments

Cognitive impairments in memory, attention, executive functioning, language or perception cause many of the day-to-day problems after head injury. Rehabilitation interventions for cognitive impairments will usually be just one component of a broader programme aimed at enabling the head-injured person to achieve agreed functional goals. Nevertheless, there is an emerging evidence base relating to how best to manage specific cognitive impairments. Following a brief discussion of the importance of assessment, this section will describe the approaches that are recommended in relation to each of the major cognitive domains.

## Cognitive assessment and rehabilitation planning

The aim of assessment is to determine the nature of any impairment in cognitive, emotional, behavioural or physical functioning and identify the functional consequences in terms of the patient's ability to participate in activities of daily living, work, education, social and leisure activities. Several members of the rehabilitation team contribute to the assessment of cognitive functioning, including clinical psychologists, speech and language therapists and occupational therapists. All of the team members should contribute to the identification of problems with functional everyday activities, but occupational therapists have a particularly important role to play through direct observation/assessment of patients carrying out activities of daily living and, if appropriate, vocational tasks.

The patient's awareness of his or her impairment and the consequences for everyday life should also be examined. The factors that may contribute to impaired insight/awareness after brain injury are many and varied. Clare presents a biopsychosocial model of awareness in Alzheimer's disease, though the principles apply to most neurological conditions.[1,2] Another useful model is the hierarchical model of Crosson *et al.* which suggests that awareness may be *intellectual, emergent* or *anticipatory*.[3] Intellectual awareness refers to knowing that you have an impairment, but not necessarily recognizing the occurrence of problems as they occur. Emergent awareness refers to 'online' awareness of problems as they occur, whilst anticipatory awareness refers to using knowledge of deficits to anticipate problems and taking steps to prevent problems occurring. The Self-Regulation Skills Interview can be used to examine the patient's level of awareness of problems at each of these levels.[4]

Assessment of mood, emotion and behaviour is critical to rehabilitation planning for several reasons. Firstly, mood disorders are common after brain injury and so represent an important therapeutic target in their own right. Secondly, mood disorders may have an impact

*Head Injury: A Multidisciplinary Approach*, ed. Peter C. Whitfield, Elfyn O. Thomas, Fiona Summers, Maggie Whyte and Peter J. Hutchinson. Published by Cambridge University Press. © Cambridge University Press 2009.

on cognition and so assessment of mood is important for the interpretation of performance on cognitive tests. Finally, mood disorder rather than cognitive impairment may be the major limiting factor in terms of the patient's ability to participate in activities of daily living and it is therefore important to establish this, so that therapeutic efforts can be appropriately directed.

The task then is to formulate or map the relationship between the pathology, the impairments and their functional consequences. One way of doing this is for team members, in a summary of assessment meeting, to use a standard template where all elements of the assessment are listed, and a preliminary formulation of the causal relationships between impairment and functional elements can begin to be drawn out (see Fig. 22.2, p. 230).

Perhaps the most critical aspect of planning for rehabilitation is setting the rehabilitation goals. In most circumstances it is best if goals are written in terms of functional outcomes, but under each of the goals for which it is relevant, there should be documentation of plans of action relating to the management of cognitive impairments that are obstacles to the achievement of the long-term goal.

## Approaches to rehabilitation for cognitive impairments

Rehabilitation for cognitive impairments can be approached in several ways. Wilson presents a comprehensive model of cognitive rehabilitation.[5] She highlights how, when planning a rehabilitation intervention, one must consider whether the focus will be on addressing impairments, disabilities or handicaps (impairments, activities and participation in the ICF). She goes on to note that one might try to restore lost functioning, encourage anatomical reorganization, use residual skills more efficiently, find an alternative to the final goal, modify the environment or use a combination of these. Let us imagine that we have a patient who has memory problems that cause difficulties in his daily life including work activities. If we can improve his memory functioning in a general way, then improvement in all aspects of his functioning which have been affected by impaired memory should follow. However, if we cannot improve memory *per se*, we may need to look at the specific tasks (one by one if necessary) that are affected and enable the patient to compensate for impaired memory in relation to each task. The former approach, if effective, would be more efficient, but if we cannot improve memory in a very general way, then the latter approach will be more likely to bring about real improvements in everyday functioning, albeit potentially limited to those specific situations that are targeted in the rehabilitation context.

Wilson rightly emphasizes that it is important to refer to the evidence base in relation to the treatment of specific cognitive impairments. This evidence base remains limited, but is large enough that several systematic reviews have been conducted.[6–11] In the sections below, the evidence as it relates to the cognitive domains of memory, attention, executive functioning, language and perception will be considered. However, before turning to the specific cognitive domains it is important to return to the issue of insight and awareness.

As noted, awareness is a critical issue in rehabilitation, much of which is dependent upon the patient independently implementing strategies to compensate for deficits in everyday life. If a patient lacks insight, then careful attention should be paid to the factors that are likely to be responsible. For some, insight difficulties arise from poor attention that prevents self-monitoring and hence the patient fails to notice problems as they occur (something that is particularly relevant in relation to poor social communication). Similarly, impaired memory may mean that the patient cannot remember the nature or frequency of errors. Deficits in executive functioning may mean that the patient cannot anticipate the consequences of actions. For some there may be a lack of demand on cognitive skills – think how little responsibility patients in an inpatient rehabilitation ward have for independent organizing, planning, remembering and initiation of activities. The patient who has not yet returned to work may find it hard to appreciate the cognitive demands that are made in the course of everyday work until actually placed in that situation (or a closely analogous one). For others, denial of disability may represent a means of coping with the overwhelming consequences of injury. The intervention will vary depending on the cause of the insight problem. However, for most patients with insight difficulties, some combination of education about brain injury, supported exposure to functional difficulties and psychological support emphasizing positive coping will be appropriate.[12] Work aimed at improving insight must be clearly set in the context of positive, functional goals, though it is often the case that the patient's ultimate goal may not be achievable. For some patients it may not be possible to improve insight and it will be necessary to focus on modifications to the environment that have the effect of reducing cognitive demands on the patient.

Let us turn then to the specific cognitive domains and discuss, with reference to the evidence base, the approaches that are recommended.

## Memory

There is very little evidence that memory can be improved through simple mental exercise or practice at remembering (e.g. practising remembering lists or objects, playing computer games) – people can get better at memory exercises, but this may not translate into improvements in everyday functioning. There is much stronger evidence to support the use of strategies/aids that act as cognitive prostheses, compensating for memory impairment. Cicerone et al. and Cappa et al. concluded that, for those with mild impairment, training in the use of 'internal' memory strategies as well as the use of external memory aids such as notebooks or diaries should be standard practice.[6,7,10] Internal strategies include the use of visual imagery and other mental association strategies aimed at improving the encoding of information.[13] For those with more severe impairment, external memory aids including the use of electronic reminding devices are recommended. The most extensively evaluated electronic reminding system is NeuroPage.[14] This system uses a standard pager, worn by the patient. Reminder messages are entered on to a central computer and at the appropriate time automatically sent to the patient's pager. Wilson et al. studied the efficacy of NeuroPage in a randomized controlled trial and showed that it was very effective in improving everyday functional performance.[14] Analysis of just the head injury data from this study confirmed its effectiveness in this specific patient group.[15] In memory rehabilitation, one size does not fit all. It is important to work with the patient/family to construct a system of memory aids/strategies designed to meet the range of specific everyday remembering demands the patient has placed upon them (or wants to take on).

## Attention

There is some evidence that training specific attentional functions using computerized cognitive training programmes might be beneficial, though there is less evidence as to whether such training programmes generalize to performance on functional activities.[16] Evidence that training in the use of strategies to manage, or compensate for, attentional problems is stronger.[7] A meta-analysis by Park and Ingles suggested that there is good evidence to support the hypothesis that the performance of individuals with attentional impairments on functional activities can be improved through training.[17] By working directly on functional activities, patients may develop strategies to compensate for attentional difficulties or, in some cases, become skilled at a particular task such that the task requires less conscious attention and is less subject to errors caused by poor attention. Often strategies learned in relation to one functional situation can be applied in other situations. For example, using a 'speak aloud' strategy to manage attention when performing a task sequence could be applied to several situations.[18]

### Executive functioning

The term 'executive functions' relates to the cognitive skills required to plan, problem solve and achieve intended goals effectively. Several studies suggest that problem-solving training can be useful, at least for some patients.[19] It is likely that this would only be beneficial for those who are more mildly impaired, though the question of who can benefit has not been systematically examined. The training involves patients being taught to follow a sequence of stages involved in problem solving (recognizing problem, defining goal, identifying possible solutions, choosing solution, making plan, implementing plan, monitoring progress). Goal Management Training (GMT) uses a self-instructional approach and is based on teaching the patient the concept of using a 'mental blackboard' to write intended goals/tasks on, and then to develop a mental checking routine to more effectively maintain attention to tasks and intended goals.[20] The use of external alerting (via SMS text messaging) in combination with GMT has been shown to be beneficial in improving functional performance on an everyday prospective remembering task.[21] The NeuroPage system referred to above has also been shown to be useful at prompting action in a patient with an initiation deficit.[22] Careful consideration of the nature of the deficit that is contributing to poor problem solving or task management can be helpful in selecting the appropriate intervention approach.

### Visuo-spatial functions

Very few disorders of visual or spatial perception have been subject to rehabilitation studies with the exception of unilateral neglect, which is much less common after head injury than after stroke. It does, however, provide a good example of how theories of attention, perception and action are coming together to influence the development of rehabilitation interventions. Visual scanning training is now recommended as a practice standard. Recent studies have also suggested that limb-activation training should also be considered. This involves training the patient to make at least minimal movements of the left limb in left hemispace, an intervention that is hypothesized to reduce neglect as a result of activating right hemisphere representations of left personal and peri-personal space and reducing the inhibitory activation of the intact left hemisphere.[7,10]

### Language and communication

Rehabilitation for language deficits has the longest tradition and the most extensive database upon which to draw conclusions regarding the effectiveness of rehabilitation, though there has been considerable variation in the conclusions that have been drawn by those who have reviewed the evidence. As with unilateral neglect, much of the aphasia therapy research relates to people after stroke; however, most recent reviews conclude that aphasia therapy can be effective.[7,23] Aphasia therapy refers to interventions for specific language deficits identified from careful assessment of precise areas of impairment sometimes based on cognitive-neuropsychological models of language. One of the criticisms of such approaches has been that they do not necessarily bring about changes in people's ability to participate in everyday activities requiring language (e.g. social conversation). It has been argued therefore, that rehabilitation should focus on the broader concept of functional communication (i.e. the activities and participation level of the ICF framework). This is particularly relevant for people who have suffered a head injury, as after head injury a range of impairments other than specific language deficits may impact on communication. Difficulties such as impulsivity, impaired perception of emotion in others, poor attention and monitoring leading to poor turn-taking or tangential speech can all impact on communication even when basic language skills are intact and therefore need to be addressed as part of the rehabilitation programme.[24]

## Conclusions

We live in exciting times when it comes to neuropsychological rehabilitation. The evidence base concerning the effectiveness of treatment approaches is beginning to be substantial enough to provide recommendations on what standard clinical practice should be for each of the major domains of cognitive impairment. Treatments based on sound theoretical models of normal cognition are emerging. But equally important, awareness is growing that any treatment for a specific cognitive impairment must also have a clear relationship with improvements in the ability to participate in activities of everyday life.

## Neurorehabilitation of challenging behaviour

Rehabilitation is 'a problem-solving educational process aimed at reducing disability and handicap…'.[25] The term 'challenging behaviour' has its origins in the field of learning disability and thus many of the techniques used in its remediation also have their basis here.[26] As 'behaviour of such intensity, frequency, or duration that the physical safety of the person or others is likely to be placed in serious jeopardy', or 'behaviour which is likely to limit or delay access to and use of ordinary community facilities', challenging behaviour is socially defined.[27] The implied difficulties represent challenges not only to the individual but to services. An extreme challenge in one set of circumstances may not be defined as such in any other. For this reason and prior to any intervention, it is worth considering the comments of Ylvisaker et al. suggesting that when needs are met and quality of life is enhanced, problem behaviours will decrease spontaneously.[28] Similarly, where intervention is necessary, focus should ideally be on a comprehensive lifestyle change rather than on the isolated and fragmented reduction of behaviours deemed unacceptable by others.

In the field of brain injury, challenging behaviours can be a direct result of injury, a reaction to it or entirely unrelated. Each individual requires different rehabilitation and the same individual can require different rehabilitation, depending on the basis of their difficulty and stage in the process of recovery and adjustment. Assessment and formulation have a crucial and evolving role.

Behavioural approaches form the basis of treatments of choice for challenging behaviour as there is good evidence that associative learning can occur even in the face of severe brain damage.[29] Behaviour does not occur in a vacuum.[30] It has a context, antecedents and consequences and is *maintained* by any combination of these factors, which should be systematically and exhaustively evaluated and explored. Such an evaluation represents a *functional analysis*.

Accurate behavioural assessment involves the initial collation of information from all possible sources and perspectives. Behaviours are then precisely and comprehensively defined to ensure accuracy in observation and recording. It should be clear whether it is the behaviour itself which is posing a problem or its frequency/quality. Suitable methods of observing and recording behaviour will be dependent on the environment as well as the availability and motivation of staff.[31] Prior to the implementation of any intervention, a *baseline* should be established – that is a record of the frequency and severity of the behaviour without input.

Variations in interventional approaches place greater or lesser emphasis on modifications of either antecedents or consequences on the basis of their hypothesized roles in the maintenance of the problem. Thus one might consider environmental cues or settings in which behaviours are expected to occur.[28] Alternatively, one might focus on the removal of reinforcement thereby 'extinguishing' a particular behaviour[32], the positive reinforcement of a desired behaviour or one incompatible with the behaviour which one is attempting to eliminate[33] or introduce a cost response linked to the undesired behaviour.[34,35] Positive procedures are selected wherever possible.[36] Quite aside from their inherent appeal in delivery, there are important ethical considerations associated with either extinction or punishment.

A profile of patient strengths and weaknesses should be incorporated into the functional assessment and, ideally collaboratively and on this basis, meaningful and clearly specified long- and short-term goals are identified, which reflect the overlap between needs and wants and are achievable in terms of resources and context. Goal setting suggests a clear direction and facilitates the assessment of progress.[37] Tasks or steps required to reach a goal can be broken down and if necessary, by the process of 'shaping', each individual step can be reinforced *en route* to achieving the greater task.[37] Where possible, self-management should prevail. A projected timescale for achieving the goals, certainly for reviewing them, is essential. Where possible, planned interventions should be rehearsed prior to implementation. Once implementation is underway, it is no less important to keep accurate records of events for the purposes of evaluating progress and outcome.[38]

Rehabilitation of challenging behaviour can be challenging in itself and failure is not uncommon. The most frequently encountered difficulty is inconsistency in implementation of plans. Structured communication amongst involved individuals is crucial. Other than this, there may be a fundamental mismatch between individual and professional priorities and additionally, staff behaviour and attitudes are pivotal.[39,40]

# Neuropsychological rehabilitation of children with Acquired Brain Injury: a brief overview

Over 500 000 young people under the age of 16 attend a hospital in the United Kingdom every year as a result of a traumatic brain injury. It is the most common cause of death and acquired disability in childhood. If one also considers the other common causes of acquired brain injury (ABI), i.e. encephalitis and other neurological diseases, over 3000 previously healthy children acquire a significant disability every year in the United Kingdom and require rehabilitation.

The vast majority of these children return home to their families and schools, and on the surface may appear to have made remarkable recoveries. However, ABI causes 'invisible injuries', and the nature of the damage to the child's cognitive, social and emotional ability is much harder to assess accurately when compared to adult brain injuries.

Some children with focal brain injuries may acquire age appropriate skills and be free from the problems associated with a corresponding injury that has occurred in adulthood. Unfortunately, this tends to happen at a price. For instance, particular skills may well be preserved, but other neuropsychological abilities may be compromised. It is also important to note that generalized cerebral injuries in children appear to be more devastating than in adults: the earlier the injury, the smaller the store of learned knowledge and skills, and therefore the greater the global impairment.

Crucially, the age of the child, the nature of the injury and the stage of skills development all interact to determine the eventual outcome for the child. The pre-injury cognitive ability of the child, the social context and family functioning also play an important part in the recovery process.

The bulk of the work involved in the successful rehabilitation of the child usually falls to relatives and teachers. Too few of the families and schools supporting these children have sufficient knowledge about the cognitive, social and emotional problems, which can emerge at a much later date when the skills mediated by specific areas do not develop as expected. For example, the ability to plan and organize is mediated by the frontal lobes which mature throughout adolescence. An injury in this area in a pre-school child would not become apparent for a further 10 or 15 years, and in many cases the reason for a teenager being chaotic and disorganized may be misattributed to age and personality rather than to a disability. In other words, children gradually grow into their deficits. This last point highlights the need for long-term monitoring of children's development.

Bearing this in mind, every child with a moderately severe ABI should undergo a neuropsychological assessment in order to guide the planning for the rehabilitation of the child. An important part of the work of the Neuropsychologist is to prepare an individualized 'passport', which should describe clearly the child's current cognitive profile of strengths and weaknesses, and detail what this means in real-life situations in the classroom and at home. It should also list all the other behaviours that may be secondary effects of the injury (e.g. frustration, loss of self esteem and social difficulties which can become more problematic over time). The family should also have written information detailing the potential difficulties the child might reasonably be expected to encounter in the future, taking into consideration the site of the injury and the age at which the child was injured.

A more recent development has been to train children to use the discrete skills most often disrupted in ABI (i.e. attention, impulse control and memory functioning). This work is promising and initial results indicate that improvements made are maintained 6 months later.[41] However, by far the most important aspect of rehabilitation at present is to increase the knowledge base of all those in contact with the child so that the child's behaviour is understood sympathetically, and appropriate measures are put in place to maximize the child's potential and minimize the impact of the injury.

## Occupational therapy

Occupational therapy assists people to achieve health and life satisfaction by improving their ability to carry out the activities that they need to do or choose to do in their daily lives (College of Occupational Therapists).[42]

Molineux affirmed that occupational therapists 'view humans as occupational beings, not merely that occupation is an important part of human life' and refers us to current assumptions which underpin the practice of occupational therapy described by Kielhofner.[43,44] The assumptions are that, humans have an occupational nature; humans can experience occupational dysfunction (difficulty engaging in daily activities); and that occupation can be used as a therapeutic agent.

Following brain injury, people may experience difficulties performing everyday activities. The varied and often complex nature of occupational dysfunction experienced requires specialized assessment and treatment, provided by an occupational therapist with expertise in brain injury.

Analysis of a person carrying out selected activities can determine where performance is limited, and can ascertain a person's potential for returning to previous occupations. This also enables the therapist to identify abilities and deficits, and forms the basis of a goal-orientated treatment plan.

## Post-acute rehabilitation

Intervention by the occupational therapist at this stage focuses on improving occupation and independence. A variety of standardized assessments and behavioural observations are used to build a functional performance profile. At this stage occupational therapy assists the person with a brain injury to learn new ways of carrying out occupations which they find difficult, and to find new occupations which are meaningful and/or satisfying to them. This may involve incorporating strategies into daily routines to compensate for performance skills deficits, for example, schedules to structure and pace daily routines if fatigue is an issue, use of external aids (diary/electronic organizers/alarms) for memory and executive deficits, coloured markers on the cooker controls for visual difficulties or using checklists to facilitate independence in personal care. The occupational therapist will also facilitate practice of daily living activities to relearn essential skills, such as dressing, meal preparation, budgeting and shopping. This may include community mobility practice such as learning to use public transport, if driving is not possible. Therapy may incorporate strategies to compensate for cognitive deficits and guidance on social skills. Occupational therapists can provide aids and adaptive equipment to support independent living, e.g. adapted feeding utensils, toilet rails, shower and bath seats and give advice on positioning including the provision of splints, prescription of appropriate seating, wheelchairs and pressure relieving equipment. They may undertake brain injury education and emotional support for patients, families and carers to assist in the development of awareness regarding the problems that affect daily living and participation in life roles.

For those people with profound brain injury, the occupational therapist will, alongside the interdisciplinary team, evaluate levels of awareness using a detailed multisensory evaluation. Once cognitive functions are identified, they will support the person in a minimally conscious or locked in state to engage with their environment in an appropriate manner. This may include the provision of electronic assistive technology and environmental control systems. Assessment can also help to determine whether a person remains in a vegetative state, in which case interventions will focus on disability management and maintaining basic care needs through, for example, the provision of appropriate positioning and pressure care aids.

The occupational therapist plays a major role in facilitating the transition of care from hospital to community and will coordinate home and environmental assessments to identify any equipment, adaptation and support needs for discharge.

## Community rehabilitation

The primary focus of occupational therapy in the community setting is to maximize the person's ability to function in their own environment, and participate in their life roles. There is an emphasis on adjusting to limitations, improving quality of life and family and carer support. Resumption and participation in previous life roles (family, friends, social and work) can be affected by a number of consequences of brain injury including cognitive impairment, psychosocial issues and physical impairments. People may experience difficulties with self-confidence, self-esteem, emotional issues, anxiety and social reintegration. Opportunity to practise tasks and incorporate them into a daily routine is essential for learning. Consistency of approach and learning strategies is gained through close multidisciplinary working and family and carer liaison. Restorative and adaptive approaches are used by occupational therapists. Individually tailored treatment programmes may be introduced to extend activities of daily living (e.g. shopping, and domestic tasks) through facilitated practice, develop skills in the use of computers and information technology for learning, education and communication and to maintain participation in leisure activities – either old or new. The occupational therapist may provide education and support for behavioural, emotional and sexual issues and may assist social reintegration through support, social and interest groups. They may provide advice on the person's capacity to return to driving and any adaptations to vehicles that may be required. If driving is not possible, the occupational therapist will enable access to community facilities and the use of alternative transport options. For those people who have more severe physical difficulties, the occupational therapist will have a role in evaluating their abilities and making recommendations for assistive equipment and environmental adaptations, including electrical assistive technology and environmental control systems.

Work is an essential and valued role in many people's lives. It may fulfil the occupational needs of those who wish to have paid employment, social integration and personal satisfaction. Occupational therapists will integrate vocational rehabilitation into the person's rehabilitation programme, and increasingly occupational therapists are found working in specialized vocational rehabilitation programmes. Vocational rehabilitation focuses on raising awareness of the impact of brain injury on work-related skills, and facilitating a realistic exploration of vocational options. The occupational therapist may carry out functional capacity evaluations, and establish a retraining programme, which reduces the impact of impairments and increases independence, awareness and insight. The retraining programme will include strategies to compensate for difficulties and will develop functional performance, insight, attention, stamina, confidence and social skills to ensure effective integration to the workplace.

Brain injury can affect all areas of daily living and prevent participation. As described, occupational therapy, using occupation as an assessment tool and therapeutic medium, is essential at all stages of the person's journey in their recovery and adjustment to life following a brain injury.

# Physiotherapy

Physiotherapy plays a pivotal role in both the acute and later phases of rehabilitative care. Whilst airway and respiratory issues normally take precedence in the early stages following trauma (see Chapter 23), early attention to the musculoskeletal system is important in promoting recovery of head control and limb function.

## Musculoskeletal care

Spasticity results from any lesion in the upper motor neurone pathway causing impaired extra-pyramidal inhibitory influence on $\alpha$ and $\gamma$ motor neurones. Reflex arcs are disinhibited giving rise to hyper-reflexia and increased tone, typically in the antigravity muscles of the upper limb flexors and lower limb extensors. The velocity-dependent increase in tonic stretch is seen as a greater resistance to faster stretch. Spasticity can occur early following TBI and may result in limb deformities compromising patient care and delaying early rehabilitation.[44–47]

Muscle stretch/lengthening is resisted by hypertonia. As a consequence, muscles remain in a shortened position for prolonged periods of time, which results in changes to the physical properties of muscle and associated soft tissues. Sarcomeres in series, responsible for determining distance and force of muscular contraction, are reduced, thereby decreasing muscle length and extensibility.[44,48,49,50–53] These muscular and soft tissue changes result in loss of joint range and movement.[49,54–57] Muscle function can also be compounded by pain associated with heterotrophic ossification and the presence of skeletal fractures in the multiply injured.[58]

Active or passive stretching is recommended to prevent contracture formation. The optimum degree and frequency is unknown; however, prolonged stretch has been shown to reduce spasticity.[46,47,59,60] This is achieved by casting, which is now an established means of controlling contractures and spasticity in both adults and children.[55-57,61] Proactive casting is frequently employed early in the course of treatment for TBI patients. This provides the prolonged stretch required to maintain joint range during the initial unconscious period and is commonly applied prior to weaning from mechanical ventilation.[54-57,62] The optimum method of casting remains debatable. Removable casts are custom fashioned to allow passive range of movement exercises to maintain tissue and joint extensibility. Potential drawbacks of non-removable serial casting include muscle atrophy, pain, deep venous thrombosis and pressure ulceration. The most suitable method of casting depends on the patient cohort, cognition and conscious level.[46,48,62,63]

From a patient management perspective, spasticity has two components amenable to treatment – biomechanical and neuronal.[45,51,64,65] The biomechanical aspect is managed by physiotherapy – passive movements, positioning, splinting and casting are all commonplace.[64] Alleviation of the neuronal component of spasticity is achieved by antispasmodic drugs. Baclofen and tizanidine are drugs commonly used, others include sodium dantrolene and clonidine. All these drugs have potential side effects and some have been implicated in possibly delaying cognitive recovery following brain injury.[64,66,67] In cases of focal spasticity or severe spasticity, Botulinum Toxin A (BTX-A) can be used. BTX-A is a powerful neurotoxin, which inhibits pre-synaptic acetylcholine release at the neuromuscular junction producing a localized temporary muscle weakness.[64,68] Its effects can be seen within 24–72 hours and lasts on average 3–4 months. Used in conjunction with passive movements and casting, it has been shown to significantly reduce tone, allow toleration of the cast and improve functional recovery.[69]

## Motor control

The wide variety of treatment approaches in rehabilitation have their foundations in an array of motor control theories.[70,71] The challenge for the physiotherapist is to develop their own model of practice, where the treatment methods they select have a scientific, physiotherapeutic and practical knowledge base.

Movement of patients between different positions (postural sets) aims to stimulate proprioceptive input and thereby enhance efferent activity.[72] Excitation of the vestibulo-spinal tract involves recruitment of lower limb extensors, proximal musculature and head movement.[73] This is closely linked with reticulospinal tract activity, influencing extensor tone and involving the cerebellum in maintaining equilibrium. Since the feet afford afferent input into the vestibulospinal tract, standing can be used as a therapeutic means of activation. The tilt-table is a useful adjunct to facilitate early, safe standing. It is particularly useful for patients who are unconscious and require total support.[74] Additionally, the use of weight bearing helps maintain length in the plantar flexors.[61,75,76] Brain-injured recumbent patients have impaired autonomic orthostatic responses; initially, only small angles of tilt should be used with continued monitoring of BP, $SaO_2$, heart rate, respiratory rate and skin colour. Malalignment should be avoided as this impairs normal proprioceptive input.[74-78]

Trunk control is as important as respiratory care and spasticity management in the rehabilitation of the head injured. The role of the trunk is fundamental to head control and limb function via the shoulder and pelvic girdles.[56] Physiotherapy treatment of the trunk therefore needs to be incorporated into a patient's treatment plan; for this reason alternating sessions of standing (tilt-table initially, therapist facilitated later) and work in sitting are often used. Positioning, attained by the tilt-table and sitting, enables normal head–neck alignment, stimulates visual and vestibular facilitated pathways and promotes dynamic stability of anterior neck muscles.[56,74,78] The anterior neck muscles are important for tongue movements and swallowing as they help stabilize the hyoid bone.[56,74] Early active and passive orofacial movements are encouraged as this helps with respiratory care, nutrition and communication recovery.[56]

Movement modulation mediated by the cerebellum can be targeted to assist motor learning by means of task(s) repetition.[71,79] Movement and control of movement against gravity encourages balance control. As improvements in proximal trunk control, head control and selective lower limb movements occur, treatments gradually incorporate facilitation of gait. The therapist should continually strive to rehabilitate patients beyond their present functional ability in order to attain their maximal future functional status.

## Posture and seating

Posture and seating are important in normalizing proprioceptive feedback; postural stability is necessary for functional activity.[80] Seating systems are frequently used for patients with severe neurologic impairment and are used as adjuncts to the previously mentioned treatments.[81] Ankle range of movement and tone management are fundamental to wheelchair dependent patients, the ability to achieve plantigrade position contributes to ease and safety of transfer into the chair, and also reduces the risk of pressure areas associated with poor alignment.[62]

By applying external supports to the patient in the most functional and least restrictive positions, a stable posture can be attained.[51,80] Appropriate orientation of the trunk in space is important to consider. Rearward tilting is used in many seating systems.[82,83] The use of gravity to assist stability is considered vital in the severely posturally incompetent patient but used with caution to limit any further detrimental effects of social, visual and environmental isolation.[84] Additionally, a wedge cushion, bilateral thoracic supports and head support along with the inclusion of a table can be used to build a stable posture.[51,80] Stability in the sitting position confers better orofacial control, swallowing and speech; social interaction and communication are enhanced reinforcing recovery of function and improving the patient's quality of life.[51,75,80,81]

The demands/priorities of the brain-injured patient frequently change and therefore treatment regimes should be consistently reviewed and updated. Close observation and assessment must continue even when medical stability is achieved. Early and timely rehabilitation is vital to limit and promote recovery from any neurological deficit.

## Speech and language therapy

The speech and language therapist working in brain injury rehabilitation is faced with the challenge of teasing out the communication deficits from any co-existing impairments and attempting to assist the patient towards regaining an acceptable level of interaction.

## Disorders of communication

Until the early 1970s, language dysfunction was not considered to be one of the main consequences of closed head injury, in contrast with impairments of memory and concentration.[85,86] Many authors agree that classical aphasic syndromes are relatively rare following TBI although the presence of word finding difficulties is recognized and Wernicke's aphasia has been reported in one or two papers.[85–88] Although many patients do perform reasonably well on traditional tests of aphasia, deficits of basic language processing are by no means uncommon in brain injury. In addition to word finding difficulties, other characteristics of aphasia, such as paraphasias, impaired comprehension and reading and writing deficits are frequently encountered. Verbal fluency deficits are also common. Linguistic disorders tend to be more prevalent during the earlier stages of the patient's recovery and have frequently resolved by the time of discharge from hospital.

The ability to communicate verbally and non-verbally in a social context is often impaired following a TBI.[89–92] Difficulties with pragmatic communication skills, or how language is *used*, can persist long after any associated linguistic deficits. Deficiencies are frequently evident in: turn-taking in conversation; initiating, maintaining and terminating conversation; and using (and comprehending) facial expression, eye contact, tone of voice and gesture.[93–95] Patients are also reported as responding slowly or not at all, and appearing uninterested in the other speaker or their point of view.[90,96] Disorders of discourse are also very common. Discourse can be described as a series of related sentences used in communication interchanges, mainly in conversation but also in, for example, narrative discourse such as story-telling, and procedural discourse during which a process is described, such as how to make spaghetti bolognaise. Impaired discourse skills can be characterized by: an over-abundance of talk that is tangential and contains irrelevant and unrelated details, or a meagre amount with little information content; difficulty staying on topic; difficulties generating questions or comments to sustain conversation; disordered sequencing of information, with disorganized stories, sequences of events and descriptions of procedures which are difficult to follow; difficulties understanding or manipulating abstract language such as sarcasm, puns or metaphors[89,91,92,97–99].

Verbal output can also be 'inaccurate and confabulatory', which is usually attributable to cognitive dysfunction rather than to a deficiency of linguistic processing or pragmatics.[100]

'Cognitive communication disorder' is often used as a diagnostic label to cover any or all of the non-linguistic communication disorders following traumatic brain injury. The presence of additional cognitive deficits will have an adverse effect on communicative competence. Poor planning and impaired concentration can reduce the efficacy of sequencing and inclusion of relevant information in conversation or narrative; reduced listening skills can impact upon the ability to absorb and integrate spoken language; visual neglect and visuo-perceptual disorders affect reading and writing; lowered arousal can diminish the available resources and energy to process complex communicative tasks; and poor self-monitoring influences how well the person engages with others.[90,101]

Some authors attribute disorders of pragmatics and discourse following TBI to cognitive dysfunction, in particular to executive dysfunction.[85,101,102] Where communication disorders are non-linguistic in origin and are a direct consequence of other cognitive deficits, as above, the expectation is that the ability to communicate will improve when cognitive functioning does. Disorders of pragmatics and discourse are extensively described in the literature as a consequence of damage to the right cerebral hemisphere.[103,104] The characteristic features are more or less identical whether social communication is damaged by a TBI or a right hemisphere stroke. As disorders of basic language processing following TBI can reasonably be linked to trauma in the language centres of the dominant (usually left) hemisphere or their connections, it seems fitting that, in at least some cases, pragmatic disorders following TBI could result from damage to the functions of the right hemisphere.[105]

Disorders of speech, especially dysarthria, are common after a TBI, although there is disagreement in the literature regarding prevalence and recovery.[106] Depending on the neuropathology, any of the main subgroups of spastic, flaccid, ataxic, hypo- and hyper-kinetic, or a mixed dysarthria, can be identified, with spastic dysarthria most common due to the regularity with which bilateral upper motor neurone damage occurs. There is considerable variability with regard both to the severity and the extent to which articulation, respiration, rate, resonance, volume and prosody are implicated. An additional complication is the possibility of dyspraxia affecting the articulation of speech sounds.

## Assessment of communication skills

There is no universally recommended single method of assessing communication disorders following TBI. The population is a heterogeneous one and requires an individual approach. The patient's clinical presentation will change over time as a result of treatment, spontaneous recovery or a combination of both. A flexible approach to assessment of communication disorders is essential, as test selection and the timing of assessment will be influenced by a range of factors. Variables such as level of consciousness and arousal, agitation and restlessness, fatigue, concentration, emergence from PTA, levels of co-operation, insight, the extent of co-occurring cognitive deficits, and the presence of identifiable specific communication deficits, will determine whether the patient has reached the stage of being able to cope with the often lengthier and more demanding formal standardized tests or whether a more informal approach, which can be more easily adapted to cope with the patient's changing condition, is preferred.

## Rehabilitation of communication disorders

Rehabilitation of communication disorders following TBI is a highly individualized, dynamic process. A multi-disciplinary team approach is essential, as patients with a TBI frequently present with a range of disorders requiring input from several disciplines. Where possible, patients are encouraged to identify their own communication difficulties, highlighting those which they perceive to be the most disabling, although poor insight frequently inhibits this. The speech and language therapist will attempt to design a rehabilitation plan in accordance with the patient's needs, possibly focusing on or prioritizing those deficits which would be most responsive to therapy. Techniques are often employed with the aim of remediating or restoring previous functions, as in word finding tasks and language therapy in general, or in articulation drills for dysarthria. Attempts are made to incorporate materials which are of personal interest or value to the patient in order to maximize motivation and participation. Compensatory techniques and assistive technology might be explored where further improvement is unlikely, for example, in cases of severe dysarthria. For such patients a practical approach would be to train family members and friends as 'communication partners' in order to help them find optimal ways of conversing with and eliciting information from the person with a TBI. Detailed descriptions of approaches which have been used in the rehabilitation of impairments of pragmatic communication and discourse are provided elsewhere in the literature.[103,107–109]

There is scant information available on the efficacy of treatment methods.[110] The response to rehabilitation generally tends to be better in those who are motivated, have insight into their difficulties and the goals of therapy, and who have a supportive family and/or social network.

The consequences of enduring communication impairments can be more devastating than those of physical deficits and are associated with failure to return to or maintain employment,[111] the gradual disintegration of family dynamics, often resulting in divorce,[90,112] and social isolation.[90,113] The importance of rehabilitation for communication disorders, and continued support for patients and their families, cannot be overstated.

## Case management

A brain injury case manager can facilitate rehabilitation, particularly community-based rehabilitation, and also organize the support needed to enable the injured person to live in the community. A case manager, often from a relevant profession such as occupational therapy, psychology, social work or special education, acts as a coordinator.[114] Their role may include:

- Identifying the needs and goals of the injured person
- Referring to a mix of existing services – each may be able to meet *some* of the injured person's needs
- Exploring social/employment possibilities, including supported or voluntary work
- Supporting and educating the patient and family to help with adjustment
- Where necessary, finding appropriate housing, and setting up a care/support regime including recruiting and training carers.

The case manager therefore provides the overall coordination of continuing rehabilitation and care, identifying local resources and activities to help the brain-injured individual.[115]

Individuals who are struggling to adapt to their limitations due to cognitive deficits, behavioural problems, and other sequelae of injury may benefit from case management. Examples include individuals who would benefit from a move to a home of their own with a support package, re-entering education or finding employment including voluntary work, and ongoing support with maintaining a safe and structured lifestyle which may include access to therapy services from time to time. Often hard-to-place individuals with behavioural problems, cognitive limitation, and whose families struggle to cope are referred for case management, but many others with less obviously pressing problems can also benefit.

Rehabilitation is often funded through the legal system as part of compensation claims. Defenders' and Plaintiffs' representatives are under an obligation to consider what may be achieved under the Rehabilitation Code.[116] This requires the parties to be pro-active in minimizing the disability suffered by the injured party, which is potentially of benefit to both defender and injured party.

Case managers are often funded by this route and, where there may be a right of legal action, it is important for patients and families to seek advice from a specialized firm of lawyers at a reasonably early stage. Many firms in the UK will provide an initial consultation free of charge. Advice on suitably experienced firms may be obtained from the relevant Law Society or, in the UK, from:

- Headway (the brain injury association) www.headway.org.uk free helpline 0808 800 2244
- Association of Personal Injury Lawyers (APIL) www.apil.com helpline 0870 609 1958

This is not the only route to funding a case manager and in some cases funding is by a health authority and/or social services.

## Return to work

Return to work (RTW) is an important marker of the outcome of injury. Loss of the ability to work will, for most adults, represent a loss of status, position, financial well-being and self-esteem and may induce loss of feelings of worth.

The reported rates of return to work after TBI vary between studies. A recent study found only 14% in full-time work 30 months' post-injury compared to 93% before injury.[117] It is generally agreed that it is cognitive and behavioural factors, including memory/concentration difficulties, and reduced social skills and temper control, which are the main impediments to return to work.[111] Malec reported that the percentage *not* employed after rehabilitation was 29% compared with 47% in those without rehabilitation.[118] Ben-Yishay's group in New York reported a reduction in unemployed rates from 100% to 22% after rehab, although in other centres the reductions have been less dramatic.[119]

It would be wrong to assume that people just get back to work with the passage of time after brain injury. A UK study of patients who had not had specialist vocational rehabilitation showed a low level of return to work (29% compared with 86% working before injury) with no improvement in that figure between 2- and 7-year follow-ups.[111] General practitioners encounter patients with serious brain injury relatively infrequently and may not be aware of the range of services, so specialists involved in acute management should make referrals where they can. Specialist (RTW) rehabilitation can be very effective. Wehman *et al.* in Virginia have developed the job coaching approach and in a 2000 study the per-client costs (of the order of $10k) were modest compared to the costs of unemployment and dependence on benefits.[120]

Practical steps that health professionals should take are:

1. Caution the patient against premature return to work. Returning while cognitively impaired and/or still showing obvious emotional lability may damage the individual's relationships and reputation at work. It is better to allow time to recover and, where appropriate, for specialists to assess whether the individual should return to full or restricted duties.

2. Where appropriate, refer for rehabilitation. Rehabilitation directed towards minimising the effects of memory and other cognitive failures, and improving social skills and anger management should be the first step before return to work is attempted.

3. Referral should be considered to a specialist return-to-work (RTW) programme. In the UK some services, such as those provided by Rehab UK and Momentum, are generally free at the point of delivery. For others, funding will need to be arranged on a case-by-case basis. The points noted about legal representation in the 'Case Management' section of this book are relevant in relation to funding for such programmes. Some Colleges of Further Education have programmes intended for those aiming to return to employment or re-enter education after brain injury (or other forms of injury). Such programmes can be a useful step back into employment. In the UK, 'Jobcentre Plus' will have a Disability Employment Adviser (DEA), whose role is to help those returning to work after a health-related absence. The DEA can potentially provide access to training and suitable employment.

4. A further alternative to returning to work, which can be an excellent first step to building a work routine and confidence, is to undertake voluntary work. There are many websites, for example, www.do-it.org.uk for England and Volunteer Centre Network www.volunteerscotland.org.uk for Scotland.

In conclusion, the consequences of brain injury are wide ranging and affect a person's cognitive, physical, emotional, social and functional abilities. This has an impact on family, occupational, educational and social life. The care of the post-acute head-injured patient involves consideration of a complexity of needs requiring a holistic multidisciplinary approach to rehabilitation. This approach should not only consider the needs of the patient but also the needs of their family. Brain injury is a life-long condition, and the needs of a person with brain injury will change not only according to their stage of recovery but also with their stage and goals in life. As a result, the level of treatment and support required from the rehabilitation team may vary; however, in many cases it will be long term and in some cases for the lifetime of the person with brain injury.

# References

1. Clare L. The construction of awareness in early stage Alzheimer's disease: a review of concepts and models. *Br J Clin Psychol* 2004; **43**: 155–75.

2. Ownsworth T, Clare L, Morris R. An integrated biopsychosocial approach to understanding awareness deficits in Alzheimer's disease and brain injury. *Neuropsychol Rehabil* 2006; **16**: 415–38.

3. Crosson B, Barco PP, Velozo CA, Bolesta MM, Werts D, Brobeck T. Awareness and compensation in post-acute head injury rehabilitation. *J Head Trauma Rehabil* 1989; **4**: 46–54.

4. Ownsworth T, McFarland K, Young R McD. Development and standardisation of the self-regulation skills Interview (SRSI): a new clinical assessment tool for acquired brain injury. *Clin Neuropsychol* 2000; **14**: 76–92.

5. Wilson BA. Towards a comprehensive model of cognitive rehabilitation. *Neuropsychol Rehabil* 2002; **12**: 97–110.

6. Cicerone KD, Dahlberg C, Kalmar K *et al.* Evidence-based cognitive rehabilitation: recommendations for clinical practice. *Arch Phys Med Rehabil* 2000; **81**: 1596–614.

7. Cicerone KD, Dahlberg C, Malec JF *et al.* Evidence-based cognitive rehabilitation: updated review of the literature from 1998 through 2002. *Arch Phys Med Rehabil* 2005; **86**: 1681–92.

8. Chesnut RM, Carney N, Maynard H, Mann NC, Patterson P, Helfand M. Summary report: evidence of the effectiveness of rehabilitation for persons with traumatic brain injury. *J Head Trauma Rehabil* 1999; **14**(2): 176–88.

9. Carney N, Chesnut RM, Maynard H, Mann NC, Patterson P, Helfand M. Effect of cognitive rehabilitation on outcomes for persons with traumatic brain injury: a systematic review. *J Head Trauma Rehabil* 1999; **14**(3): 277–307.

10. Cappa SF, Benke T, Clarke S, Rossi B, Stemmer B, van Heugten CM. EFNS guidelines on cognitive rehabilitation: report of an EFNS task force. *Europ J Neurol* 2005; **12**: 665–80.

11. Halligan P, Wade D (eds) *The Effectiveness of Rehabilitation for Cognitive Deficits*. Oxford, Oxford University Press, 2005.

12. Prigatano GP. *Principles of Neuropsychological Rehabilitation*. Oxford, Oxford University Press, 1999.

13. Craik FIM, Winocur G, Palmer H *et al.* Cognitive rehabilitation in the elderly: effects on memory. *J Int Neuropsych Soc* 2007; **13**: 132–42.

14. Wilson BA, Emslie H, Quirk K, Evans JJ. Is Neuropage effective in reducing everyday memory and planning problems? A randomised control crossover study. *J Neurol, Neurosurg Psychiatry* 2001; **70**: 477–82.

15. Wilson BA, Emslie H, Quirk K, Evans JJ, Watson P. A randomized controlled trial to evaluate a paging system for people with traumatic brain injury. *Brain Inj* 2005; **19**: 891–4.

16. Sturm W, Fimm B, Cantagallo A *et al.* Computerised training of specific attention deficits in stroke and traumatic brain injury patients: a multicentre efficacy study. In: Leclecq M, Zimmerman P, eds. *Applied Neuropsychology of Attention*. Hove, Psychology Press, 2002; 365–80.

17. Park N, Ingles JL. Effectiveness of attention rehabilitation after acquired brain injury: a meta-analysis. *Neuropsychology* 2001; **15**: 199–210.

18. Park N, Barbuto E. Treating attention impairments. In: Halligan P, Wade, D, eds. *The Effectiveness of Rehabilitation for Cognitive Deficits*. Oxford, Oxford University Press, 2005; 81–90.

19. Evans JJ. Can executive impairments be effectively treated? In: Halligan P, Wade D, eds. *The Effectiveness of Rehabilitation for Cognitive Deficits*. Oxford, Oxford University Press, 2005; 247–56.

20. Levine B, Robertson IH, Clare L *et al.* Rehabilitation of executive functioning: an experimental-clinical validation of goal management training. *J Int Neuropsychol Soci* 2000; **6**: 299–312.

21. Fish J, Evans JJ, Nimmo M *et al.* Rehabilitation of executive dysfunction following brain injury: 'Content-free cueing' improves everyday prospective memory performance. *Neuropsychologia* 2007; **45**: 1318–30.

22. Evans JJ, Emslie H, Wilson BA. External cueing systems in the rehabilitation of executive impairments of action. *J Int Neuropsychol Soci* 1998; **4**: 399–408.

23. Basso A. Language deficits: the efficacy of the impairment-based treatment. In: Halligan P, Wade D, eds. *The Effectiveness of Rehabilitation for Cognitive Deficits*. Oxford, Oxford University Press, 2005; 185–94.

24. Marshall J. Can speech and language therapy with aphasic people affect activity and participation levels? In: Halligan P, Wade D, eds. *The Effectiveness of Rehabilitation for Cognitive Deficits*. Oxford, Oxford University Press, 2005; 195–207.

25. Wade DT. *Measurement in Neurological Rehabilitation*. Oxford, Oxford University Press, 1992.

26. Miller E. *Recovery and Management of Neuropsychological Impairments*. Chichester: John Wiley, 1984.

27. Emerson E, Barrett S, Bell C *et al. Developing services for people with severe learning disability and challenging behaviour: report of the early work of the Special Development Team in Kent*, Institute of Social and Applied Psychology, University of Kent at Canterbury, 1987.

28. Ylvisaker M, Jacobs HE, Feeney T. Positive supports for people who experience behavioural and cognitive disability after brain injury. *J Head Trauma Rehabil* 2002; **18**: 7–32.

29. Goldstein L. Behaviour problems. In: Greenwood RJ, Barnes MP, McMillan TM, Ward CD, eds. *Handbook of neurological rehabilitation*. Hove, Psychology Press, 2003; 419–32.

30. Yule W. Functional analysis and observation and recording techniques. In: Yule W, Carr, J, eds. *Behaviour Modification for People with Mental Handicaps*, 2nd edn. London, Croom Helm, 1987; 8–27.

31. Barker C, Pistrang N, Elliott R. *Research Methods in Clinical and Counselling Psychology*. Chichester, John Wiley & Sons Ltd, 1994; 112–31.

32. Wood RLI, Burgess P. The psychological management of behaviour disorders following brain injury. In: Fussey I, Giles GM, eds. *Rehabilitation of the Severely Brain-injured Adult. A Practical Approach*. London, Croom Helm, 1988; 43–68.

33. Wood RLI, Eames P. Application of behaviour modification in the treatment of traumatically head-injured adults. In: Davey G, ed. *Applications of Conditioning Theory*. London, Methuen, 1981; 81–101.

34. Wood RLI. *Brain Injury Rehabilitation: A Neurobehavioural Approach*. London, Croom Helm, 1987.

35. Didden R, Duker R, Korzilius H. Meta-analytic study on treatment effectiveness for problem behaviours with individuals who have mental retardation. *Am J Ment Retard* 1997; **101**: 387–99.

36. Donnellan AM, La Vigna GW, Negri-Shoultz N, Fassbender LL. Progress without punishment. In: *Effective Approaches for Learners with Behavior Problems*. New York, Teachers College Press, 1988.

37. Wilson BA, Herbert CM, Shiel A. Behavioural approaches in neuropsychological rehabilitation. In: *Optimising Rehabilitation Procedures*. Hove, Psychology Press, 2003; 27–31.

38. Oddy M. Taking the lead in brain injury services. *Psychol* 2000; **13**: 21–3.

39. Van den Broek MD. Why does neurorehabilitation fail? *J Head Trauma Rehabil* 2005; **20**: 464–73.

40. Ager A, O'May F. Issues in the definition and implementation of 'best practice' for staff delivery of interventions for challenging behaviour. *J Intell Developm Disabil* 2001; **26**: 243–56.

41. van't Hooft I. Cognitive rehabilitation. *In: Children with Acquired Brain Injuries.* Published thesis. Karolinska University Press. Stockholm, Sweden, 2005 (http://diss.kib.ki.se/2005/91-7140-380-9/thesis.pdf).

42. Definitions and Core Skills for Occupational Therapy. *College of Occupational Therapists.* London, 2006 (http://www.cot.org.uk/members/profpractice/briefings/pdf/23Definitions&CoreSkills.pdf).

43. Molineux M. *Occupation for Occupational Therapists.* Oxford, Blackwell Publishing, 2004.

44. Kielhofner, G. *Conceptual Foundations of Occupational Therapy*, 2nd edn. Philadelphia, F.A. Davis, 1997.

45. Verplancke D, Snape S, Salisbury CF, Jones PW, Ward AB. A randomized controlled trial of botulinum toxin on lower limb spasticity following acute acquired severe brain injury. *Clin Rehabil* 2005; **19**: 117–25.

46. Mortenson PA, Eng JJ. The use of casts in the management of joint mobility and hypertonia following brain injury in adults: a systematic review. *Phys Ther* 2003; **83**: 648–58.

47. Moseley AM. The effect of casting combined with stretching on passive ankle dorsiflexion in adults with traumatic head injuries. *Phys Ther* 1997; **77**: 240–7.

48. Pohl M, Mehrholz J, Ruckriem S. The influence of illness duration and level of conciousness on the treatment effect and complication rate of serial casting in patients with severe cerebral spasticity. *Clin Rehabil* 2003; **17**: 373–9.

49. Williams PE. Use of intermittent stretch in the prevention of serial sarcomere loss in immobilised muscles. *Ann Rheum Dis* 1990; **49**: 316–17.

50. Gossman MR, Sahrmann SA, Rose SJ. Review of length-associated changes in muscle. Experimental evidence and clinical implications. *Phys Ther* 1982; **62**: 1799–808.

51. Herbert R. The passive mechanical properties of muscle and their adaptation to altered patterns of use. *Aust J Physiother* 1988; **34**: 141–8.

52. Rose S, Rothstein JM. Muscle mutability. Part 1. General concepts and adaptations to altered patterns of use. *Phys Ther* 1982; **62**: 1773–87.

53. Goldspink G, Williams PE. Muscle fibre and connective tissue changes associated with use and disuse. In: Ada L, Canning C, eds. *Key Issues in Neurological Physiotherapy [Physiotherapy: Foundations for Practice].* Oxford, Butterworth-Heinemann, 1990; 197–218.

54. Campbell M. *Rehabilitation for Traumatic Brain Injury; Physical Therapy Practice in Context.* Edinburgh, Churchill Livingstone, 2000; 169–205.

55. Edwards S, Charlton P. Splinting and the use of orthosis in the management of patients with neurosurgical disorders. In: Edwards S, ed. *Neurological Physiotherapy: A Problem Solving Approach.* London, Churchill Livingstone, 1998; 161–88.

56. Davies P. *Starting Again: Early Rehabilitation After Brain Injury and Other Severe Brain Lesions.* Berlin, Springer-Verlag, 1994.

57. Conine TA, Sullivan T, Mackie T, Goodman M. Effect of serial casting for the prevention of equinus in patients with acute head injury. *Arch Phys Med Rehabil* 1990; **71**: 310–12.

58. Hurvitz E, Mandac BR, Davidoff G, Johnson JH, Nelson VS. Risk factors for heterotopic ossification in children and adolescents with severe traumatic brain injury. *Arch Phys Med Rehabil* 1992; **73**: 459–62.

59. Al-Zamil ZM, Hassan N, Hassan W. Reduction of elbow flexor and extensor spasticity following muscle stretch. *J Neurol Rehabil* 1995; **9**: 161–5.

60. Schmit BD, Dewald JP, Rymer WZ. Stretch reflex adaptation in elbow flexors during repeated passive movements in unilateral brain-injured patients. *Arch Phys Med Rehabil* 2000; **81**: 269–78.

61. Ada L, Canning C, Paratz. J. Care of the unconscious head-injured patient. In: Ada L, Canning C, eds. *Key Issues in Neurological Physiotherapy [Physiotherapy: Foundations for Practice].* Oxford, Butterworth-Heinemann, 1990; 249–89.

62. Singer BJ, Jegasothy GM, Singer KP, Allison GT. Evaluation of serial casting to correct equinovarus deformity of the ankle after acquired brain injury in adults. *Arch Phys Med Rehabil* 2003; **84**: 483–91.

63. Yarkony GM, Sahgal V. Contractures: a major complication of craniocerebral trauma. *Clin Orthop Relat Res* 1987; **219**: 93–6.

64. Barnes MP. An overview of the clinical management of spasticity. In: Barnes MP, Johnson GR, eds. *Upper Motor Neurone Syndrome and Spasticity: [Clinical Management and Neurophysiology].* Cambridge, Cambridge University Press, 2001; 1–11.

65. Sheehan G. Neurophysiology of spasticity. In: Barnes MP, Johnson GR, eds. *Upper Motor Neurone Syndrome and Spasticity: [Clinical Management and Neurophysiology].*

Cambridge, Cambridge University Press, 2001; 12–78.

66. Dobkin BH. Functional rewiring of brain and spinal cord after injury: the three Rs of neural repair and neurological rehabilitation. *Curr Opin Neurol* 2000; **13**: 655–9.

67. Jackson-Friedman C, Lyden PD, Nunez S, Jin A, Zweifler R. High dose baclofen is neuroprotective but also causes intracerebral hemorrhage: a quantal bioassay study using the intraluminal suture occlusion method. *Exp Neurol* 1997; **147**: 346–52.

68. Davis EC, Barnes MP. The use of botulinum toxin in spasticity. In: Barnes MP, Johnson GR, eds. *Upper Motor Neurone Syndrome and Spasticity: [Clinical Management and Neurophysiology]*. Cambridge, Cambridge University Press, 2001; 206–19.

69. Kay RM, Rethlefsen SA, Fern-Buneo A, Wren TA, Skaggs DL. Botulinum toxin as an adjunct to serial casting treatment in children with cerebral palsy. *J Bone Joint Surg Am* 2004; **86**: 2377–84.

70. Mathiowetz V, Haugen JB. Motor behaviour research: implications for therapeutic approaches to central nervous system dysfunction. *Am J Occup Ther* 1994; **48**: 733–45.

71. Horak FB, Henry SM, Shumway-Cook A. Postural perturbations: new insights for treatment of balance disorder. *Phys Ther* 1997; **77**: 517–33.

72. Allum JH, Bloem BR, Carpenter MG, Hulliger M, Hadders-Algra M. Proprioceptive control of posture: a review of new concepts. *Gait Posture* 1998; **8**: 214–42.

73. Kandel ER, Shwartz JH, Jessel TM. *Essentials of Neural Science and Behaviour.* Connecticut, Appleton and Lange, 1995.

74. Edwards S, Carter P. General principles of treatment. In: Edwards S, ed. *Neurological Physiotherapy: A Problem Solving Approach.* London, Churchill Livingstone, 1998; 87–113.

75. Richardson DLA. The use of the tilt-table to effect passive tendo-achilles stretch in a patient with head injury: *Physiother Theory Pract* 1991; **7**: 45–50.

76. Bohannon RW, Larkin P. Passive ankle dorsiflexion increases in patients after a regimen of tilt table – wedge board standing:

a clinical report. *Phys Ther* 1985; **11**: 1676–78.

77. Chang AT, Boots RJ, Hodges PW, Thomas PJ, Paratz JD. Standing with the assistance of a tilt table improves minute ventilation in chronic critically ill patients. *Arch Phys Med Rehabil* 2004; **85**: 1972–6.

78. Squires AJ. Using the tilt table for elderly patients. *Physiotherapy* 1983; **69**: 150–2.

79. Frank JS, Earl M. Coordination of posture and movement. *Phys Ther* 1990; **70**: 855–63.

80. Pope PM, Bowes CE, Booth E. Advances in seating the severely disabled neurological patients. *Physio Ireland* 1994; **15**: 9–14.

81. Kirkwood CA, Bardsley GI. Seating and positioning in spasticity. In: Barnes MP, Johnson GR, eds. *Upper Motor Neurone Syndrome and Spasticity: [Clinical Management and Neurophysiology]*. Cambridge, Cambridge University Press, 2001; 122–41.

82. Pountney TE, Mulcahy CM, Clarke SM, Green EM. *The Chailey Approach Posture Management – An Explanation of the Theoretical Aspects of Posture Management and Their Practical Application Through Treatment and Equipment.* Birmingham, Active Design Ltd, 2000.

83. Nwaobi OM. Seating orientations and upper extremity function in children with cerebral palsy. *Phys Ther* 1987; **67**: 1209–12.

84. Andersson BJ, Ortengren R, Nachemson A, Elfstrom G. Lumbar disc pressure and myoelectric back muscle activity during sitting. I: studies on an experimental chair. *Scand J Rehabil Med* 1974; **6**: 104–14.

85. McDonald S. Pragmatic language skills after closed head injury: ability to meet the informational needs of the listener. *Brain Lang* 1993; **44**: 28–46.

86. McDonald S. Putting communication disorders in context after traumatic brain injury. *Aphasiology* 2000; **4**: 339–47.

87. Cools C, Manders E. Analysis of language and communication function in traumatic brain injured patients. *Int J Rehabil Res* 1998; **21**: 323–9.

88. King KA, Hough MS, Walker MM, Rastatter M, Holbert D. Mild traumatic brain injury: effects on naming in word retrieval and discourse. *Brain Inj* 2006; **20**: 725–32.

89. Togher L. Giving information: the importance of context on communicative

opportunity for people with traumatic brain injury. *Aphasiology* 2000; **14**: 365–90.

90. MacLennan DL, Cornis-Pop M, Picon-Nieto L, Sigford B. The prevalence of pragmatic communication impairments in traumatic brain injury. *Proceedings from the Brain Injury Association Conference* 2002. (http://www.premier-outlook.com/pdfs/article_archive/winter_2002/PRAGMATICCOMWINTER2002.pdf).

91. Hough MS, Barrow I. Descriptive discourse abilities of traumatic brain-injured adults. *Aphasiology* 2003; **17**: 183–91.

92. Dahlberg C, Hawley L, Morey C, Newman J, Cusick CP, Harrison-Felix C. Social communication skills in persons with post-acute traumatic brain injury: three perspectives. *Brain Inj* 2006; **20**: 425–35.

93. Pimental PA, Kingsbury NA. The injured right hemisphere: classification of related disorders. In: Pimental PA, Kingbury NA, eds. *Neuropsychological Aspects of Right Brain Injury.* Austin, Texas, Pro-Ed, 1989; 19–64.

94. Snow P, Ponsford J. Assessing and managing changes in communication and interpersonal skills following TBI. In: Ponsford J, Sloan S, Snow P, eds. *Traumatic Brain Injury: Rehabilitation for Everyday Adaptive Living.* Sussex, UK, Psychology Press Ltd, 1995; 137–64.

95. Galski T, Tompkins C, Johnston MV. Competence in discourse as a measure of social integration and quality of life in persons with traumatic brain injury. *Brain Inj* 1998; **12**: 769–82.

96. Togher L, McDonald S, Code C. Communication problems following traumatic brain injury. In: McDonald S, Togher L, Code C, eds. *Communication Disorders Following Traumatic Brain Injury.* Sussex, UK, Psychology Press Ltd, 1999; 1–14.

97. Douglas JM, Bracy CA, Snow PC. Measuring perceived communicative ability after traumatic brain injury: reliability and validity of the La Trobe Communication Questionnaire. *J Head Trauma Rehabil* 2007; **22**: 31–8.

98. Drummond SS, Boss MR. Functional communication screening in individuals with traumatic brain injury. *Brain Inj* 2004; **18**: 41–56.

99. Borgaro SR, Prigatano GP, Kwasnica C, Alcott S, Cutter N. Disturbances in affective communication following brain injury. *Brain Inj* 2004; **18**: 33–9.

100. Hagan C. Language disorders in head trauma. In: Holland A, ed. *Language Disorders in Adults.* San Diego, CA, College Hill Press, 1984; 245–81.

101. Body R, Perkins M, McDonald S. Pragmatics, cognition, and communication in traumatic brain injury. In: McDonald S, Togher L, Code C, eds. *Communication Disorders Following Traumatic Brain Injury.* Sussex, UK, Psychology Press Ltd, 1999; 81–109.

102. Martin I., McDonald S. Weak coherence, no theory of mind, or executive dysfunction? Solving the puzzle of pragmatic language disorders. *Brain Lang* 2003; **85**: 451–66.

103. Tompkins CA. *Right Hemisphere Communication Disorders: Theory and Management.* San Diego: Singular Publishing Group, 1995.

104. Myers PS. Profiles of communication deficits in patients with right cerebral hemisphere damage: Implications for diagnosis and treatment. *Aphasiology* 2005; **19**(12): 1147–60.

105. Snow P, Douglas J, Ponsford J. Conversational discourse abilities following severe traumatic brain injury: a follow-up study. *Brain Inj* 1998; **12**: 911–35.

106. Murdoch BE, Theodoros DG. Dysarthria following traumatic brain injury. In: McDonald S, Togher L, Code C, eds. *Communication Disorders Following Traumatic Brain Injury.* Sussex, UK, Psychology Press Ltd, 1999; 211–28.

107. Braverman SE, Spector J, Warden DL *et al.* A multidisciplinary TBI inpatient rehabilitation programme for active duty service members as part of a randomized clinical trial. *Brain Inj* 1999; **13**: 405–15.

108. Cicerone KD, Mott T, Azulay J, Friel JC. Community integration and satisfaction with functioning after intensive cognitive rehabilitation for traumatic brain injury. *Arch Phys Med Rehabil* 2004; **85**: 943–50.

109. Myers PS. *Right Hemisphere Damage.* San Diego, CA, Singular Publishing Group, Inc, 1999.

110. Cope DN. The effectiveness of traumatic brain injury rehabilitation: a review. *Brain Inj* 1995; **9**: 649–70.

111. Brooks N, McKinlay W, Symington C, Beattie A, Campsie L. Return to work within the first seven years of severe head injury. *Brain Inj* 1987; **1**: 5–19.

112. Brooks N, Campsie L, Symington C, Beattie A, McKinlay W. The effects of severe head injury on patient and relative within seven years of injury. *J Head Trauma Rehabil* 1987; **2**: 1–13.

113. Hammond FM, Hart T, Bushnik T, Corrigan J, Sasser H. Change and predictors of change in communication, cognition and social function between 1 and 5 years after traumatic brain injury. *J Head Trauma Rehabil* 2004; **19**: 314–328.

114. British Association of Brain Injury Case Managers (BABICM). Principles and guidelines for case management best practice. http://www.babicm.org/guidelines.htm.

115. McKinlay WW, Watkiss AJ. Long-term management. In: Rose FD, Johnson DA, eds. *Brain Injury and After: Towards Improved Outcome*. Chichester, John Wiley & Sons Ltd, 1996; 119–41.

116. The Rehabilitation Code (Code of Best Practice on Rehabilitation, Early Intervention and Medical Treatment in Personal Injury Claims) http://www.justice.gov.uk/civil/procrules_fin/contents/protocols/prot_pic.htm#6174089.

117. Murphy L, Chamberlain J, Weir A, Berry D, Nathaniel-James D, Agnew, R. Effectiveness of vocational rehabilitation following acquired brain injury: preliminary evaluation of a UK specialist rehabilitation programme. *Brain Inj* 2006; **20**: 1119–29.

118. Malec JF, Basford JS. Postacute brain injury rehabilitation. *Arch Phys Med Rehabil* 1996; **77**: 198–207.

119. Ben-Yishay Y, Silver SM, Piasetsky E, Rattok J. Relationship between employability and vocational outcome after intensive holistic cognitive rehabilitation. *J Head Trauma Rehabil* 1987; **2**: 35–48.

120. Wehman P, Kregel J, Keyser-Marcus L *et al.* Supported employment for persons with traumatic brain injury: A preliminary investigation of long-term follow-up costs and program efficiency. *Arch Phys Med Rehabil* 2003; **84**: 192–6.

# Chapter 25

# Neuropsychology and head injury

Maggie Whyte, Fiona Summers, Camilla Herbert, William W. McKinlay, Lorna Torrens, Roisin Jack and Jane V. Russell

Clinical neuropsychology is defined by Lezak as 'an applied science concerned with the behavioural expression of brain function and dysfunction'.[1] Clinical neuropsychologists in the UK undertake practical and academic doctoral training in clinical psychology, giving them the experience and knowledge required to identify a psychological disorder which is key in differentiating between organic and psychological factors in neurological disorder. Recognition by the British Psychological Society as a clinical neuropsychologist requires a further academic qualification, 2 years supervised practice and demonstration of research skills.

The reasons for neuropsychological assessment and consultation in brain injury are wide ranging and include diagnosis, prognosis, treatment and research. Neuropsychological assessment may be used to differentiate between the psychological or organic causes of presenting behaviours and identify co-existing disorders such as dementias, psychiatric conditions or toxicity. Assessment can establish the extent and nature of the brain injury and make predictions about likely recovery. This may inform decisions about return to work, rehabilitation or future care needs. Assessment can monitor recovery in a brain-injured patient and measure the effects of intervention. It may be used to inform on the most appropriate intervention for cognitive, behavioural or emotional difficulties. Finally, neuropsychological assessment is used in research to further knowledge about functional neuroanatomy, the consequences of brain injury and the mechanisms of recovery as well as investigations into the validity and reliability of assessment tools and methods.

The above is certainly not exhaustive and neuropsychological assessment has a wide range of applications both in clinical settings and in wider practice e.g. forensic, educational.

## Process of neuropsychological assessment

The process of neuropsychological assessment involves the complex integration of information gathered about the patient and their difficulties from medical notes, interview with the patient and others, observation and formal assessment. Pre-morbid factors influencing cognition in the person's medical, psychiatric, developmental, educational and occupational history are considered. The history of the injury and subsequent recovery, including measures of PTA and GCS, can give an initial impression of severity of injury. Consultation with the family may reveal important information about pre-morbid personality, abilities and lifestyle, and comments by family and staff on their observations of the patient's behaviour and abilities can usefully inform assessment. The neuropsychologist will observe the patient during the interview and formal assessment in order to gather information on the presentation of difficulties, e.g. insight, processing speed or those which may influence performance on formal assessment including anxiety, motivation and secondary gain.

*Head Injury: A Multidisciplinary Approach*, ed. Peter C. Whitfield, Elfyn O. Thomas, Fiona Summers, Maggie Whyte and Peter J. Hutchinson. Published by Cambridge University Press. © Cambridge University Press 2009.

Formal cognitive assessment covers the main domains of cognitive functioning however the focus and choice of assessment is likely to vary, depending on the presentation of the patient and the impression of likely difficulties. Pre-morbid functioning is also tested and assessment results interpreted in view of this. The neuropsychologist must be aware of the limitations of the tests which are used, including information on the development of the assessments, the validity and reliability.

Following assessment, the neuropsychologist draws the information together to construct a formulation identifying which aspects of the patient's presentation are as a result of the primary consequences of the brain injury, which are secondary consequences and which are a result of other influences, pre-morbid or co-existing.

There is much evidence to support the validity of neuropsychological assessment in predicting functional outcome after TBI and return to work.[2,3] Neuropsychological assessment has been shown to be a reliable diagnostic and prognostic indicator when compared with neuroimaging.[4,5] However, there is general agreement about the utility of using a combination of neuro-imaging and neuropsychological assessment when answering diagnostic or other clinical questions.[6]

# Cognitive functioning

Impairments in cognitive functioning as a result of brain injury can be diffuse or focal depending on the nature of the injury. Diffuse brain injury, affecting many, although rarely all, areas of cognition, is common following closed brain injuries involving rapid acceleration or deceleration. Focal impairments in cognition are common following cerebrovascular accidents, penetrating traumatic brain injuries, localized infections and space-occupying lesions. The type and extent of any impairment is influenced by the site, size and depth of any lesion. Whilst diffuse brain injury affects many aspects of cognition, focal deficits can also have a significant deleterious effect upon day-to-day functioning and quality of life. Areas of cognitive impairment commonly reported in the literature following brain injury include memory, attention, processing speed, executive functioning, perception and language.

## Memory

Impairment in memory functioning is the most common complaint following brain injury and is associated with medial temporal lobe, medial and midline thalamic structures, the basal forebrain and frontal network systems.[7] There are many different types of memory functioning. Short-term memory, more commonly referred to as *working memory*, involves the temporary storage and manipulation of a limited amount of information for a short period of time (seconds). The term short-term memory is often misunderstood and confused with *episodic memory* which involves long-term storage of events and personal experiences that have occurred over the past few hours, days or weeks. *Long-term memory* also includes *semantic memory* of facts and knowledge; for example, mathematical equations and knowledge of the world, *procedural memory* of motor and cognitive skills, such as driving or riding a bike and *remote memory* for events that have occurred years before during childhood and early adulthood.

The distinction between anterograde and retrograde amnesia is important in clinical settings. *Anterograde or post-traumatic amnesia (PTA)* refers to the inability, or limited ability, to learn new information and knowledge from the point at which injury has occurred, whereas *retrograde amnesia* refers to the inability to recall events preceding the onset of brain injury. Retrograde amnesia can range from a few seconds to decades and consequently can cause significant distress for the patient and family members. Anterograde amnesia can cause considerable problems with return to work, academic study and simply remembering to do something (*prospective memory*). An important concept in memory functioning is the distinction between the registration of information, encoding and retrieval. Patients need to be able to attend to information (be this verbal, visual or tactile) for this to be encoded and stored for it then to be retrieved when necessary. The distinction between recall (uncued retrieval involving an active search process) and recognition (familiarity) is therefore important as impaired recall with intact recognition suggests deficits in retrieval rather than encoding. Impairments in both suggest deficits in the encoding of information.

## Attention

Impairment in attention is also common following brain injury and is associated with multiple brain systems including the inferior parietal cortex, the frontal cortex and limbic system structures.[8,9] Although there are many different types of attention, the most common described are focused/selective attention, sustained attention/vigilance, divided attention and alternating attention. Focused or selective attention, also commonly referred to as concentration, is the capacity to highlight important stimuli while suppressing awareness of competing distractions.[1] Sustained attention refers to the ability to maintain attention over an extended period of time, whilst divided attention involves the ability to respond to more than one task at a time for example talking on the telephone whilst writing. Alternating attention, also called set shifting, involves the ability to move attentional focus from one task to another. It is important to acknowledge that attentional abilities have limited capacity and impairments in attention have significant effects on other areas of cognition, particularly memory and executive functioning.

## Processing speed

Processing speed, the rate at which mental activities are performed, is commonly impaired following brain damage. Patients often describe slow processing speed as feeling as if they are one step behind everyone else in conversations. Patients with slow processing speed commonly take longer to respond to questions displaying delayed reaction times, which are important to consider during clinical interview.

## Executive functioning

Executive functioning refers to a range of functions associated with the ability to establish behaviour patterns and ways of thinking and to introspect upon them.[10] Impairments in executive functioning (often called dysexecutive syndrome) were initially thought to be related solely to damage to the frontal lobes (hence the old termed 'frontal lobe syndrome'); however, research now suggests wider network brain involvement, although the frontal lobes still remain important. Executive functioning encompasses a wide and varied range of behaviours, including planning and organizing, problem solving and reasoning (required in decision making), the ability to achieve goals effectively, control of impulsivity (when impaired can result in aggression, inappropriate behaviour and excitability), confabulation (unintentional production of a false memory), mental flexibility (when impaired can result in rigid inflexible thinking) and sequencing. Lack of concern, apathy and lack of insight are also associated with impaired executive functioning and cause considerable problems for families and in rehabilitation.

## Perception

Perceptual processes, the elaborations and interpretations of neural signals in different parts of the brain, which enable one to become aware of external stimulations, are associated more commonly with damage to the occipital and parietal lobes, although research suggests some involvement of the temporal lobes and subcortical regions.[11] Impaired perceptual processes include agnosias (the inability to recognize the meaning, identity and nature of sensory stimuli presented either by touch, sight or sound), neglect and visual inattention. This includes structural perception and semantic processing of faces (prosopagnosia).

## Language

Language and communication disorders following brain injury are frequent and include dysphasia, dysarthria, impairments in pragmatic communication and discourse, and the secondary effect of other cognitive impairments such as executive functioning on communication.

## Bedside testing

Clinical neuropsychologists have in-depth expertise in assessing cognitive functioning; however, it is acknowledged that cognitive screening may usefully be conducted by other professionals. The most common and widely used assessment tool to screen for cognitive impairment is the Mini Mental Status Examination (MMSE).[12] However, this tool lacks the scope and sensitivity required for diagnostic assessment. The MMSE focuses mainly on memory functioning and neglects executive functioning, lacking the specificity to identify some subtle focal impairments. In addition, it is strongly influenced by age, education and ethnicity. It can be useful for monitoring change over time particularly in patients with moderate and severe impairments. The Addenbrooke's Cognitive Examination (Revised) (ACE-R) provides a more in-depth yet brief assessment, including aspects of executive functioning. ACE-R can be easily downloaded from www.pentorch.net/ACEfinal-v05-A1.pdf and is proving to be a reliable and sensitive measure. Like the MMSE, it was originally designed for the detection of dementia.[13] Snyder et al.[7] and Hodges[13] provide useful guides to conducting bedside examinations of cognitive performance.

## Epilepsy and cognitive functioning

Individuals with epilepsy tend to report and demonstrate cognitive dysfunction compared to age-matched controls in the general population.[14,15] Cognitive profiles demonstrate great diversity and are probably as heterogeneous as the epileptic syndromes themselves.[16,17] However, common complaints often include memory problems, decreased levels of attention and concentration, slowness in thinking and lack of motivation. Cognitive dysfunction in epilepsy can be a major contributor to the burden of the disease and can significantly disrupt many aspects of a person's life. Early-onset epilepsy may result in more generalized cognitive impairment, since the maturing brain is affected and organizational processes encumbered. Later onset is often associated with greater partial impairment especially in memory.[18] Cognition can be affected by multiple factors including seizure aetiology, severity, frequency and duration. Hereditary factors, psychosocial conditions and anti-epileptic drug effects may all influence the level of cognitive functioning.[19–21]

## Assessment of capacity

Cognitive deficits following brain injury can affect a person's capacity to make decisions. The definition of incapacity varies between different legal frameworks. In essence, a person is incapable if they are deemed not to be able to understand, remember or communicate a decision. Laws usually state that incapacity to make one decision does not infer incapacity to make another. The decisions covered by these acts refer to financial, medical and welfare matters. Ideally, decisions about capacity should include all of those central to the individual's care and may include neuropsychological input.

When assessing capacity, relevant information about the patient's current functioning and previous wishes should be gathered in consultation with other staff members, family members and carers. Consideration should be given to any barriers to capacity such as communication difficulties, mood disorder or drug and alcohol influence and steps taken to address these where practically possible. The reasons for assessment should be discussed with the individual and it should be ensured that they have received appropriate information about the situation in a way that they are able to understand. Interview should establish whether the patient is able to describe the decision to be made, able to state their opinion, can give the pros and cons of their decision and identify any risks and consequences for themselves and others. The patient would also be expected to be aware of the alternatives and be able to give the pros and cons for these. Formal cognitive assessment may be used to assist in identifying particular deficits that might impact on decision making including attention, executive functioning and memory. Assessment will also consider the influence of mood and whether the person is susceptible to the undue influence of others.

Insight is very commonly affected by brain injury, particularly frontal injuries, and is important to consider in capacity assessment. For example, a person must have sufficient awareness and understanding of their difficulties and how this impacts on their situation and care needs to be able to make decisions about their welfare needs. Executive functioning difficulties are a common consequence of TBI and may include difficulties with reasoning, problem solving, self-monitoring and mental flexibility. It is important to be aware of the likely changes in capacity in a patient with a brain injury. Capacity may change with improvement in cognition or emergence from PTA and therefore the possibility of delaying a decision should be considered.

There are a number of resources available to assist with making judgements about capacity and understanding the law. British Psychological Society guidelines on assessing capacity are available at www.bps.org and the BMA offers guidance at www.bma.org.uk. Information on the Adults with Incapacity Act (Scotland) 2000 is available at www.scotland.gov.uk/Topics/Justice/Civil/awi and for the Mental Capacity Act at www.dca.gov.uk/menincap/legis.htm.

## Mood disorders

Estimates of depression in traumatic brain injury range from 24% in Australia to 42% in the US.[22,23] This is considerably higher than the estimated 8.6% for the population of five European countries.[24] Studies have shown risk of suicide is between 2.7 and 4.1 times higher than the non-brain-injured population[25] and have estimated the prevalence of attempted suicide at 18%.[26] People with brain injury are also more at risk from anxiety disorders including post-traumatic stress disorder which, until recently, was not recognized as occurring in the absence of conscious recollection of the event.[27] Higher levels of psychiatric disorders are reported following brain injury including psychosis, personality disorder, major depression and alcohol abuse.[28,29]

A combination of current and pre-morbid psychosocial and anatomical factors influences the development of post-traumatic mood disorder. The likelihood of developing depression is influenced by many of the social consequences of brain injury including changes in occupation, social support, family circumstances, loss of activities and marital breakdown. Pre-morbid factors such as poor social functioning, alcohol abuse, inadequate coping mechanisms and psychological disorder may increase the risk.

The contribution of neuroanatomical factors of injury to mood disorder is not fully understood, although laterality of injury, proximity to dorsal frontal systems and an effect on serotonergic activity are likely to be an influence.[30] Brain injury may have an effect on processing anxiety and fear reactions and lesions to the temporo-limbic areas have been associated with anxiety disorders.[31]

## Assessment of mood disorders

Care needs to be taken not to confuse the symptoms of mood disorder and the consequences of brain injury. Depression can be over-estimated in TBI due to the overlap in symptoms including physical, motivation and cognitive impairment.[32] Irritability, frustration, fatigue, poor concentration and apathy may be a direct result of organic damage rather than depression.[33] Many of the standard rating scales for depression are unsuitable for patients with TBI, since some of the questions relate to physical symptoms or limitations on activity, which may be a result of the injury rather than psychological disorder. Normal adjustment in acute stages of the disorder may be mistaken for depression.

## Treatment of mood disorders

Treatment of mood disorders in brain injury is complex and it is unlikely that one treatment in isolation will be effective.[33] Intervention might involve a combination of psychological and pharmacological intervention and may require the context of a comprehensive overall rehabilitation package for the individual to be effective.

*Cognitive behavioural therapy* (CBT) is currently the most commonly practised and evidence-based psychological intervention for mood disorder. Many of the consequences of brain injury may affect a person's ability to participate in psychological therapy and adjustments to take into account cognitive difficulties such as processing speed, memory, executive function-ing and attention deficits may require adapted approaches and be more time-consuming. Very few studies have looked at the effectiveness of psychological therapy in people with brain injury, although CBT has been shown to be an effective treatment of social anxiety in people with brain injury.[34] CBT-based group intervention has also been shown to improve levels of depression in individuals with TBI.[35] Studies looking at the effectiveness of CBT in other neurological populations associated with cognitive deficits show encouraging preliminary findings.[36,37]

Alternative approaches such as psychotherapy, behavioural therapy and solution-focused therapy may be appropriate for intervention with a brain-injured population.

*Antidepressant medication* has been shown to be effective following stroke; however, there is little research on pharmacological treatment of mood disorder in traumatic brain injury.[37] Interactions with other drugs and effect on seizure threshold need consideration.[37]

## Changes in behaviour following brain injury

Behavioural changes are frequently cited by families as being harder to cope with, and more likely to lead to family breakdown, than physical or cognitive problems.[38] They represent an important challenge in rehabilitation and can present either as excesses or deficits. They commonly include apathy, irritability, anger and aggression, impulsivity, poor social judge-ment, emotional lability and an exaggeration of pre-morbid personality characteristics.[39] By their very nature, brain injuries frequently occur in individuals with a history of behavioural difficulty. Such individuals are predisposed to exhibit behavioural problems post-injury and presentation should be considered with regard to the pre-morbid status.[40] Nevertheless, each individual represents a unique combination of factors.[41] A considerable range of behavioural changes may well emerge at different stages during recovery requiring a fluid and flexible approach to both assessment and management.

In the immediate aftermath of a head injury, a period of post-traumatic amnesia typically follows. Individuals present as confused, disorientated and agitated. They may be experiencing the effects of alcohol/drug withdrawal.[42] Agitation can present considerable risks to the individual and others and thus the use of restraint and pharmacological interventions may be required.[43] Sedatives such as haloperidol, lorazepam and procyclidine may suppress the challenging behaviour, but do not address the underlying cause and may be detrimental to the person's progress in rehabilitation through further impairing cognitive functioning and motivation.[44] There may be a role for neuroleptics where changes in behaviour are shown to be associated with electrophysiological disturbance.[44] Many TBI patients demonstrate extreme sensitivity to behaviour-modifying drugs. Neuropsychiatric advice should be sought at an early stage.

Patients in PTA are difficult to manage in acute services, which characteristically involve conditions likely to aggravate the situation. Ideally, they should be supervised on a one-to-one basis in a simplified environment by a non-confrontational individual, sensitive to the fluctuant nature of the condition. Reassurance and redirection, minimization of distractions and promotion of a simple but predictable routine, facilitate orientation. In this regard, it is suggested that the preparation of an orientation 'script' (including succinct statements about the injury, current placement and staff role as helpers) may be more beneficial than a question and answer session, which would invite erroneous responses thereby adding to confusion.[45] Inappropriate management at this stage can actually create behavioural problems via the unwitting reinforcement of unhelpful patterns of behaviour. There is a strong case for transfer to specialist services at the earliest opportunity.[46,47]

As the patient emerges from PTA, they become more capable of meaningful interaction. They may present as aggressive, lacking in insight and uncooperative. Regarding insight, it is important to make a distinction between anosognosia (lack of awareness thought to have a neurological basis), and the more emotionally laden lack of insight arising in a context of denial of deficit during a process of adjustment. The question of whether or not to promote insight is not clear-cut, since to do so may be to invite depression. Furthermore, there is some suggestion that patients with limited insight, manifesting itself as over-estimation of their abilities, may, in fact, benefit more from rehabilitation than more realistic individuals.[48]

Lack of cooperation is more likely to manifest itself as passive rather than active resistance.[45] It may point to limitations in cognitive ability, initiation difficulties, fatigue or emotional problems. Remediative strategies might include encouragement, prompting or the provision of forced (as opposed to open) choices.

In the longer term, behavioural difficulties might arise on discharge particularly where there are no follow-up or support systems in place. Faced with a loss of hospital routine and structure and a return to routine daily stressors and typically increased expectations and demands, new difficulties can come to the fore. Unless patients and their families have been forewarned about what to expect, how they might cope and how to access support, behavioural problems can re-emerge.

At all times, it is essential to consider the meaning and significance of behaviour, be this as an expression of needs or emotional state, a source of stimulation/occupation or a means of exerting control. 'Difficult' behaviour can affect the comfort of fellow patients, present danger or a barrier to optimum ultimate placement or community rehabilitation.[49] Equally, however, it may be inconvenient in terms of staff or ward routines and could be accommodated, or modified, with a degree of flexibility, innovative thinking and the desire to make a real difference.

# Family and brain injury

Families experience high levels of distress, anger and denial in the early post-traumatic phase. These features are followed by increasing social isolation, depression and anxiety about the future.[50-53] Injury-related factors and socio-demographic variables have consistently been found to be poor predictors of psychological adjustment of both the injured person and their relatives.[54-56] Cognitive and personality changes are more related to family distress than other consequences such as physical deficits or difficulties with activities of daily living.

## Process of family adjustment

Families often struggle to cope with the initial shock and distress of trauma and all the uncertainties this brings. With patient relocation to a rehabilitation centre, family members are often able to resume a more normal life pattern, but can feel excluded as they juggle practical problems such as return to employment and child care. However, it is important to involve family members and keep them informed as the brain-injured person themselves is more likely to opt out of rehabilitation if his or her family is not supportive of the programme.

In the longer term, families continue to report high levels of distress, with emotional problems often emerging only as the hope of natural recovery or significant improvement recedes. Coping abilities can diminish, especially with regard to emotional and behavioural changes. However, most studies that assess the long-term impact on families focus on those who have struggled to adjust, and there is some evidence to suggest that a significant proportion of families cope remarkably well. The reasons for this are not fully understood and there is a need for more research into resilience and successful coping.[57]

Many, but not all, studies suggest that spouses experience different levels of stress and burden in caring for a partner or adult child with traumatic brain injury. There can be tensions within families, commonly between a spouse or a partner and the brain-injured person's parents. Some of these are long-standing but exposed or exacerbated by the brain injury. It is often the case that the parents live separately from the brain-injured person and do not fully appreciate the situation faced by the spouse/partner. Rates of marital breakdown following brain injury are twice as high as the national average.[58]

Impact on the children of a parent's brain injury is an under-researched area, and most evidence is anecdotal or based on clinical experience rather than on research findings. This evidence suggests that most children will experience at least some problematic behavioural change following a parent's brain injury, and that there are negative changes in the ability of many head-injured adults to parent.[59] There is even less research on the impact on siblings, including adult siblings, who tend to be isolated from both the patient and access to information during the period of acute hospitalization, but who may be key people in the longer-term support network.

## Intervention and treatment with families

Few families have experience of brain injury and they require information to help them participate in decisions about ongoing care and rehabilitation. Families benefit most from intervention, education and advice from people who understand the nature of brain injury and have experience in the field.[60] Family support groups offer education and/or emotional support, with a popular format being a guest speaker followed by informal discussion. Parents tend to attend such groups for longer than spouses. Families of the less severely brain-injured also attend for longer.[61] The timing of group meetings, their location and frequency needs careful consideration to avoid increasing the pressure on relatives.

Family dynamics pre- and post-injury are often complex and family therapy is sometimes recommended, but it is important to adjust the nature of the therapy to compensate for possible cognitive difficulties, with greater use of logbooks, memory aids and visible reminders.[62]

Working with individual families or with groups of families to help them modify their behaviour and gain knowledge and skills necessary to address their situation is one successful way forward. Timing is important as in the early stages families are often not ready to adapt their own behaviour, since the hope and expectation is of recovery rather than adjustment. However, in the medium to longer term many families do need to modify the way they interact or manage the home situation and a programme of education, advice and problem-solving training can be very effective.[63]

Sexual problems are common following brain injury but are rarely discussed.[64] Given the sensitivity of the topic, couple counselling is best left to later stages in rehabilitation as people are often extremely anxious initially and focusing on the problem too early can increase rather than reduce anxiety.[65] Useful guides for sexual matters for people with brain injury are available.[66,67]

## Post-concussion symptoms

Post-concussional syndrome (PCS) refers to a collection of physical, cognitive and affective symptoms commonly reported following fairly mild head trauma. These include headache, dizziness, fatigue, irritability, poor concentration and memory, insomnia, noise intolerance, reduced stress tolerance and sometimes anxiety and low mood.[68] Although these symptoms usually resolve, they may persist for months or years in some patients. The aetiology of PCS is controversial and the roles of organic psychological and motivational factors have been the forum for much debate.

It was formerly the view that post-concussional symptoms were linked to claims for compensation.[69] However, evidence of brain insult has been found in patients with 'concussion'.[70] Delays in auditory brainstem evoked potentials[71] and reduced speed of processing on neuropsychological assessment have been reported in the early post-injury stages.[72] Neuropsychological deficits and failure to resume work are common at 3 months post-injury in people with 'minor' head injuries.[73]

The nature of the symptoms can change over time. Headache and dizziness have been found to be present both immediately after regaining consciousness and several weeks post-injury. Other somatic symptoms (vomiting, nausea, drowsiness, blurred vision) are commonly reported in the early stages of recovery, whereas later complaints include irritability, anxiety, depression, poor memory, poor concentration, insomnia and fatigue.[74] Ponsford et al. found that post-concussional symptoms declined from 1-week to 3-month follow-up.[75] Although 24% still complained of ongoing problems at 3 months, their neuropsychological scores were not abnormal. They did not differ in injury severity from those who had recovered. Alves et al. calculated the frequency with which lasting symptoms arose after uncomplicated mild head injury.[76] They found that 'persistent multiple symptom constellations' (i.e. headaches, memory problems and dizziness plus other symptoms) were rare at 12 months' post-injury. They estimated an incidence of around 1.9% taking into account those lost to follow-up. Later complaints may be caused by interplay of organic and psychological factors leading to amplification and perpetuation of clinical features.[74]

For many patients the symptoms appear genuine, although it has been suggested that between a third and a half of patients seeking compensation after mild head trauma show malingering or sub-optimal motivation on testing.[77] Neuropsychological 'effort testing' can be a key to separating those who have genuine limitations from those who are over-playing their symptoms.[78,79]

Post-concussional symptoms are sometimes confused with the symptoms of post-traumatic stress disorder.[68] There is some overlap in symptoms including fatigue, irritability, poor concentration, insomnia, reduced stress tolerance, etc., although patients with post-concussional symptoms alone do not report the intrusive recollections that characterize PTSD.[80]

Overall, most patients make a full recovery after minor head injury, but a minority continue to complain of symptoms which may be attributable to a residue of organic brain damage, but probably mainly reflect psychological functioning or secondary gain (e.g. compensation, state benefits).

Management after mild head injury should include:

1. Recognition that there may be organically driven symptoms, at least early on in the recovery process. Reassure the patient accordingly, including advising against premature return to work, which may result in failure and distress.

2. Follow-up for those mild head injury cases with symptoms. Timely review to advise on an appropriate point at which to return to work. Neuropsychological assessment, if available, can help with these decisions, although an extensive, detailed assessment may not be necessary. Tests which require speed and concentration are sensitive to the limitations patients have at this stage and typically will show resolution over the weeks that follow injury.

3. Patients who have symptoms should be advised that their resumption of normal activities should be gradual, in particular, resuming exercise and return to work.

# References

1. Lezak MD, Howieson DB, Loring DW. *Neuropsychological Assessment*, 4th edn. New York, Oxford University Press, 2004.

2. Wood RLL, Rutterford NA. Demographic and cognitive predictors of long-term psychosocial outcome following traumatic brain injury. *J Int Neuropsychol Soc* 2006; **12**(3): 350–8.

3. Sherer M, Novack TA, Sander AM, Struchen MA, Alderson A, Thompson RN. Neuropsychological assessment and employment outcome after traumatic brain injury: a review. *Clin Neuropsychol* 2002; **16**(2): 157–78.

4. Galton C, Erzinclioglu S, Sahakian BJ, Antoun N, Hodges JR. A comparison of the Addenbrooke's Cognitive Examination (ACE), conventional neuropsychological assessment, and simple MRI-based medial temporal lobe evaluation in the early diagnosis of Alzheimer's disease. *Cogn Behav Neurol* 2005; **18**(3): 144–50.

5. Scheid R, Walther K, Guthke T, Preul C, von Cramon DY. Cognitive sequelae of diffuse axonal injury. *Arch Neurol* 2006; **63** (3): 418–24.

6. Markowitsch HJ, Calabrese P. Commonalities and discrepancies in the relationships between behavioural outcome and the results of neuroimaging in brain-damaged patients. *Behavi Neurol* 1996. **9**(2): 45–55.

7. Snyder P, Nassbaum PD, Robins DL, eds. *Clinical Neuropsychology: A Pocket Handbook for Assessment*, 2nd edn. Washington, DC, American Psychological Association, 2006.

8. Cohen RA. *Neuropsychology of Attention*. New York, Plenum, 1993.

9. Heilman KM, Watson RT, Valenstein E. Neglect and related disorders. In: Heilman, KM Valenstein E, eds. *Clinical Neuropsychology*,

3rd edn, New York, Oxford University Press, 1993; 279–336.

10. Burgess PW. Assessment of executive function. In: Halligan PW, Kischka U, Marshall JC, eds. *Handbook of Clinical Neuropsychology*. Oxford, Oxford University Press, 2003.

11. Kartsonunis LD. Assessment of perceptual disorders. In Halligan PW, Kischka U, Marshall JC, eds. *Handbook of Clinical Neuropsychology*. Oxford, Oxford University Press, 2003.

12. Folstein MF, Folstein SE, McHeugh PR. Mini-mental state: a practical method for grading the cognitive state of outpatients for the clinician. *J Psychiatric Res* 1975; **12**: 189–98.

13. Hodges J. *Cognitive Assessment for Clinicians*. 2nd edn. New York, Oxford University Press, 2007.

14. Smith DB, Craft BR, Collins J, Mattson RH, Cramer JA. Behavioural characteristics of epilepsy patients compared with normal controls. *Epilepsia* 1996; **27**: 760–8.

15. Trimble MR, Ring HA, Schmitz B. Neuropsychiatric aspects of epilepsy. In: BS Fogel, ed. *Neuropsychiatry*. Baltimore, MD, Williams & Wilkins, 1996.

16. Elger CE, Helmstaedter C, Kurthen M. Chronic epilepsy and cognition, *Lancet Neurol* 2004; **3**: 663–72.

17. Mameniskiene R, Jatuzis D, Kaubrys L, Budrys V. The decay of memory between delayed and long term recall in patients with temporal lobe epilepsy. *Epilepsy Behav* 2006; **8**(1): 278–88.

18. Helmstaedter C, Gates, J. Syndromes III: 'Nonidiopathic' (cryptogenic and symptomatic) focal epilepsies with special consideration of Temporal Lobe Epilepsy (TLE). *Epilepsia* 2006; **47**: 90.

19. Lesser RP, Luderss H, Wyllie E, Dinner DS, Morris HH. Mental deterioration in epilepsy. *Epilepsia* 1986; **27**: 105–23.

20. Loring DW, Meador KJ. Cognitive and behavioural effects of epilepsy treatment. *Epilepsia* 2001; **42**: 24–32.

21. Meador KJ. Cognitive effects of epilepsy and antiepileptic medications. In: Wyllie E. ed. *The Treatment of Epilepsy*, 3rd edn. Baltimore, Williams & Wilkins, 2001; 1215–27.

22. Kersel DA, Marsh NV, Havill JH, Sleigh JW. Psychosocial functioning during the year following severe traumatic brain injury. *Brain Inj* 2001; **15**(8): 683–96.

23. Kreutzer JS, Seel RT, Gourley E. The prevalence and symptom rates of depression after traumatic brain injury: a comprehensive examination. *Brain Inj* 2001; **15**(7): 563–76.

24. Ayuso-Mateos JL, Vazquez-Barquero JL, Dowrick C *et al*. Depressive disorders in Europe: prevalence figures from the ODIN study. *Br J Psychiatry* 2001; **179**(4): 308–16.

25. Teasdale TW, Engberg AW. Suicide after traumatic brain injury: a population study. *J Neurol, Neurosurge Psychiatry* 2001; **71**: 436–40.

26. Simpson G, Tate R. Suicidality after traumatic brain injury: demographic, injury and clinical correlates. *Psych Med* 2002; **32**(4): 687–97.

27. Glaesser J, Neuner F, Lutgehetmann R, Schmidt R, Elbert T. Posttraumatic Stress Disorder in patients with traumatic brain injury. *BMC Psychiatry* 2004; **4**: 5.

28. Deb S, Lyons I, Koutzoukis C, Ali I, McCarthy G. Rate of psychiatric illness 1 year after traumatic brain injury. *Am J Psychiatry* 1999; **156**: 374–9.

29. Koponen S, Taiminen T, Portin R *et al*. Axix I and II psychiatric disorders after traumatic brain injury: a 30-year follow-up study. *Am J Psychiatry* 2002; **159**: 1315–22.

30. Alderfer BS, Arciniegas DB, Silver JM. Treatment of depression following traumatic brain injury. *J Head Trauma Rehabil* 2005; **20**(6): 544–62.

31. Williams WH, Evans J, Fleminger S. Neuro-rehabilitation and cognitive-behaviour therapy of anxiety disorders after brain injury: an overview and a case illustration of obsessive-compulsive disorder. *Neuropsychol Rehabil* 2003; **13**: 133–48.

32. Khan-Bourne N, Brown RG. Cognitive behavioural therapy for the treatment of depression in individuals with brain injury. *Neuropsychol Rehabil* 2003; **13**: 89–90.

33. Fleminger S, Oliver DL, Williams WH, Evans J. The neuropsychiatry of depression after brain injury. *Neuropsychol Rehabil* 2003; **13**: 65–87.

34. Hodgson J, McDonald S, Tate R, Gertler P. A randomised controlled trial of a cognitive-behavioural therapy program for managing

social anxiety after acquired brain injury. *Brain Impairm* 2005; **6**(3): 169–80.

35. Anson K, Ponsford J. Who benefits? Outcome following a coping skills group intervention for traumatically brain injured individuals. *Brain Inj* 2006; **20**(1): 1–13.

36. Lincoln NB, Flannaghan T, Sutcliff L, Rother L. Evaluation of cognitive behavioural treatment for depression after stroke: a pilot study. *Clin Rehabi* 1997; **11**: 114–22.

37. Larcombe NA, Wilson PH. An evaluation of cognitive behavioural therapy for depression in patients with multiple sclerosis. *Br J Psychiatry* 1984; **145**: 366–71.

38. Wood RL, Yurdakel LK. Change in relationship status following traumatic brain injury. *Brain Inj* 1997; **11**: 491–502.

39. Morton MV, Wehman P. Psychosocial and emotional sequelae of individuals with traumatic brain injury: a literature review and recommendations. *Brain Inj* 1995; **9**: 81–92.

40. Prigatano GP. Personality disturbances associated with traumatic brain injury. *J Cons Clin Psychol* 1992; **60**: 360–8.

41. Warriner EM, Rourke BP, Velikonja D, Metham L. Subtypes of emotional and behavioural sequelae in patients with traumatic brain injury. *J Clin Exp Neuropsycho* 2003; **7**: 904–17.

42. British Psychological Society Division of Neuropsychology. *Clinical Neuropsychology and Rehabilitation Services for Adults with Acquired Brain Injury*. Leicester, The British Psychological Society, 2005.

43. Eames P, Haffey WJ, Cope DN. Treatment of behavioural disorders. In: Rosenthal, M Griffith ER, Bond MR, Miller JD, eds. *Rehabilitation of the Adult and Child with Traumatic Brain Injury*, 2nd edn. Philadelphia, FA, Davis, 1990; 410–32.

44. Alderman N. Managing challenging behaviour. In: Wood RLl, McMillan TM, eds. *Neurobehavioural Disability and Social Handicap Following Traumatic Brain Injury*. East Sussex, Psychology Press; 2001.

45. Wilson BA, Herbert CM, Shiel A. Behavioural approaches in neuropsychological rehabilitation. In: *Optimising Rehabilitation Procedures*. Hove and New York, Psychology Press, 2003.

46. Johnson R, Balleny H. Behaviour problems after brain injury: incidence and need for treatment. *Clin Rehabili* 1996; **10**: 173–81.

47. McMillan TM, Greenwood RJ. Models of rehabilitation programmes for the brain injured adult. II. Mode; services and suggestions for change in the UK. *Clin Rehabil* 1993; **7**: 346–55.

48. Herbert CM, Powell GE. Insight and progress in rehabilitation. *Clin Rehabil* 1989; **3**: 125–30.

49. McMillan TM. Young adults with acquired brain injury in nursing homes in Glasgow. *Clin Rehabil* 2004; **18**: 132–8.

50. Kreutzer JS, Serio C, Berquist S. Family needs after brain injury: a quantitative analysis. *J Head Trauma Rehabil* 1994; **9**(3): 104–15.

51. Wallace CA, Bogner J, Corrigan JD, Clinchot D, Mysiw WJ, Fugate LP. Primary caregivers of persons with brain injury: life change 1 year after injury. *Brain Inj* 1998; **12**(6): 483–93.

52. Kinsella G, Ford B, Moran C. Survival of social relationships following head injury. *Int Disabil Stud* 1989; **11**: 9–14.

53. Knight RG, Devereux RT, Godfrey HPD. Caring for a family member with a traumatic brain injury. *Brain Inj* 1998; **12**(6): 467–81.

54. Oddy M, Humphrey M, Uttley D. Stresses upon the relatives of head-injured patients. *Br J Psychiatry* 1978; **133**: 507–13.

55. Gervasio AH, Kreutzer JS. Kinship and family members' psychological distress after traumatic brain injury: a large sample study. *J Head Trauma Rehabil* 1997; **12**(3): 14–26.

56. Gillen R, Tennen H, Affleck G, Steinpreis R. Distress, depressive symptoms and depressive disorder among caregivers of patients with brain injury. *J Head Trauma Rehabil* 1998; **13**(3): 31–43.

57. Perlesz A, Kinsella G, Crowe S. Impact of traumatic brain injury on the family: a critical review. *Rehabil Psych* 1999; **44**(1): 6–35.

58. Stilwell JHC, Stilwell P. *National Traumatic Brain Injury Study*. Warwick, University of Warwick, 1997.

59. Pessar LF, Coad ML, Linn RT, Willer BS. The effects of parental traumatic brain injury on the behaviour of parents and children. *Brain Inj* 1993; **7**(3): 231–40.

60. Palmer S, Herbert CM. *Poster presented at International Neuropsychology Conference*, Zurich, 2006.

61. Whitehouse AM, Carey JL. Compostion and concerns of a support group for families of

individuals with brain injury. *Cogn Rehabil* 1991; (Nov/Dec): 26–9.

62. Solomon CR, Scherzer BP. Some guidelines for family therapists working with the traumatically brain injured and their families. *Brain Inj* 1991; **5**(3): 253–66.

63. Jacobs HE. Family and behavioural issues. In: Williams JM and Kay T eds. *Head Injury: A Family Matter.* Baltimore, PH Brookes, 1991; 239.

64. Oddy M. Sexual relationships following brain injury. *Sexual Relationship Ther* 2001; **16**(3): 247–59.

65. Price JR. Promoting sexual wellness in head injured patients. *Rehabil Nurs* 1985; **10**: 12–13.

66. Griffiths ER, Lemberg S. *Sexuality and the Person with a Traumatic Brain Injury: A Guide for Families.* Philadelphia, FA Davis Company, 1993.

67. Simpson R. Sex after brain injury. *Headway News*, 1999.

68. World Health Organization. The ICD-10 classification of mental and behavioural disorders: clinical descriptions and diagnosis guidelines, 1992.

69. Miller H. Accident neurosis. *Br Med J* 1961; **1** (5230): 919–25.

70. Oppenheimer, DR. Microscopic lesions in the brain following head injury. *J Neurol Neurosurg Psychiatry* 1968; **31**: 299–306.

71. Noseworthy JH, Miller J, Murray, TJ, Regan D. Auditory brainstem responses in postconcussion syndrome. *Arch Neurol* 1981; **38**: 275–8.

72. Gronwall D, Wrightson P. Delayed recovery of intellectual function after minor head injury. *Lancet* 1974; **2**(7881): 605–9.

73. Rimmel RW, Giordani B, Barth JT, Boll TJ, Jane JA. Disability caused by minor head injury. *Neurosurgery* 1981; **9**(3): 221–8.

74. Rutherford WH, Merrett JD, McDonald JR. Symptoms at one year following concussion from minor head injuries. *Injury* 1975; **10**: 225–30.

75. Ponsford J, Willmott C, Rothwell A *et al.* Factors influencing outcome following mild traumatic brain injury in adults. *J Int Neuropsych Soc* 2000; **6**: 568–79.

76. Alves W, Macciocchi SN, Barth JT. Postconcussive symptoms after uncomplicated mild head injury. *J Head Trauma Rehabil* 1993; **8**(3): 48–59.

77. Binder LM. A review of mild head trauma. Part II: Clinical implications. *J Clin Exp Neuropsychol* 1997; **19**(3): 432–57.

78. Green P, Allen LM, Astner K. *The Word Memory Test: A User's Guide to the Oral and Computer-administered Forms.* Durham, NC, CogniSyst, 1996.

79. Tombaugh TN. *Test of Memory Malingering.* Toronto, MHC, 1996.

80. Sbordone RJ, Liter JC. Mild traumatic brain injury does not produce post-traumatic stress disorder. *Brain Inj* 1995; **9**(4): 405–12.

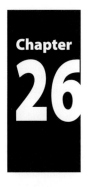

# Outcome and prognosis after head injury

Helen M. K. Gooday, Brian Pentland, Fiona Summers and Maggie Whyte

Head injury remains a major cause of disability and death, especially in young people. In survivors, the extent of recovery depends largely on the severity of the injury. Residual disabilities include both mental and physical defects. The most rapid recovery often occurs within the first 6 months after injury, but improvement may continue for years.

## Severity measures

A wide variety of measures have been used to assess the severity of the head injury. Some of the most commonly described ones are detailed below.

### Coma/level of awareness

The longer the duration of coma (as measured by the time to follow commands) the more likely a worse outcome. In particular, a duration of coma greater than 4 weeks makes a good recovery unlikely. Loss of consciousness for 30 minutes or less is often associated with mild head injury. Although a low initial Glasgow Coma Scale (GCS) score is correlated with worse outcomes, specificity is lacking indicating that some patients with a low GCS can achieve a good recovery and vice versa.

### Post-traumatic amnesia (PTA)

PTA is defined as a period of time from the initial brain injury until the individual's memory for ongoing events becomes reliable, consistent and accurate. In general, a longer duration of PTA correlates with a worse outcome. A PTA of less than an hour is regarded as a mild brain injury and a PTA exceeding 4 weeks reflects an extremely severe injury.

### MRI scan

MRI scanning sequences have been utilized to try and offer prognostic information at an early stage (see Chapter 5). Deep lesions and possibly the total lesion burden do correlate with a worse long-term outcome. In particular, the presence of bilateral brainstem lesions makes the possibility of a good recovery very unlikely.[1]

### CT scan

The presence of subarachnoid haemorrhage, cisternal effacement, significant midline shift, extradural haematoma or subdural haematoma on an acute care CT scan are all associated with worse outcomes. Owing to individual patient factors, including the burden of secondary insults, more specific conclusions about the implications of the lesions cannot be drawn.[2]

## Outcome measures

A range of different tools are also used to assess outcome after head injury. These are discussed below.

*Head Injury: A Multidisciplinary Approach*, ed. Peter C. Whitfield, Elfyn O. Thomas, Fiona Summers, Maggie Whyte and Peter J. Hutchinson. Published by Cambridge University Press. © Cambridge University Press 2009.

**Table 26.1.** The Glasgow Outcome Scale[4]

| GOS | GOSE | |
|-----|------|---|
| 1 | 1 | *Death* |
| 2 | 2 | *Vegetative State* (see text) |
| 3 | | *Severe disability; conscious but dependent* |
| | 3 | Communication is possible, minimally by emotional response; total or almost total dependency with regards to activities of daily life. |
| | 4 | Partial independence in activities of daily life, may require assistance for only one activity, such as dressing; many evident post-traumatic complaints and/or signs; resumption of former life and work not possible. |
| 4 | | *Moderate disability; independent but disabled* |
| | 5 | Independent in activities of daily life, for instance can travel by public transport; not able to resume previous activities either at work or socially; despite evident post-traumatic signs, resumption of activities at a lower level is often possible. |
| | 6 | Post-traumatic signs are present; however, resumption of most former activities either full-time or part-time. |
| 5 | | *Good recovery* |
| | 7 | Capable of resuming normal occupation and social activities; there are minor physical or mental deficits or complaints. |
| | 8 | Full recovery without symptoms or signs. |

Reproduced with permission from the BMJ Publishing Group.

## The Glasgow Outcome Scale (GOS)[3–5]

The GOS was commonly used before other scales were developed, and is the most widely used outcome measure in head injury research. The five categories of the original scale are dead, vegetative, severely disabled, moderately disabled and good recovery. An extended version of the scale (GOSE) divides each of the latter three categories into two providing a scale from 1 to 8 (Table 26.1).[4]

## The Disability Rating Scale (DRS)[6]

The DRS measures disability levels following severe head injury from coma to the community (Table 26.2). The measure is commonly employed in the brain injury outcome literature. The total score ranges from 30 (death) to 0 (no disability) with a range of intermediary levels including mild, partial, moderate and severely extreme limitation and two grades of vegetative state. These all have numerical values derived from summation of individual components of the scale.

Other more functionally based measures include the Barthel Index,[7] the Functional Independence Measure (FIM) and the Functional Assessment Measure (FAM).[8,9] For specific rehabilitation programmes, use of *goal achievement* often provides a more reliable and sensitive outcome measure.

## Threshold values

A 'threshold value' is a value of a predictor variable above or below which a particular outcome is especially unlikely. For example, several studies have reported that no patients

**Table 26.2.** The Disability Rating Scale[6]

| Arousability, awareness and responsibility | | |
| --- | --- | --- |
| **Eye Opening** | **Communication ability (verbal, written, letterboard or sign)** | **Best motor response** |
| 0 Spontaneous | 0 Orientated | 0 Obeying |
| 1 To speech | 1 Confused | 1 Localizing |
| 2 To pain | 2 Inappropriate | 2 Withdrawing |
| 3 None | 3 Incomprehensible | 3 Flexing |
| | 4 None | 4 Extending |
| | | 5 None |
| **Cognitive ability for self-care activities (Does patient know how and when? Ignore motor disability?)** | | |
| **Feeding** | **Toileting** | **Grooming** |
| 0 Complete | 0 Complete | 0 Complete |
| 1 Partial | 1 Partial | 1 Partial |
| 2 Minimal | 2 Minimal | 2 Minimal |
| 3 None | 3 None | 3 None |
| *Level of functioning (consider both physical and cognitive disability)* | | *'Employability' (as a full-time worker, homeworker or student)* |
| 0 Completely independent | | 0 Not restricted |
| 1 Independent in special environment | | 1 Selected job, competitive |
| 2 Mildly dependent | | 2 Sheltered workshop, non-competitive |
| 3 Moderately dependent | | 3 Not employable |
| 4 Markedly dependent | | |
| 5 Totally dependent | | |
| **Categorization of outcome scores (limitations, severity)** | | |
| 0 None | 4–6 Moderate | 17–21 Extremely severe |
| 1 Mild | 7–11 Moderately severe | 22–24 Vegetative state |
| 2–3 Partial | 12–16 Severe | 25–29 Extreme vegetative state |
| | | 30 Dead |

Reproduced with permission from Elsevier © 1982.

with PTA exceeding 3 months achieved a good recovery as defined by the GOS. Thus, 3 months would be considered a threshold value for the duration of PTA, at least in terms of excluding the possibility of a good recovery on the GOS. As the length of a patient's PTA extends beyond 3 months, clinicians can counsel family members about realistic expectations for the future. On the other hand, if 2 months have not yet elapsed since the injury, clinicians can give hope to families even if the patient is still in PTA. Threshold values can be seen as 'milestones' in a patient's recovery.[2]

# Outcome after severe head injury

After severe injury many patients regain an independent existence and may return to pre-morbid social and occupational activities. Inevitably, some remain severely disabled requiring long-term care, including a very small proportion (<2%) who are left in a vegetative state.

## Vegetative and minimally conscious states

The vegetative state is a clinical condition of complete unawareness of the self and the environment accompanied by sleep–wake cycles with either complete or partial preservation of hypothalamic and brainstem autonomic functions.[10]

The persistent vegetative state (PVS) can be judged to be permanent 12 months after traumatic injury in adults and children. Permanency is recognized after 3 months for non-traumatic injury in adults and children. In adults who are in a vegetative state at 1 month post-injury, 33% will die by 12 months, 15% will remain in PVS, and 52% will recover consciousness, although only 7% will make a good recovery as defined by the GOS.[11]

The Minimally Conscious State (MCS) is a condition of severely altered consciousness in which there is minimal but definite behavioural evidence of self- or environmental awareness.[12] The natural history and long-term outcome have not yet been fully characterized.

# Outcome after moderate head injury

Outcomes after moderate TBI are less uncertain than after severe TBI. More than 90% of individuals with moderate TBI will achieve either moderate disability or good recovery.[13,14] There are certain risk factors associated with the poorer outcomes: lower GCS scores (e.g. 10 or lower), older age and abnormalities on the CT scan.[13,14] When these are present, patients are more likely to harbour moderate or severe degrees of disability. However, the above studies have shown that even individuals who make a good recovery often have residual neuro-behavioural problems.

# Outcome after mild head injury

There is no universally agreed definition of mild head injury. In 1993 the American Congress of Rehabilitation Medicine Head Injury Special Interest Group on Mild Traumatic Brain Injury defined mild traumatic brain injury as an injury to the head or mechanical forces applied to the head involving loss of consciousness for less than 30 minutes (possibly no loss of consciousness) with post-traumatic amnesia for less than 24 hours.[15] Some researchers have differentiated complicated and uncomplicated mild TBI.[16] A complicated mild TBI is diagnosed if the person has a GCS score of 13–15 but shows some brain abnormality (e.g. oedema, haematoma or contusion) on a CT scan.

Patients who sustained a mild head injury were previously believed to have no organic sequelae, and symptoms of post-concussion syndrome were considered to be psychiatric or psychological in nature, or due to malingering.[17,18] It is now known that a small proportion of patients who have had a mild TBI do have long-lasting neurological and cognitive impairment. Post-concussional syndrome is discussed in more detail in Chapter 25.

More than 150 000 patients with a head injury are known to be admitted to hospital each year in the United Kingdom. Estimates of the frequency of subsequent disability in such patients previously ranged from two or three to 45 per 100 000 population per year.[19–22] This variation reflected limitations in previous studies, particularly the lack of data on patients with an apparently mild injury, who account for 80% of admissions.[19] A prospective study conducted in Glasgow showed that increased severity of injury on admission was associated with increased rate of death or vegetative state, and a decreased rate of good recovery.[23] In contrast, the initial severity of injury was not related to late disability, which occurred in almost half of each group. Survival with moderate or severe disability was common after mild head injury (47%) and similar to that after moderate (45%) or severe injury (48%). By extrapolation from the population identified (90% of whom had mild injuries), it was estimated that annually in Glasgow (population 909 498 in 2000) 1400 young people and adults were still disabled 1 year after head injury. The incidence of disability in young people and adults admitted with a head injury was therefore 100–150 per 100 000 population, much greater than previously anticipated.

## Compounding effects of secondary insults

Primary traumatic damage to the brain may be made worse by the superimposition of 'secondary insults'. These can occur soon after the injury, during transfer to the hospital and during the subsequent treatment of the brain-injured patient. Such insults may be of either intracranial or systemic origin (i.e. hypotension, hypoxaemia, pyrexia) and may arise during initial management or later in intensive care. Secondary insults were characterised in the 1970s and 1980s, when a number of researchers reported that in severely brain-injured patients hypoxia was found in 30% and arterial hypotension in 15% on arrival in the emergency department. Secondary insults also occur within the intensive care environment. Gopinath *et al.* used a jugular venous catheter to identify episodes of jugular venous desaturation and reported that episodes of desaturation were strongly associated with a poor neurological outcome. Just a single desaturation increased the incidence of poor outcome from 55% to 75%.[24] Much of the focus of modern head injury management is therefore directed at minimizing the incidence and severity of such insults. These are discussed in detail in other chapters of this book.

## Long-term outcome

### Risk for Alzheimer's disease

For the past 20 years there has been considerable interest in the relation between traumatic brain injury and the future development of Alzheimer's disease (AD). It has been suggested that traumatic brain injuries reduce 'cognitive reserve', resulting in increased vulnerability to developing the disease.[25] The literature is conflicting, but it would appear that patients who sustain severe TBIs may be at a slightly increased risk of developing AD.[26–28] There is no evidence that patients who have mild TBIs are at increased risk.

### Progressive neurological disease, including punch drunk syndrome

The effects of repeated neuronal damage are cumulative; when this exceeds the capacity for compensation, permanent evidence of brain damage ensues. It is well recognized that repeated concussive or subconcussive blows as experienced by various athletes, and partic-ularly boxers, sometimes induces the development of neurological signs and progressive dementia.[29] This condition, known as 'dementia pugilistica', may develop some years after the last injury and is most likely to develop in boxers with long careers who have been dazed, if not knocked out, on many occasions. In a detailed study of the brains of 15 ex-boxers, one of the characteristic patterns of damage was the presence of many neurofibrillary tangles diffusely throughout the cerebral cortex and the brainstem.[30] These tangles broadly con-formed to the topographic pattern found in Alzheimer's disease.

More recently, other athletes involved in contact sports who have sustained repeated minor concussion have been studied using neuroimaging and neuropsychological assessment. There is evidence that three or more concussions in high school and university athletes are associated with small but measurable cumulative effects, and increased risk for future concussions. This subject has recently been reviewed.[31]

## Genetic factors and outcome from head injury

Apolipoprotein E4 (APOE 4) is a lipid transporter in the brain and cerebrospinal fluid.[32] It is the product of a single gene. The presence of APOE 4 alleles, especially in the homozygous condition, appear to be associated with worse outcome after TBI, [33] although other studies have had contradictory results. APOE 4 is believed to play a role in the inflammatory response and neuronal repair following trauma. It has been associated with age-related cognitive impairment, decreased synapse–neurone ratio, increased susceptibility to neurotoxins and hippocampal atrophy.[34]

## Special populations: older age

Older patients have a worse outcome after a TBI, and the lower the admission GCS, the more likely an unfavourable outcome. In particular, in patients over 65, the chances of a good recovery after severe TBI are unlikely. There are many potential reasons for this, ranging from the nature of the injuries in the elderly (e.g. subdural haematomas) to age-related changes in the brain (e.g. decreased functional reserve, less elasticity of blood vessels, etc.). Several authors have noted that, in terms of outcome, a moderate TBI in the elderly resembles a severe TBI in a younger person.[35–37] Even the outcomes of mild TBI in the elderly are much worse, with many never returning to their pre-morbid functional status.[38]

## Special populations: penetrating injuries

The early mortality rate after penetrating injury is much higher than that of closed head injury.[39] Lower GCS scores and CT findings of bilaterality or transventricular injury are associated with worse outcomes. Owing to the high early mortality rate, proportionally fewer survivors are left vegetative or severely disabled compared with the closed severe head injured cohort.[39] The incidence of post-traumatic epilepsy is substantially higher in patients who have a penetrating head injury, compared with those who have a severe closed head injury.

## Communication with families after TBI

Families have identified information about prognosis as one of their most important needs in the aftermath of TBI.[40–42] Clinicians have an important role in providing information about prognosis to patients and families after head injury. Unfortunately, this need often goes unmet, as families' report they are rarely provided with adequate prognostic information.[41,42]

Despite its clear importance, clinicians are often reluctant to have a discussion regarding prognosis. Some reasons for this reticence apply specifically to the delivery of poor prognosis: a lack of training in the delivery of 'bad news', the emotionally demanding nature of providing a poor prognosis, a fear of extinguishing hope, and the fact that a poor prognosis highlights the limits of professional help.[43] Other barriers can affect discussion of prognosis such as the difficulty in extracting clinical guidelines from a large body of literature.[43]

It is important to be aware that family responses to brain injury vary and commonly include denial, shock, anger, helplessness, guilt, bereavement and a sense of loss.

## Setting the scene

There have been several useful reviews on improving the process by which information is communicated, especially in the case of 'bad news'.[44-46] The following points are useful to consider:

- Find a quiet, comfortable room without interruptions (i.e. bleep free).
- Sit close and speak face to face.
- Have the family member's support network present, if wanted.
- Present the information at a pace the family can follow.
- Periodically summarize the discussion to that point.
- Periodically ask a family member to repeat or summarize what was said.
- Keep the language simple and direct, without euphemism or jargon.
- Allow time for questions.

## General guidelines for communicating prognostic information

There is now a considerable amount of literature regarding the discussion of prognosis with patients and families.[8] Below are some suggestions on how to communicate information:

- Begin with the family's desire for information. By asking family members what they already know and what their current perceptions are, it is possible to build on the knowledge they already have. This also allows correction of any misinformation that might distort their understanding of the information to follow.
- Ensure that the meaning and content of the outcomes are understood.
- Present quantitative information in a manner that can be understood:
  - Try to use 'natural frequencies' when communicating probabilistic information (e.g. 'Eight out of ten people with this type of injury will make a good recovery').
  - Attempt to 'frame' information in both a positive and negative manner (e.g. 'That is the same as saying that two out of ten people with this type of injury will not make a good recovery').
  - Present information both qualitatively as well as quantitatively (e.g. 'There is a very good chance of a good recovery').
  - When possible, consider presenting the information visually.
  - Ask person to restate, in their own words, their understanding of the information provided.

## Conclusion

A variety of parameters can be used to measure the nature of the outcome following a head injury. The severity of the primary injury is of paramount importance, but other factors including age and the burden of secondary insults are important. Repeated trauma and genetic factors may contribute to long-term sequelae, as may co-morbidities such as alcohol and substance abuse.

# References

1. Firsching R, Woischneck D, Klein S. Classification of severe head injury based on magnetic resonance imaging. *Acta Neurochir* 2001; **143**: 263–71.

2. Kothari S. Prognosis after severe TBI: a practical, evidence based approach. In: Zasler ND, Katz DI, Zalfonte RD, eds. *Brain Injury Medicine, Principles and Practice*. New York, Demos Medical Publishing, 2007; 169–99.

3. Jennett B, Bond M. Assessment of outcome after severe brain damage: a practical scale. *Lancet* 1975; **1**: 480–4.

4. Jennett B, Snoek J, Bond MR, Brooks N. Disability after severe head injury: observations on the use of the Glasgow Outcome Scale. *J Neurol Neurosurg Psychiatry* 1981; **44**: 285–93.

5. Maas AIR, Braakman R, Schouten HJA, Minderhoud JM, Van Zomeren AH. Agreement between physicians on assessment of outcome following severe head injury. *J Neurosurg* 1983; **58**: 321–5.

6. Rappaport M, Hall KM, Hopkins K, Belleza T &, Cope DN. Disability Rating Scale for severe head trauma: coma to community. *Arch Phys Med Rehabil* 1982; **63**: 118–23.

7. Mahoney FI, Barthel DW. Functional evaluation: the Barthel Index. *Maryland State Med J* 1965; **14**: 61–5.

8. Uniform Data Systems. *The Functional Independence Measure*. New York, State University of Buffalo, 1987.

9. Uniform Data System for Medical Rehabilitation. *Guide for the Uniform Data State for Medical Rehabilitation (Adult FIM)*, version 4.0. Buffalo, State University of New York at Buffalo, 1993.

10. American Academy of Neurology. Practice parameter: assessment and management of patients in the persistent vegetative state. *Neurology* 1995; **45**: 1015–18.

11. The Multi-Society Task Force on PVS. Medical aspects of the persistent vegetative state (part 2). *N Engl J Med* 1994; **330**: 1572–9.

12. Giacino J, Ashwal S, Childs N *et al*. The minimally conscious state: definition and diagnostic criteria. *Neurology* 2002; **58**: 349–53.

13. van der Naalt J. Prediction of outcome in mild to moderate head injury: a review. *J Clin Exp Neuropsychol* 2001; **23**: 837–51.

14. Stein SC. Outcome from moderate head injury. In: Narayan RK, Wilberger JE, Povlishock JT, eds. *Neurotrauma*. New York, McGraw-Hill, 1996; 755–65.

15. Mild Traumatic Brain Injury Committee American Congress of Rehabilitation Medicine, Head Injury Interdisciplinary Special Interest Group. Definition of mild traumatic brain injury. *J Head Trauma Rehabil* 1993; **8**: 86–7.

16. Williams DH, Levin HS, Eisenberg HM. Mild head injury classification. *Neurosurgery* 1990; **27**: 422–8.

17. Miller H. Accident neurosis. *Br Med J* 1961; **1**: 919.

18. Miller H. Mental after-effects of head injury. *Proc Roy Soc Med* 1966; **59**: 257–61.

19. McMillan R, Strang I, Jennett B. Head injuries in primary surgical wards in Scottish hospitals: Scottish head injury management study. *Health Bull* 1979; **37**: 75–81.

20. Field JH. *Epidemiology of head injuries in England and Wales*. London, Research Division, Department of Health and Social Security, 1975.

21. Bryden J. How many head injuries? The epidemiology of post head injury disability. In: Wood R, Eames P, eds. *Models of Brain Injury Rehabilitation*. Baltimore, Johns Hopkins University Press, 1989; 17–26.

22. Kraus JF. *Epidemiology of head injury*. In: Cooper PL, ed. *Head Injury*. 3rd edn. London, Williams and Wilkins, 1993; 1–25.

23. Thornhill S, Teasdale GM, Murray GD *et al*. Disability in young people and adults one year after head injury: prospective cohort study. *Br Med J* 2000; **320**: 1631–5.

24. Gopinath SP, Robertson CS, Constant CF *et al*. Jugular venous desaturation and outcome after head injury. *J Neurol Neurosurg Psychiatry* 1994; **57**: 717–23.

25. Lye TC, Shores EA. Traumatic brain injury as a risk factor for Alzheimer's disease: a review. *Neuropsychol Rev* 2000; **10**: 115–29.

26. Starkstein SE, Jorge R. Dementia after traumatic brain injury. *Int Psychogeriatr* 2005; Suppl 1: S93–107.

27. Jellinger KA. Head injury and dementia. *Curr Opin Neurol* 2004; **17**: 719–23.

28. Fleminger S, Oliver DL, Lovestone S, Roabe-Hesketh S, Giora A Head injury as a risk factor for Alzheimer's disease: the evidence 10 years

on; a partial replication study. *J Neurol Neurosurg Psychiatry* 2003; **74**: 857–62.

29. Corsellis JAN. Boxing and the brain. *Br Med J* 1989; **289**: 105.

30. Corsellis JAN, Bruton CJ, Freeman-Browne D. The aftermath of boxing. *Psychol Med* 1973; **3**: 270.

31. Collins MW, Iverson GL, Gaetz M *et al.* Sport-related concussion. In: Zasler ND, Katz DI and Zalfonte RD, eds. *Brain Injury Medicine, Principles and Practice*. New York, Demos Medical Publishing, 2007; 407–23.

32. Coleman M, Handler M, Martin C. Update on apolipoprotein E state of the art. *Hosp Phys* 1995; **31**: 22–4.

33. Teasdale GM, Nicoli JA, Murray G *et al.* Association of apolipoprotein E polymorphism with outcome after head injury. *Lancet* 1997; **350**: 1069–71.

34. Nathoo N, Chetty R, van Dellen JR, Barnett GH. Genetic vulnerability following traumatic brain injury: the role of apolipoprotein E. *Mol Pathol* 2003; **56**: 132–6.

35. Ross AM, Pitts LH, Kobayashi S. Prognosticators of outcome after major head injury in the elderly. *J of Neurosci Nurs* 1992; **24**: 88–93.

36. Pentland B, Jones PA, Roy CW *et al.* Head injury in the elderly. *Age Aging* 1986; **15**: 193–202.

37. Rothweiler B, Temkin NR, Dikmen SS. Ageing effect on psychosocial outcome in traumatic brain injury. *Arch Phys Med Rehabil* 1998; **79**: 881–7.

38. Maurice-Williams RS. Head injuries in the elderly. *Br J Neurosurg* 1999; **13**: 5–8.

39. Pruitt, Jr BA. Part 2: Prognosis in penetrating brain injury. *J Trauma* 2001; **51**: S44–86.

40. NIH Consensus Development Panel on Rehabilitation of Persons with Traumatic Brain Injury: rehabilitation of persons with traumatic brain injury. *J Am Med Assoc* 1999; **282**: 974–83.

41. Holland D, Shigaki CL. Educating families and caretakers of traumatically brain injured patients in the new health care environment: a three-phase model and bibliography. *Brain Inj* 1998; **12**: 993–1009.

42. Junque C, Bruna O, Mataro M. Information needs of the traumatic brain injury patient's family members regarding the consequences of the injury and associated perception of physical, cognitive, emotional, and quality of life changes. *Brain Inj* 1997; **11**: 251–8.

43. Christakis NA. *Death Foretold*. Chicago, The University of Chicago Press, 1999.

44. Buckman R. *How to Break Bad News: A Guide for Healthcare Professionals*. Baltimore, The Johns Hopkins University Press, 1992.

45. Ptacek JT, Eberhardt TL. Breaking bad news: a review of the literature. *J Am Med Assoc* 1996; **276**: 496–502.

46. Girgis A, Sanson-Fisher RW. Breaking bad news: consensus guidelines for medical practitioners. *J Clin Oncol* 1995; **13**: 2449–56.

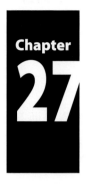

# Chapter 27

# Medico-legal aspects of head and neck injury

Peter J. Hutchinson and Peter C. Whitfield

The medico-legal consequences of head and neck injury fall broadly into two categories: personal injury and medical negligence. This chapter will discuss liaison with the various authorities that require medico-legal input relevant to head injury and whiplash. Although focusing on UK practice, the principles discussed also apply to other countries.

## Personal injury

Authorities requesting medical reports include solicitors (personal injury claims), insurance companies, the police and coroner. Reports need to be tailored to address the specific requirements of the requesting authority, for example, an opinion on the mechanism of injury for the police /coroner, or an opinion on the degree of disability and whether it is likely to be permanent for insurance companies.

## Personal injury reports

Medico-legal personal injury reports for solicitors need to be comprehensive covering a wide range of issues of both fact and opinion. Instructions can be received from solicitors representing the claimant, defendant or may be jointly instructed by both parties. Medico-legal reports should be addressed to the court and need to acknowledge that it is the duty of an expert to help the Court on matters within his/her own expertise, and that this duty is paramount and overrides any obligation to the person from whom the expert has received instructions, or by whom he/she is paid.

The date of report and accompanying persons should be recorded. In head injury and whiplash reports the background is critical. Accurate recording of pre-event history and relationship with post-event symptoms is essential. Specific pre-event neurological, psychological and psychiatric symptoms should be determined. The patient's description of past medical history should be placed in the context of the medical records, from both primary care physician and hospital records. The patient's social and in particular employment status should also be included.

The mechanism of injury should be explained in detail and include the duration of loss of consciousness, retrograde and post-traumatic amnesia. Differentiation is required between the patient's recollection of events and what they have been subsequently told (often on many occasions). Specific points, such as whether a seat-belt was in place, may also need to be addressed. The acute symptoms experienced by the patient in the immediate aftermath of the injury should be documented in detail. Both physical symptoms such as headache, dizziness, focal deficits and psychological symptoms such as short-term memory problems should be described. These symptoms can then be compared with the current status of the patient. The treatment administered should be clearly described. Prognosis in terms of on-going symptoms and future pattern, and the effect on lifestyle is crucial. The impact on activities of daily

*Head Injury: A Multidisciplinary Approach*, ed. Peter C. Whitfield, Elfyn O. Thomas, Fiona Summers, Maggie Whyte and Peter J. Hutchinson. Published by Cambridge University Press. © Cambridge University Press 2009.

living, hobbies, family relationships and employment should be described. A statement on dependence on others and capacity both now and in the future is required. Specific factors in terms of prognosis include risk of seizures and life expectancy. Recommendations for on-going treatment should be given and finally a summary and opinion. This can be characterized as what would have happened to the patient in the absence of the index event (the 'but for' test) and what has happened to the patient as a consequence of the index event. If there is a range of medical opinion regarding the diagnosis, prognosis or significance of the injury to the constellation of symptoms and signs, this should be stipulated.

The risk of seizure depends on the severity of injury as defined by the Glasgow Coma Score and, in addition, there are specific risk factors, which include depressed skull fracture, intracranial haematoma and post-traumatic amnesia greater than 24 hours.[1] Population-based studies provide data on the cumulative probability of seizures. Annegers et al.[2] in a sample of 4541 patients with traumatic brain injury quote the 5-year cumulative probability of seizures as 0.7% in patients with mild injuries, 1.2% with moderate injuries and 10% with severe injuries. The equivalent figures for 30-year cumulative incidence are 2.1% (mild), 4.2 % (moderate) and 16.7% (severe) The literature, however, can only provide guidance based on population figures and the incidence for an individual can be extremely difficult to determine. The risk of seizures has major implications for driving, particularly Group 2 licence holders.

The issue of life expectancy is often also very difficult to establish for an individual. It is well recognized that patients in vegetative state have reduced life expectancy. Patients with less severe degrees of disability are also at risk, for example, due to the complications of aspiration and pneumonia, or sudden death following seizure. Recent evidence indicates that the overall death rate is increased for at least 7 years after head injury,[3] and that the primary causes of death after head injury are the same as those in the general population. However, on an individual basis, patients who had made a good recovery may well have a normal life expectancy.

Predicting outcome can also be notoriously difficult, particularly in the acute stages following injury. Patients who are deemed to have made a good recovery at the time of discharge are at risk of on-going physical, psychological and psychiatric symptoms with potentially major implications for domestic life and employment. For patients with severe disability, it is usually difficult to be objective until a minimum period of 6 months has elapsed following injury and the patients may change for 2 years (often regarded as or near finality) or beyond. Serial assessment of objective outcome measures such as the Extended Glasgow Outcome Score,[4] or SF-36 quality of life questionnaire,[5] may be helpful in such situations. More detailed assessment with imaging (e.g. MRI) and neuropsychological testing may also be indicated.

## Police and coroner reports

Reports for the coroner and police should commence with full name, medical qualifications, status and length of tenure. Reports should be detailed and factual, not assume any additional knowledge, and be written in terms that can be understood by those outside the medical profession. Police reports may require no more than a factual statement of the injuries. However, information on the mechanism of injury and prognosis may also be required. One of the commonest questions is whether the alleged mechanism of injury is consistent with the nature of the injuries sustained. Statements should begin with the sentence 'I am writing this statement in my capacity as the doctor responsible for the treatment of the said patient following his/her alleged assault on the particular date in question.' Accurate documentation particularly with regard to external signs of injury is essential in cases of alleged assault. While CT scans provide long-term evidence of the nature of skull fractures and cerebral injury, external signs of bruising and lacerations heal with time. Photography of such injuries should be undertaken to provide a permanent record.

Reports for the coroner need to provide a factual chronology of events, with particular regard to the mechanism of injury, description of the presenting symptoms and examination findings. In addition to recording positive examination findings, relevant negative findings should also be noted. It is also necessary to differentiate which parts of your report are based in the medical records compared with your memory of events.

## Driving licence authorities

In terms of driving licences, requirements differ between countries. In the United Kingdom, the Driving Vehicle Licensing Authority (DVLA) is responsible for issuing and revoking licences. Reports for the UK DVLA are usually straightforward, particularly with regard to Group 1 (car, motorcycle) licences. Such reports comprise the answers to specific questions on a template. The situation with regards to Group 2 licences (heavy goods vehicle, bus, coach) is much more complex, particularly with regards to the risk of seizures. The DVLA produces an 'At a glance guide to driving in terms of medical conditions,' which is regularly updated and available on the internet.[6] In terms of head injury these relate to on-going symptoms and the risk of seizures.

Current guidelines from the DVLA (Group 1 licence) state that, for a serious head injury with a compound depressed fracture requiring surgical treatment, a 6–12 month period off driving should exist. The duration of the recommendation depends upon features (PTA, dural tear, focal signs and seizures) and clinical recovery. Patients with serious head injury and no neurosurgical intervention, if free from seizures, may require up to 6 months off driving, depending on recovery and features that predispose to seizures. If there is loss of consciousness with no history of intracranial haematoma, depressed fracture or seizures and clinical recovery is full and complete, driving may resume without notifying the DVLA. Extradural haematomas requiring craniotomy, but with no cerebral damage, and acute sub-dural and intracerebral haematomas treated with burr hole drainage, require 6 months off driving. Extradural haematomas with cerebral damage requiring craniotomy and acute sub-dural clots and intracerebral haemorrhage treated with craniotomy require 1 year off driving. For chronic subdural haematomas treated surgically, driving may resume on recovery.

Current guidelines for the DVLA (Group 2 licence) are far more stringent, indicating that a Group 2 licence may be returned when the risk of seizure is deemed to be less than 2% per annum. While there is some evidence in the literature that may assist in the making of the decision, personal opinion for the individual case is required.

## Medical negligence

Opinions on medical negligence, defined as a lack of proper care and attention (*Oxford Dictionary*), following the treatment of head injury and whiplash should remain in the domain of experts with extensive experience. A clear understanding of the role of the court, judge, solicitor, barrister and medical experts is required. A list of definitions is provided in Table 27.1. The role of the medical expert is to provide a highly detailed account of the circumstances surrounding the assessment and treatment of the patient. The principle underlying the assessment of medical negligence dates back to 1957 and is known as the Bolam test[7,8] (Case *Bolam v Friern Hospital Management Committee*):

**Table 27.1.** Definitions

| **Defendant** |
|---|
| The person against whom a legal case is filed. |
| **Plaintiff or complainant** |
| The person, corporation or other legal entity that initiates a legal case. |
| **Duty of care** |
| The administration of the appropriate treatment by a health care professional. |
| **Breach of duty of care** |
| Treatment falling below the acceptable standard of a competent health care professional |
| **Causation of injury** |
| The demonstration that, if a breach of duty can be proved, it either directly caused the injuries or materially contributed to the injuries. |
| **Burden of proof** |
| The burden of proof is on the claimant. It is for the claimant to prove the case to the Court |
| **Standard of proof** |
| The test for assessing causation of injury is 'on the balance of probabilities' (i.e. more likely than not). This is a much less rigorous standard of proof than that used in the criminal courts ('beyond reasonable doubt') |

> A doctor is not guilty of negligence if he has acted in accordance with a practice accepted as proper by a responsible body of medical men skilled in that particular art. Putting it another way round the doctor is not negligent if he is acting in accordance with such a practice, merely because there is a body of opinion that takes a contrary view.

In essence, therefore, an opinion as to whether standard practice was followed is required. Whether current guidelines, e.g. the UK National Institute for Health and Clinical Excellence Guidelines on the initial management of adults and children with head injury NICE,[9] have been followed or not is one such example. However, the relationship between evidence-based guidance and the determination of medical negligence is complex.[10] It is generally recognized that guidelines set standards (such that non-adherence may require explanation) but they do not constitute a *de facto* legal standard of care. They can be used, however, to provide a benchmark for the Courts to assist in the judgement of clinical conduct.

Medical negligence may apply if incorrect treatment has been administered or if appropriate treatment has not been undertaken. The case of *Bolitho v City and Hackney*[11] relates to causation where there is an omission as opposed to action. The issue to be considered was whether a doctor who delegated seeing a patient to a junior doctor, whose bleep failed to work, would have administered a particular treatment (in this case intubation of a child in respiratory distress *if* she had attended the child).

The consequence to the patient covers a wide spectrum from minor (of no or little consequence to the patient) to major (failure in duty to do the best for the patient resulting in harm). The cause and consequences, i.e. what has happened to the patient as a result of the action, needs to be established. Overall, the process needs to address whether negligence has, or has not, occurred and whether the action or lack of action has resulted in harm. Many negligence claims follow from miscommunication or issues regarding consent. Accurate documentation in the medical records is essential at all stages in the assessment and treatment process.

Consent is a particularly difficult issue in the context of head injury. Patients with minor injuries may be confused and not comprehend the rationale for the treatment strategy. Patients with major injuries will not be in a position to give consent. If next-of-kin are not available, accepted practice is to act in the best interest of the patient. The degree of information to be given for neurosurgical procedures in general is the subject of strong debate but on a background of the cases of *Sidaway v Board of Governors of the Bethlem Royal Hospital [1985]*[12] and *Chester v Afshar [2004]*,[13] which relate to spinal surgery, the doctrine of fully informed consent as opposed to valid consent indicates the need to inform patients and their relatives of all risks to the fullest possible extent.

Many patients with head injury and whiplash are assessed and treated by trainee junior doctors. In terms of decision making from the legal perspective, the courts do not make allowance for lack of experience. Junior doctors are required to apply the same standard of care as their seniors.[8]

# Cervical spine injuries

The focus of this book has been to describe the principles of the management of head injury. Head injury is often associated with cervical spine injury. Injuries to the cervical spine carry a particularly high burden of risk from a medico-legal perspective.

Thorough assessment of the cervical spine is mandatory in any patient who has sustained a head injury. The incidence of cervical spine fracture varies with the severity of the head injury. In a series of intubated blunt trauma patients in the UK, 14% had cervical spine injuries.[14] In the NEXUS study of North American patients with head injury of any severity, the cervical fracture rate was 2.4%.[15] The Canadian study of head-injured patients with GCS of 15, reported a 2% incidence of concurrent cervical spine injury.[16] Missed cervical spine injuries can lead to devastating neurological deficits that should be considered avoidable.

The identification of cervical spine injuries requires clinical evaluation, radiological imaging and careful interpretation of the findings. A systematic approach is provided by Advanced Trauma Life Support Courses.[17] The NICE guidelines provide recommendations derived mainly from a consensus view of the Canadian clinical prediction rules regarding the evaluation of the cervical spine.[4] The aim of the guidelines is to reduce the risk of missed injuries using a safe, cost-effective strategy. Even with the availability of guidelines, clinical judgement must prevail. Cervical spine immobilization should be a treatment standard until a neck injury has been excluded in all head-injured patients with an initial GCS less than 15, and also in any patient with neck pain or symptoms and/or signs referable to the cervical spine. Different strategies are recommended for children and adults (Table 27.2). For adults a plain film series (AP/ lateral and odontoid peg views) remains the cardinal investigation in ruling out cervical spine injury. The addition of oblique views does not enhance the predictive value and a single lateral view approach is inferior, missing a significant proportion of injuries detected by a three-view series.[18] The sensitivity of plain films is inferior to that of CT scans.[19] For patients with high risk injuries (GCS 3–12; also see Table 27.2) around 15% of fractures would be missed using plain films alone. Although many of these are not of clinical importance, CT scanning with multiplanar sagittal and coronal reformatting is recommended and should be performed concurrently with the initial CT head scan. There is no evidence to suggest that CT scans of the cervical spine must be performed in all

**Table 27.2.** Summary of NICE recommendations: the cervical spine

*NICE cervical spine recommendations for children*

- In general, CT scans should be avoided.
- Children aged 10 years or more can be treated as adults for the purposes of cervical spine imaging.
- Children under the age of 10 years should receive A/P and lateral plain films without an A/P peg view. (The guidelines do not clearly state whether all children under 10 years with head injury should receive such imaging or only those with clinical signs or dangerous mechanism of injury; clinical judgement should prevail.)
- In children under 10 years CT of the cervical spine should only be used in cases where patients have a severe head injury (GCS <9) or where there is a strong suspicion of injury despite normal plain films (e.g. neurological symptoms) or where plain films are inadequate. This imaging should be within 1 hour of presentation or when they are sufficiently stable.

*NICE cervical spine recommendations for adults and children aged 10 years and over*

- All patients who have sustained a head injury and present with any of the following risk factors should have full cervical spine immobilization attempted:
  - GCS less than 15 on initial assessment by healthcare worker
  - Neck pain or tenderness
  - Focal neurological deficit
  - Paraesthesia in the extremities
  - Any other clinical suspicion of cervical spine injury
- Cervical spine immobilization should be maintained until full clinical (and radiological if deemed necessary) assessment indicates it is safe to remove the immobilization device.
- Safe clinical assessment can be carried out if the patient:
  - Was involved in a simple rear-end motor vehicle collision
  - Is comfortable in a sitting position in the emergency department
  - Has been ambulatory at any time since injury with no midline cervical spine tenderness
  - Presents with delayed onset of neck pain
- Indications for immediate cervical spine imaging request in adults:
  - Neck pain or midline tenderness with:
    - Age 65 or older, or
    - Dangerous mechanism of injury (fall >1 m or five stairs; axial load to the head, e.g. diving, roll-over crash, high speed MVA, ejection from vehicle, bicycle collision, motorized recreational vehicle)
  - Considered unsafe to assess the range of movement of the cervical spine for reasons other than those above.
  - The patient cannot actively rotate 45° to the left and right.
  - A definitive diagnosis of cervical spine injury is required urgently (e.g. before surgery).
- Patients who are considered at low risk for clinically important brain and/or cervical spine injury should be re-examined within a further hour.
- The initial investigation of choice for the detection of cervical spine injuries is a three-view plain radiograph series, however…
  - Adult patients should have CT imaging of the cervical spine requested immediately if:
    - GCS below 13 on initial assessment
    - Has been intubated

293

**Table 27.2** (*cont.*)

- Technically inadequate plain films
- Suspicious or abnormal plain films
- Continued suspicion of neck injury despite a normal X-ray
- The patient is being scanned for multi-region trauma.

*Radiological considerations*

- Cervical spine imaging should be performed simultaneously with head imaging if this is also considered urgent.
- CT scans should cover any areas of concern or uncertainty on plain films or clinical grounds.
- The occipital condyle region of the skull should be examined on bone window settings.
- Facilities for multiplanar reformatting and interactive viewing should be available.
- MRI is indicated in the presence of neurological symptoms and signs referable to the cervical spine and if there is suspicion of a vascular lesion (e.g. fracture through the foramen transversarium; lateral masses or a posterior circulation syndrome).

From National Institute for Health and Clinical Excellence (2007) CG56 *Head injury: Triage, assessment, investigation and early management of head injury in infants, children and adults.* London: NICE. Available from www.nice.org.uk/CG056. Reproduced with permission.

head-injured patients regardless of severity. The role of MRI has been carefully studied in a series of 366 obtunded patients who underwent CT and MRI cervical spine imaging. MRI scanning added additional information to the CT scan in a few cases. These comprised cervical cord contusion (seven cases), single column ligament injury (four cases), disc injury (three cases) or a combination of injuries (one case). None of these injuries was considered unstable. The authors concluded that CT scanning of the entire cervical spine was an appropriate technique for the exclusion of unstable neck injuries in all obtunded trauma patients without the need for MR imaging.[20]

Once a cervical spine injury has been identified, several management options exist, including conservative management alone, internal fixation and external fixation using a Halo jacket.

## Whiplash associated disorders

The Quebec Task Force (QTF) defined 'whiplash' as 'an acceleration–deceleration mechanism of energy transfer to the neck [that] may result from rear-end or side-impact motor vehicle collisions, but can also occur during diving or other mishaps. The impact may result in bony or soft tissue injuries (whiplash injury), which may lead to a variety of clinical manifestations (whiplash associated disorders).[21] The QTF defined 6 months post-trauma as the time differentiating acute from chronic injury. A scale of injury severity for whiplash associated disorder (WAD) from Grade 0 (no symptoms or signs) to Grade IV (fracture/dislocation) was proposed (Table 27.3). Although neck pain is the key clinical feature, most patients are poly-symptomatic with any of the following: neck stiffness, headache, low back pain, shoulder pain, dizziness and non-specific visual disturbance. Risk factors for chronic WAD include older age, female sex, a high level of symptoms at onset, pre-traumatic headache, pre-existing degenerative disease and multiple symptoms.[22]

**Table 27.3.** The Quebec Classification of whiplash-associated disorders

| Grade | Clinical presentation |
|---|---|
| 0 | No symptoms or signs |
| I | Neck pain, stiffness or tenderness. No signs |
| II | Neck pain and musculoskeletal signs which may include decreased range of motion and point tenderness |
| III | Neck complaint and neurological signs |
| IV | Fracture and/or dislocation |

From: *Scientific Monograph of the Quebec Task Force on Whiplash* – Associated Disorders: Redefining 'Whiplash' and its Management. Walter O. Spitzer et al. Spine, Volume 20, Number 8S, 1995. Reproduced with permission from Lippincott, Williams and Wilkins.

When a radiologically overt bony and/or ligamentous injury has been identified, a clear explanation for neurological symptoms and signs can be assigned. In cases of lesser severity, where imaging investigations are normal, explaining the persistence of symptoms and signs is more difficult. Biomechanical studies on volunteer cases do identify predictable biophysical changes in the spine during a whiplash injury. These include straightening of the spine (loss of lordosis) followed by flexion and compressive axial forces within the upper cervical spine. Finally, extension of the head and neck occurs. During the latter phase, EMG recordings indicate that sternocleidomastoid muscle contraction attempts to counteract extension of the spine.[23] While such mechanisms can readily explain a short-lived musculoskeletal injury pattern, chronic symptoms are more difficult to explain.

The incidence of WAD has been estimated at around 70/100 000 (Canadian provinces) to 325/100 000 (the Netherlands).[24] Recovery rates from WAD differ in different countries. In general, patients who remain symptomatic at 3 months usually continue to experience symptoms at 2 years.[25,26] The broad heterogeneity of studies led to estimates that 40%–66% of cases were pain free by 3 months, increasing to 58%–82% by 6 months and then only around 55%–86% >6 months post-injury.[27] Studies from the litigation-free Lithuanian city of Kaunas reported initial neck and/or head pain in 35%–47% of whiplash cases. The maximum duration of symptoms was 20 days. 4% of the 200 cases reported neck pains at least 7 days per month after 1 year, compared with 4.1% of the control population.[28] In a retrospectively studied group, 9.4% of the whiplash cases experienced neck pains compared with 5.9% of control patients; this difference was not statistically significant. Pre-accident symptoms were reported to be important.[29] The authors concluded that cultural factors are of importance in generating the clinical picture of WAD. They postulated that a large number of WAD cases are caused by an expectation of disability and attribution of pre-existing symptoms to the neck trauma.[28,29] Owing to the methodology of this study these conclusions are open to challenge. The majority of whiplash case series identify patients from Emergency Department records whereas in Lithuania patients were identified from police accident record files. This bias selection may be sufficient to explain the findings. Other research workers have found any link between symptoms and compensation to be tenuous and have suggested that psychological factors interact with symptoms to lead to different social outcomes in patients with different psychological profiles.

The persistence of post-whiplash neck symptoms has been reviewed with clarity by an experienced medico-legal expert.[27] When compiling a report, the clinician must consider the various possible explanations that can explain a chronic state. These include:

1. **Structural damage to the spine as a result of injury**. Imaging investigations need careful scrutiny to detect injuries. In the majority of patients with WAD, investigations are normal. The QTF considered imaging unnecessary for Grade I WAD.[21]

2. **Acceleration of symptoms due to cervical spondylosis**. Radiological cervical spondylosis is considered normal in patients over 40 years of age. However, the conversion from an asymptomatic state to one with symptoms and signs is frequently cited as an explanation for WAD cases with pre-existing radiological degenerative disease. The link between radiological abnormality and clinical symptoms is usually based upon conjecture rather than by positive identification. These symptoms may be generated by muscular or ligamentous dysfunction or by intervertebral disc degeneration, and facet or zygapophysial joint arthrosis, although the exact cause of the pain is usually unknown. The nature of the injury and the temporal association between injury and symptoms are the key factors to consider when adopting this explanation.

3. **Unreported pre-accident symptoms**. Several studies indicate that pre-existing neck symptoms are commonly present in patients sustaining whiplash injuries.[27,29] In addition, some patients may have experienced pre-traumatic symptoms at a level that the claimant did not consider worthy of medical attention. A pitfall is to overlook such pre-existing symptoms and attribute their post-traumatic correlates to the index accident. Careful scrutiny of medical and physiotherapy records may be required to detect the presence of such symptoms.

4. **Psychological illness**. Patients with a WAD can develop a reactive depressive episode associated with emotional changes, a fear of travel, poor concentration and sleep disturbance. This may lead to a state of negativity, exaggerated symptomatology and catastrophizing. Symptom amplification in which the patient attributes all clinical manifestations to the accident may then lead to perpetuation of symptoms. A psychiatric report to assess the severity and cause of such features may be useful in establishing causation. A prospective study of the psychological profiles of 117 'whiplash' patients did not identify specific pre-disposing factors that correlated with somatic features.[30]

5. **Conscious exaggeration of symptoms**. Given the financial terms of compensation settlements and the attention afforded to chronic illness patients, conscious exaggeration of symptoms may occur. This is suggested by discordance between the injury and the severity and extent of symptoms and signs, inconsistencies during examination and the universal failure of treatments to afford some degree of benefit. Such behaviour may continue after settlement, due to the patient adopting chronic illness behaviour.

The management of patients with WAD is guided by a large number of small and generally poor quality clinical trials. The Cochrane Review considered the evidence too sparse to advocate either active strategies or passive treatments as the mainstay therapeutic modality.[24]

## Support services

There are several organizations that can provide support for patients and relatives. The type and availability varies between countries. In the UK the Brain and Spine Foundation produces a number of publications relevant to head injury in terms of patient and relative information booklets. Headway, the charity for the brain-injured, also publishes a number of booklets. Specific advice and carer support is also available. Headway can also provide advice on the medico-legal process with a list of approved solicitors on the Headway panel. Other sources of support include the Citizens' Advice Bureau. Patients and/or relatives who are concerned regarding treatment that has been received can contact the patient advice and liaison service, Information Complaints' Advocacy Service or Health ombudsman.

## Conclusion
Expert medical advice is increasingly being sought in relation to criminal, insurance, personal injury and negligence issues. Guidelines and the literature, both original publications, reviews and books, can assist in the preparation of such reports. However, these are based primarily on population data, and individual opinion based on the experience of the report writer is paramount in the compilation and interpretation of medical evidence.

## References

1. Jennett B. *Epilepsy after Non-missile Head Injuries*. London, England, William Heinemann Medical Books, 1975.
2. Annegers JF, Hauser WA, Coan SP, Rocca WA. A population-based study of seizures after traumatic brain injury. *N Engl J Med* 1998; **338**: 20–4.
3. McMillan TM, Teasdale GM. Death rate is increased for at least 7 years after head injury: a prospective study. *Brain* 2007; **130**: 2520–7.
4. Wilson JT, Pettigrew LE, Teasdale GM. Structured interviews for the Glasgow Outcome Scale and the extended Glasgow Outcome Scale: guidelines for their use. *J Neurotrauma* 1998; **15**: 573–85.
5. Jenkinson C, Wright L, Coulter A. Criterion validity and reliability of the SF-36 in a population sample. *Qual Life Res* 1994; **3**: 7–12.
6. www.dvla.gov.uk.
7. Bolam v Friern Hospital Management Committee (1957) 2 *A11 ER* 118.
8. Jones JW. The healthcare professional and the Bolam test. *Br Dent J* 2000; **188**(5): 237–40.
9. www.nice.org.uk/guidance/index.jsp? action=byID&o=11836.
10. Hurwitz B. How does evidence based guidance influence determinations of medical negligence? *Br Med J* 2004; **329**: 1024–8.
11. Bolitho v City and Hackney Health Authority (1997) **39** *BMLR* 1; (1998) 1 Lloyds Rep Med 26.
12. Sidaway v Bethlem Royal Hospital Governors (1985) **1** *A11 ER* 635.
13. Chester v Afshar (2004) *UKHL* 41.
14. Brohi K, Healy M, Fotheringham T *et al*. Helical computed tomographic scanning for the evaluation of the cervical spine in the unconscious, intubated trauma patient. *J Trauma* 2005; **58**(5): 897–901.
15. Hoffman JR, Mower WR, Wolfson AB, Todd KH, Zucker MI. Validity of a set of clinical criteria to rule out injury to the cervical spine in patient with blunt trauma. National Emergency X-Radiography Utilization Study Group. *N Engl J Med* 2000; **343**(2): 94–9.
16. Stiell IG, Wells GA, Vandemheen KL *et al*. The Canadian C-spine rule for radiography in alert and stable trauma patients. *J Am Med Assoc* 2001; **286**(15): 1841–8.
17. Advanced Trauma Life Support Manual. Chicago, USA, ACS, 1997.
18. Cohn SM, Lyle WG, Linden CH, Lancey RA. Exclusion of cervical spine injury: a prospective study. *J Trauma* 1991; **31**(4): 570–4.
19. Holmes JF, Akkinepalli R. Computed tomography versus plain radiography to screen for cervical spine injury: a meta-analysis. *J Trauma* 2005; **58**(5): 902–5.
20. Hogan GJ, Mirvis SE, Shanmuganathan K, Scalea TM. Exclusion of unstable cervical spine injury in obtunded patients with blunt trauma: is MR imaging needed when multi-detector row CT findings are normal? *Radiology* 2005; **237**: 106–13.
21. Spitzer WO, Skovron ML, Salmi LR *et al*. Scientific monograph of the Quebec Task-Force on whiplash-associated disorders – redefining whiplash and its management. *Spine* 1995; **20**(8): S1–73.

22. McClune T, Burton AK, Waddell G. Whiplash associated disorder: a review of the literature to guide patient information and advice. *Emerg Med J* 2002; **19**: 499–506.

23. Brault JR, Siegmund GP, Wheeler JB. Cervical muscle response during whiplash: evidence of a lengthening muscle contraction. *Clin Biomech* 2000; **15**(6): 426–35.

24. Verhagen AP, Scholten-Peeters GGGM, van Wijngaarden S, de Bie RA, Bierma-Zeinstra SMA. Conservative treatments for whiplash. *Cochrane Database of Systematic Reviews* 2001, Issue **4**. Art. No.: CD003338. DOI: 10.1002/14651858. CD003338.pub3.

25. Gargan MF, Bannister GC. The rate of recovery following whiplash injury. *Eur Spine J* 1994; **3**: 162–4.

26. Maimaris C, Barnes MR, Allen MJ. Whiplash injuries of the neck: a retrospective study. *Injury* 1998; **19**: 393–6.

27. Pearce JMS. A critical appraisal of the chronic whiplash syndrome (editorial). *J Neurol Neurosurg Psychiatry* 1999; **66**: 272–6.

28. Obelieniene D, Schrader H, Bovim G, Miseviciene I, Sand T. Pain after whiplash: a prospective controlled inception cohort study. *J Neurol Neurosurg Psychiatry* 1999; **66**: 279–83.

29. Schrader H, Obelieniene D, Bovim G *et al*. Natural evolution of the late whiplash syndrome outside the medicolegal context. *Lancet* 1996; **347**: 1207–11.

30. Radanov BP, Di Stefano G, Schnidrig A, Sturzenegger M. Common whiplash: psychosomatic or somatopsychic? *J Neurol Neurosurg Psychiatry* 1994; **57**: 486–90.

# Index